To Dad,

Happy 48th Bi

Lots of Love

Adam
xxx

SEPT '98'

SHIPWRECKS OF THE WEST OF SCOTLAND

SHIPWRECKS

OF THE

WEST OF SCOTLAND

INCLUDING WRECKS FROM
KINTYRE TO CAPE WRATH,
ALONG WITH THE INNER HEBRIDES

BOB BAIRD

NEKTON BOOKS
1995

Although reasonable care has been taken in preparing this book, the Publishers and Author respectively accept no responsibility or liability for any errors, omissions or alterations, or for any consequences ensuing upon the use of, or reliance upon, any information contained herein. Due caution should be exercised by anyone attempting dives on any wreck herein described or indicated. The maps and diagrams are intended for guidance only and are not suitable for navigation purposes. The Author and Publishers would be glad to hear of any inaccuracies or any new relevant material.

SHIPWRECKS OF THE WEST OF SCOTLAND
BY BOB BAIRD

ISBN **1 897995 02 4** Paper bound edition
ISBN **1 897995 03 2** Hard back edition

Copyright © Nekton Books 1995

All rights reserved. No part of this publication may be reproduced, stored in a retrieval system, or transmitted in any form or by any means, electronic, mechanical, photocopying, recording or otherwise , without the prior permission of the Publishers.

Published by Nekton Books,
94 Brownside Road, Cambuslang, Glasgow, G72 8AG
Telephone/Fax 0141 641 4200.

Printed by Charles Thurnam & Sons Limited, Carlisle

Cover design and internal layout grid by Ian Johnston
Maps and drawings by Bob Baird and Gordon Ridley

Cover illustration: The probable remains of the *Hyacinth* in Ardantrive Bay near Oban (photograph by Bob Baird). Upper inset:: The paddle steamer *Mountainer* aground on Lady's Rock, Firth of Lorne in 1889 (photograph courtesy of Mitchell Library, Glasgow City Libraries). Lower inset:: The burnt-out wreck of the liner *Bermuda* aground in Eddrachillis Bay, Sutherland in 1933 (photograph courtesy of the World Ship Society).

All reasonable care has been taken to trace the owners of copyright pictures. Where it has not been possible to trace copyright, the publishers will meet any reasonable request if contacted by the owners of such copyright.

The database upon which this book is based was prepared using Ashton Tate *dBase III+* running on an Apricot XEN-i 386 computer. This was coverted into *WordPerfect 5.1* files and ported into Macintosh format in Microsoft *Word 5.1* using *Apple File Exchange*. These files were imported in Aldus *PageMake 5.0* running on an Apple Macintosh *Quadra 700* computer, along with illustrations produced using Adobe *Illustrator 3.2* and photographs that were image processed within Adobe *Photoshop 2.5.1*. The text is set in *Goudy* 10 point.

Also from the team of Bob Baird and Nekton Books:

> **Shipwrecks of the Forth**, published in 1993

CONTENTS

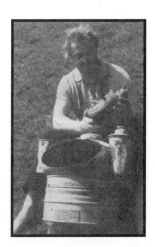

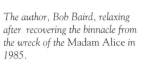

The author, Bob Baird, relaxing after recovering the binnacle from the wreck of the Madam Alice *in 1985.*
Photograph: Author's collection.

MAPS, DIAGRAMS & PHOTOGRAPHS

Maps & diagrams:

Photographs & paintings:

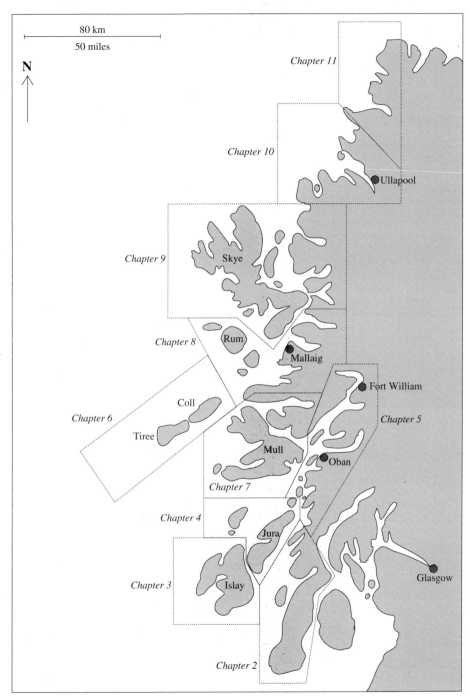

Map of the West Coast of Scotland showing the area covered by this book

CHAPTER 1

INTRODUCTION

FIRST WORDS

Shipwrecks of the West of Scotland is a reference guide to shipping losses from Sanda Island, off the Mull of Kintyre to Cape Wrath, and includes Islay, Mull, Skye and the smaller islands of the Inner Hebrides. This is the first co-ordinated work on shipwrecks to be published covering that whole area, and plugs a major gap in the documentary coverage of shipping losses around the coasts of Scotland. It is my second book in a series which, in conjunction with books already written by others about shipwrecks in the Clyde and the South west of Scotland, will eventually provide a record of shipping losses around the entire coast of Scotland, and follows the same successful format as its forerunner, *Shipwrecks of the Forth*.

Apart from two books, one about the shipwrecks of Islay (*Dive Islay Wrecks* by Steve Blackburn, 1986) and a second entitled *Argyll Shipwrecks* (by Peter Moir and Ian Crawford, 1994), there have been no other books written specifically about the ship-wrecks of the Atlantic coast of the West of Scotland. Parts of this area have been popular with divers for many years, particularly around Oban and Mull, and some of the wrecks are very well known, but published material about them has been rather scant and, with the exception of Gordon Ridley's first two dive guides (*Dive West Scotland*, 1984, and *Dive North West Scotland*, 1985), generally limited to articles about one single wreck, or a few selected wrecks in a fairly small area.

THIS BOOK

This book derives from my long-standing interest in ships, wrecks and marine salvage, and since taking up diving as a hobby some 15 years ago, my interest has been further developed and focused mainly on wrecks in Scottish waters. Over the years, I have read many books and articles, and gathered diverse pieces of information on this subject. Transferring raw snippets of information gleaned from many sources in different forms to a computer database required a standardisation of the various types of basic informa tion to enable data to be compared and assessed, and an orderly picture began to emerge. I very quickly realised that the mass of data I had collected formed the basis for a book on the subject, and all that was required to make it more than merely a list, was some further research to add meat to the bones, both for the sheer enjoyment of extending my own personal knowledge, and also to make it a more useful and enjoyable source of information to those with a similar interest.

In my quest for further information on wrecks in one area, I kept stumbling on references to wrecks in other areas, and with the discovery of each new piece of information, the area covered by my database gradually expanded to include the entire East coast of Scotland, the North coast, and the West coast from Cape Wrath down to Sanda Island off the Mull of Kintyre.

Research for a book of this nature can never be wholly complete, but one has to stop at some point to produce the first edition. This book contains details of 350 ships lost off the West of Scotland, many being described for the first time. From the latitude of the most southerly wreck in this book at 551000N to the most northerly at 585800N, the straight line distance is 228 nautical miles.

My own research is continuous, and further information will inevitably come to my attention, aided, I hope, by input from others, including readers of this book. Perhaps at some future date, if a sufficiently large amount of new information is forthcoming to justify it, an updated second edition may eventually be produced.

Most divers are keen to dive on wrecks and to learn something about them, although there is a certain amount of reluctance sometimes amongst divers to divulge jealously-guarded wreck information to other divers, who often tend to be regarded as potential competitors. I have found from personal experience, however, that being willing to share my knowledge with others generally brings its own rewards in the form of reciprocal information and friendships with fellow enthusiasts, and has vastly improved the quality of my own diving.

WRECK RESEARCH

The information in this book has been gleaned over a number of years from many sources, including newspaper files, the Admiralty Hydrographic Department, and Lloyds. In addition, many books and other publications have provided useful information, as indeed have many individuals. Wartime losses are particularly difficult to research because the strict censorship which applied during these periods suppressed information from the public domain. As a result, wartime newspapers are not very helpful. The Patrick Stephens reprint of the HMSO publication *British Vessels Lost at Sea 1914-1918 and 1939-1945* was one of the principal sources of information on wartime losses of British ships, but when referring to that source, be aware that the positions given are generally estimates of the position at the time of attack. No doubt in some instances the vessel sank almost immediately, but in others, the actual sinking may not have occurred for some considerable time after the attack, (up to several days later in some cases), during which period the damaged vessel may still have been under power, or taken in tow before sinking, or merely drifted for a time before finally foundering or being driven ashore.

It has long been a matter of regret to me that the dates of first reporting of charted wrecks are not given on the charts, as that would be a considerable aid to identifying them, or at the very least, eliminating some of the speculation regarding their possible identities. For example, a wreck first reported in 1920 is extremely unlikely to be a ship known to have sunk in 1940! For some wrecks several slightly different positions have been recorded over the years, and I have generally accepted information dated 1987, for example, as being more accurate than a 1919 position for the same wreck. This is not because the wreck has moved in the intervening period, but simply reflects the greater accuracy resulting from continuing advances in electronic navigation technology.

It used to be said that if you asked a young merchant navy officer where his ship was, he would confidently make a precise dot on the chart with a sharp pencil. A more experienced officer would draw a circle around the dot, and the older and wiser the officer, the larger the circle would be. With his years of experience in navigating across the oceans, the Captain would probably describe a fairly large circle on the chart with his finger and say "Somewhere in this area".

I have done my best to select what I consider to be perhaps the most accurate of the sometimes vague and conflicting information available. When an exact position is not known, I have endeavoured to provide as close an estimate as the information currently available to me will permit, and this is indicated in the text. By far, the most common causes of shipwrecks are running aground and collisions, while during both wars, submarine torpedoes, mines, and attack by aircraft were additional hazards which accounted for a substantial number of the wrecks.

DIVING THE WRECKS

As an aid to finding some of the wrecks I have endeavoured to provide transits where these are known to me. Some of the wrecks are too far off shore for transits to be useful, and must be located by some other means. The formula for calculating the distance in nautical miles to the radar horizon is 1.22 x the square root of height of scanner (in ft.) The eyes of someone sitting in an inflatable boat are likely to be no more than about some 4 ft. above the water surface, in which case the horizon is 2.44 nautical miles away. Even standing up, eye level will be only about 6 ft. above the water surface, and the horizon will be 2.99 nautical miles away. This means that the shore line beyond that distance is not visible, as, due to the curvature of the Earth, it will be beyond and below the horizon. Hence, objects at sea level on the shore line can not be seen from distances beyond the horizon. Only the tops of objects such as hills which stick up over the horizon will be visible, but not their bases. Anyone who has tried to position a small boat accurately over a wreck, using only hand-held compass bearings to points a long distance across open water, will know the degree of inaccuracy inherent in that method of position fixing!

Apart from seaworthy boats, echo sounders and accurate navigation and position fixing equipment such as Decca or GPS are absolutely essential for finding a great many of the wrecks. A magnetometer would also be of considerable assistance, but it is only in recent years that these electronic aids have become relatively common items of equipment for many divers. Availability of this equipment does not in itself, however, provide the complete answer to all of the problems. It is still necessary to know where to look for the wrecks, and that information is provided, to the best of my ability, in this book. To compensate for the lack of available transits for the majority of the wrecks, I have endeavoured to give Decca positions.

Boats are required to reach virtually all of the wrecks, and many of the visiting groups of divers come very well equipped in this regard. Hiring one of the specialist dive boats which operate in the area, or a local trawler, is probably still the best practical solution for many divers who wish to explore those wrecks located a long way offshore, and has the additional advantage of the skipper's local knowledge and experience, along with all the technological equipment and comfort provided by a relatively large vessel.

The area covered by this book includes Sea Areas Malin, Hebrides & Minches. The prevailing wind during the summer months is from the South west and West, and is the major factor governing diving activities. For about 10% of the time it is calm, but it can sometimes blow up to Severe Gale, Force 9, its passage across the Atlantic unhindered by any land masses. Surface conditions can vary enormously throughout the area, some places experiencing several rather sudden changes of weather and sea conditions in a single day, but from whichever direction the weather is coming, there are always sheltered areas in the lee of islands, or in the many bays created by the heavily-indented nature of the mainland coast.

Strong tidal streams run around headlands, and in the narrow sounds separating islands, or between islands and the mainland. There are no major rivers disgorging sediment or other pollutants into the seas off the West Coast, which is washed by clean Atlantic water flowing in the Gulf Stream, and is noticeably warmer than the waters of the North Sea. As a result, underwater visibility is generally very good, - gin clear in places, particularly towards the North and West, and marine life of all sorts is prolific. In early spring (March/April), the increasing sunlight causes a burst of plant activity, producing a plankton bloom which temporarily reduces underwater visibility to as little as 2-3 metres. By May, this has largely disappeared, but in September, the autumn storms bring nutrient-rich deeper waters to the surface where there is still sufficient light to allow the plankton to bloom again briefly.

Many of the wrecks in this book are not charted, but most of the charted wrecks in the area have been included, and while this book has been written primarily for the interest of fellow divers, some of the wrecks are too deep for sport diving, and are therefore likely to be only of academic interest to divers.

However, with the advent of *technical diving* and further developments which will inevitably follow in the future, there may come a time when some of the deeper wrecks will be within the reach of divers. In the meantime, it doesn't hurt to know the locations and identities of the deeper wrecks. Furthermore, it is well known that wrecks attract fish and so some of the wrecks may be of interest to fishermen and sea anglers.

Further information

To add to my own knowledge, I should be grateful for any further information which readers may be able to provide. Knowing a date for the sinking of a vessel provides a good starting point for personal research through the files of local newspapers, unless the date is during the First or Second World Wars, when censorship prevented newspapers from publishing information which would now be useful to wreck detectives.

Some of the named wrecks whose positions are not accurately known will no doubt tie up with some of the charted wrecks which have yet to be identified, while others will be the remains of vessels for which, through lack of sufficient information, I am presently unable to suggest a possible name with any degree of confidence. A good many of the wrecks are well known to divers, but many more are not. I have personally dived on only a tiny proportion of these wrecks, and should welcome information from divers visiting any of the wrecks, to let me know what was found, possibly enabling identification of an *Unknown*, or to correct any errors of fact or omission I may have made. My database contains information on many more wrecks than are included in this book, and I would be willing to have a go at identifying any wreck found which does not appear to be included herein.

Acknowledgements

I am indebted to a number of individuals who have provided useful information, and would especially like to thank Gordon Ridley and Ian Whittaker for their invaluable assistance with information, encouragement and technological support in the preparation of this book.

The wreck details

In general, the wrecks are described from South to North (i.e. in latitude order), but this is perhaps not the most useful order in which to describe the wrecks around the various islands and in the large sea lochs and bays. The shapes of these geographical features do not always lend themselves to such a strict logical sequence, and therefore it is not rigidly adhered to throughout the book. Detailed information on each wreck is given immediately under the vessel's name. This is followed by details of the circumstances of the loss of the vessel, its present whereabouts and condition (where known) and other more general information where this is known. Any wreck can be found by reference to the two indexes - a name index and a latitude index. These give both the page number and the wreck number (these are assigned sequentially throughout the book).

Maps and charts

For maximum comprehension of, and benefit from, the information provided in this book, it is recommended that it should be read in conjunction with the Admiralty charts listed opposite.

1790 - Oban and Approaches
1794 - North Minch - Southern Part
1795 - The Little Minch
1839 - (Ullapool)
2126 - Approaches to the Firth of Clyde
2168 - Approaches to the Sound of Jura
2171 - Sound of Mull and Approaches
2207 - Ardnamurchan Point to Sound
    of Sleat
2208 - Mallaig to Canna Harbour
2210 - Approaches to Inner Sound
2320 - (Crinan)
2326 - Loch Crinan to Firth of Lorne
2378 - Loch Linnhe - Southern Part
2390 - Sound of Mull

2394 - Loch Sunart
2396 - Sound of Jura - Southern Part
2474 - (Tobermory)
2475 - Sounds of Gigha and Gunna
2481 - Sound of Islay
2500 - Loch Broom and Little Loch Broom
    and Approaches
2501 - Summer Isles
2502 - Eddrachillis Bay
2509 - Rubha Reidh to Cailleach Head
2534 - (Mallaig, Portree)
2540 - Loch Alsh and Approaches
2617 - Sound of Iona
2722 - Skerryvore to St. Kilda
2798 - North Channel

The Ordnance Survey 1:50,000 Landranger series maps, (sheets 9, 15, 19, 23, 24, 32, 33, 39, 40, 46, 47, 48, 49, 55, 60, 61, 62, and 68), would also provide a useful reference guide while reading this book, particularly in respect of the many vessels which were lost through running aground.

Depths shown on the present metric series of Admiralty charts are given at a datum of LAT (Lowest Astronomical Tide), which is the lowest sea level which can be predicted to occur under average meteorological conditions and under any combination of astronomical conditions. In practice, this only occurs infrequently, and not necessarily at slack water. It can be affected by abnormal weather conditions such as strong winds, variations in barometric pressure and storm surges. The actual depth of water over a wreck is the charted depth plus the height of the tide at the time. Tidal ranges on the west coast of Scotland vary considerably.

Off theSouth east of Islay, there is an amphidromic point, around which the tides rotate, and where the difference between high and low water is virtually zero for days on end during neap tide periods. This area has the smallest tidal range in Scottish waters, although there are strong tidal streams and broken water, particularly around the headlands of the South west peninsulas. Cotidal lines, (lines joining points at which high water occurs at the same time), radiate from an amphidrome, and the tidal range increases with distance from it. Further North, the tidal range rises to between four and five metres, making the height of the tide a factor to be considered when diving the deeper wrecks.

Tide tables giving the predicted heights of the tide at low and high water, and the different times at which they will occur in various places, are also produced using LAT as a datum. The tide tables always give times in GMT (Greenwich Mean Time), and take no account of British Summer Time, which is one hour ahead of GMT. Care must be taken to adjust the times given in these tables by adding one hour during the summer months, from about the end of March to about the end of October each year, when BST (British Summer Time) applies. No adjustment is required during the winter months when GMT is in operation.

When using LAT-based tide tables with old charts which had a datum of MLWS

(Mean Low Water Springs) - which is slightly higher than LAT - the actual depth will be slightly, (perhaps about half a metre), less than the calculated depth. Tidal streams are the horizontal movement of water caused by the vertical rise and fall of the tide, which normally changes direction about every six hours.

Tidal ranges and tidal streams are at their greatest during periods of Spring Tides, and at their least during periods of Neap Tides.

THE RULE OF TWELTHS

For places where the rise and fall of the tide follows a regular pattern, a rough calculation of the height of the tide, and strength of the tidal stream, between low and high water can be made using the Rule of Twelfths. The rule assumes that the rise and fall of the tide is:

1/12 of the range during the first hour
2/12 of the range during the second hour
3/12 of the range during the third hour
3/12 of the range during the fourth hour
2/12 of the range during the fifth hour
1/12 of the range during the sixth hour

A fuller explanation of this rather complex subject is given in Nautical Almanacs.

POSITIONS OF PROMINENT POINTS

The positions of some of the more prominent navigational points included within the area covered by this book are listed opposite:

	LAT North	LONG West
Sanda Island Light	5516.50	0534.90
Mull of Kintyre Light	5518.60	0548.10
Arranman Barrels Light	5519.40	0532.80
Rudha Mail, Sound of Islay	5526.20	0607.35
Otter Rock Light Buoy, Islay	5533.92	0607.85
Mull of Oa Monument, Islay	5535.24	0619.90
Eilean a Chuirn, Islay	5540.14	0601.15
Orsay Light, Rinns of Islay	5540.38	0630.70
McArthur's Head, South, Islay	5545.85	0602.80
Dubh Artach	5606.00	0637.90
Skerryvore	5619.40	0706.75
Lismore Light, Loch Linnhe	5627.40	0536.40
Glas Eileanan, Sound of Mull	5629.80	0542.70
Ardtornish Point, Sound of Mull	5631.10	0545.10

Eileanan Glasa, Sound of Mull	5632.30	0554.70
Loch Eatharna, Coll	5636.67	0630.90
Rubha nan Gall, Mull	5638.33	0603.91
Ardmore Point, Mull	5639.40	0607.60
Cairns of Coll	5642.27	0626.70
Ardnamurchan Point	5643.64	0613.46
Neist Point, Skye	5725.40	0647.20
Waternish Point, Skye	5736.50	0638.00
Eilean Trodday	5743.60	0617.80
Cailleach Head	5755.83	0524.15
Stoer Head	5814.40	0524.00
Rubha Reidh	5814.40	0548.60
Cape Wrath	5837.55	0459.87

NOTE

Some of the wrecks listed in this book may be considered to be War Graves - notably HMS Vandal.

War Graves are covered by the Protection of Military Remains Act 1986 and include the wrecks of any Royal Navy ship or merchant vessel lost on active Government service and which have human remains aboard.

Apparently it is normally permissible to dive on these wrecks but not to disturb or remove anything from the site.

PLEASE RESPECT THESE FACTS

THE COMPASS

Modern compasses have a scale marked in degrees, with 0° at North round clockwise to 360° again at North.

Previously, the compass rose was marked in *Points* and *Quarter Points*. Some compass cards are marked with both degrees and points, the degrees being on the outside.

There are 32 compass points in a circle of 360 degrees. One point, therefore, equals 11.25°, and a quarter point, which is the smallest division shown on a card marked in that way, equals marginally under 3° (2.8125°).

The illustration shows the compass, and the names of the points and quarter points, and the table gives their equivalents in degrees.

Note that none of the by-points or quarter points takes its name from a three-letter point: For example, N by E is correct, not NNE by N, and NE by N¾N is correct, not NNE¼E.

The present metric series of Admiralty charts have compass roses marked in degrees true, on the outside of the rose, and degrees magnetic, on the inside, the difference between them being the local magnetic variation. The amount and direction of the annual change is also given within the compass rose.

If information concerning the position of a wreck includes a compass bearing, it is important to note the date from which the bearing originates, and to take account of the local magnetic variation in the area over the years which have elapsed since the date of the information.

Point	Heading	Point	Heading	Point	Heading	Point	Heading
NORTH	0	EAST	90	SOUTH	180	WEST	270
N 1/4 E	2.8125	E 1/4 S	92.8125	S 1/4 W	182.8125	W 1/4 N	272.8125
N 1/2 E	5.625	E 1/2 S	95.625	S 1/2 W	185.625	W 1/2 N	275.625
N 3/4 E	8.4375	E 3/4 S	98.4375	S 3/4 W	188.4375	W 3/4 N	278.4375
N by E	11.25	E by S	101.25	S by W	191.25	W by N	281.25
N by E 1/4 E	14.0625	E by S 1/4 S	104.0625	S by W 1/4 W	194.0625	W by N 1/4 N	284.0625
N by E 1/2 E	16.875	E by S 1/2 S	106.875	S by W 1/2 W	196.875	W by N 1/2 N	286.875
N by E 3/4 E	19.6875	E by S 3/4 S	109.6875	S by W 3/4 W	199.6875	W by N 3/4 N	289.6875
NNE	22.5	ESE	112.5	SSW	202.5	WNW	292.5
NE by N 3/4 N	25.3125	SE by E 3/4 E	115.3125	SW by W 3/4 S	205.3125	NW by W 3/4 W	295.3125
NE by N 1/2 N	28.125	SE by E 1/2 E	118.125	SW by W 1/2 S	208.125	NW by W 1/2 W	298.125
NE by N 1/4 N	30.9375	SE by E 1/4 E	120.9375	SW by W 1/4 S	210.9375	NW by W 1/4 W	300.9375
NE by N	33.75	SE by E	123.75	SW by W	213.75	NW by W	303.75
NE 3/4 N	36.5625	SE 3/4 E	126.5625	SW 3/4 W	216.5625	NW 3/4 W	306.5625
NE 1/2 N	39.375	SE 1/2 E	129.375	SW 1/2 W	219.375	NW 1/2 W	309.375
NE 1/4 N	42.1875	SE 1/4 E	132.1875	SW 1/4 W	222.1875	NW 1/4 W	312.1875
NORTH EAST	45	SOUTH EAST	135	SOUTH WEST	225	NORTH WEST	315
NE by E	47.8125	SE by S	137.8125	SW by W	227.8125	NW by N	317.8125
NE 1/2 E	50.625	SE 1/2 S	140.625	SW 1/2 W	230.625	NW 1/2 N	320.625
NE 3/4 E	53.4375	SE 3/4 S	143.4375	SW 3/4 W	233.4375	NW 3/4 N	323.4375
NE by E	56.25	SE by S	146.25	SW by W	236.25	NW by N	326.25
NE by E 1/4 E	59.0625	SE by S 1/4 S	149.0625	SW by W 1/4 W	239.0625	NW by N 1/4 W	329.0625
NE by E 1/2 E	61.875	SE by S 1/2 S	151.875	SW by W 1/2 W	241.875	NW by N 1/2 W	331.875
NE by E 3/4 E	64.6875	SE by S 3/4 S	154.6875	SW by W 3/4 W	244.6875	NW by N 3/4 W	334.6875
ENE	67.5	SSE	157.5	WSW	247.5	NNW	337.5
E by N 3/4 N	70.3125	S by E 3/4 E	160.3125	W by S 3/4 S	250.3125	N by W 1/4 N	340.3125
E by N 1/2 N	73.125	S by E 1/2 E	163.125	W by S 1/2 S	253.125	N by W 1/2 N	343.125
E by N 1/4 N	75.9375	S by E 1/4 E	165.9375	W by S 1/4 S	255.9375	N by W 3/4 N	345.9375
E by N	78.75	S by E	168.75	W by S	258.75	N by W	348.75
E 3/4 N	81.5625	S 3/4 E	171.5625	W 3/4 S	261.5625	N 3/4 W	351.5625
E 1/2 N	84.375	S 1/2 E	174.375	W 1/2 S	264.375	N 1/2 W	354.375
E 1/4 N	87.1875	S 1/4 E	177.1875	W 1/4 S	267.1875	N 1/4 W	357.1875
EAST	90	SOUTH	180	WEST	270	NORTH	360

SWEEPING OF WRECKS

Charted wrecks which have been swept are indicated on the chart by a bar with upright vertical projections at either end, immediately below the Wk symbol which contains a figure representing the depth

The word *swept*, as applied to wrecks, is commonly misunderstood, and often erroneously presumed to mean that a sweep wire has literally swept, or removed, the superstructure off a sunken vessel for the purpose of increasing the safe clearance depth. This is complete nonsense. It would require a wire of infinite breaking strain to be towed by a

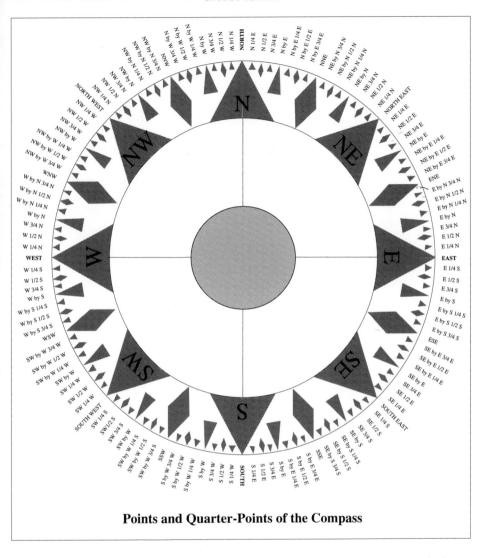

Points and Quarter-Points of the Compass

ship of infinite power and propeller efficiency, and could only apply to wrecks which were sitting upright on the bottom.

When a wreck is said to have been swept, this simply means that its minimum clearance depth has been determined by the use of one of the following two methods:

Bar-Sweep:

In this alternative, more accurate, method of measuring the minimum depth of a wreck, a rigid iron bar is suspended horizontally below a ship drifting over the wreck. The bar is hung over the side on three measured lines - one at each end, and one in the middle to

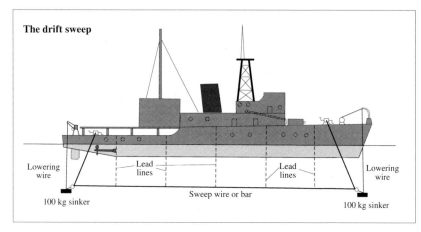

The drift sweep

Lowering wire

Lead lines

Lead lines

Lowering wire

100 kg sinker

Sweep wire or bar

100 kg sinker

The bar or drift sweep

avoid any bending effect on the bar. The depth of the bar is adjusted until the bar just avoids fouling the wreck as the ship drifts over it.

By computing the time of the measurement against tidal prediction tables, the depth is converted to chart datum.

Oropesa Sweep:

The Oropesa sweep used by mine-sweepers was named after the ship in which it was first tried out in 1918.

A heavy torpedo-shaped float took the sweep wire out on to the mine-sweeper's quarter, about 500 yards astern. An *otter* attached to the sweep wire below this float, and a *kite* attached to the wire immediately astern of the trawler, controlled the depth of the wire, working on the principle of air kites. The kite held the inboard end of the sweep wire down in the water, while the otter at the other end kept the sweep wire curving out about 250 yards on the mine-sweeper's quarter.

The mine-sweeper following behind steamed just inside the limit of the leader's curving sweep, and in larger groups, every following vessel did the same, so that only the lead ship was at risk from mines as she nosed into unswept waters.

The serrated sweep wire cut the mooring cables of the mines, which were exploded or sunk by gunfire as they bobbed to the surface.

The Single Oropesa sweep

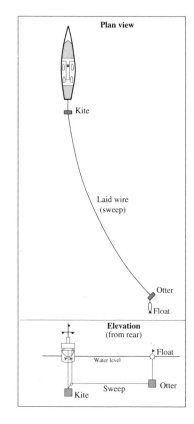

Plan view

Kite

Laid wire (sweep)

Otter

Float

Elevation
(from rear)

Float

Water level

Kite

Sweep

Otter

Side scan sonar

Hydrographic surveys are carried out by the Royal Navy using ships equipped with sonar sweeping apparatus designed specifically for the purpose of detecting dangers underwater. However, this equipment is less well suited to either finding the least depth over wrecks or for measuring their dimensions. More accurate methods are used to find the least depth over wrecks, such as the Oropesa and drift sweeps or vertical echo sounding. No equipment has been designed solely for the purpose of measuring the dimensions of wrecks although side scan sonar is normally used. This was originally developed to assist anti-submarine vessels to identify submarines sitting on the bottom. It has since been used to examine all kinds of bottom features. However, there are certain limitations (see below) when using side scan sonar to measure wreck dimensions and these should be treated cautiously.

The horizontal and vertical scales on the side scan image are different. Thus, when using this equipment to accurately measure the length of a wreck, the survey ship's course must be parallel to the orientation of the wreck, so that the wreck echo and shadow lie vertically on the recording paper.

The performance of a sideways looking sonar varies with the depth of the water, the quality of the bottom and the water conditions. Furthermore, the sonar trace is interpreted by an experienced operator, thus introducing the possibility of human error. Finally, although electronic equipment is being continuously improved, older hydrographic surveys of an area will not have used the latest, more accurate, equipment.

Tonnage

Gross Tonnage: is a measure of space, not of weight, and indicates the total permanently enclosed space of a ship - i.e. her internal volume - and is calculated on the basis of 100 cu. ft. = 1 ton.

Net Tonnage: is the Gross Tonnage less the space occupied by engines, boilers, bunkers, crew's quarters and all other space which, although essential for the working of the ship, is *non-earning*. The Net Tonnage, therefore, indicates how much revenue-earning space there is in the ship.

Tons Displacement: is the actual weight of the ship in long tons (2240 lbs. avoirdupois), as determined by the equivalent weight of water displaced by the ship when afloat.

Tons Deadweight: is the total weight of cargo, fuel, stores, crew and all other items which are not actually a part of the ship, but which the ship can carry when she is floating down to her load marks.

CHAPTER 2

THE WRECKS OF KINTYRE

INTRODUCTION

Kintyre and Knapdale together make up the longest peninsula in Scotland. (Kintyre means Lands End). By road, it is 77 miles from Inveraray to Campbeltown. From the head of Loch Fyne to the Mull of Kintyre is almost 100 miles.

The peninsula has a great deal of fabulous scenery which would delight anyone, but it does not have the same qualities of spectacular magnificence and grandeur as the North west.

From West Loch Tarbert ferries run to Jura and Islay. At Tayinloan there is also a ferry to the island of Gigha.

Campbeltown, near the extreme South east end of the peninsula, has a population of around 6000, and is 135 miles by road from Glasgow. The main road follows the West coast from Tarbert, but the narrower road down the East coast is scenically better in the panorama of the Arran hills seen across Kilbrannan Sound.

At Macrihanish, on the West coast of the peninsula, about five miles from Campbeltown, there is an RAF/NATO air base, which also handles a small number of commercial flights to and from Glasgow and Islay.

The lighthouse at the Mull of Kintyre sits on top of 90 metre sheer cliffs, and is only twelve miles across the North Channel from Northern Ireland.

Sanda Island is the largest of a group of rocky islets two miles off the south eastern tip of Kintyre. Sheep Island and Glunimore island, two others of the group, are the main breeding places in the Clyde for puffins.

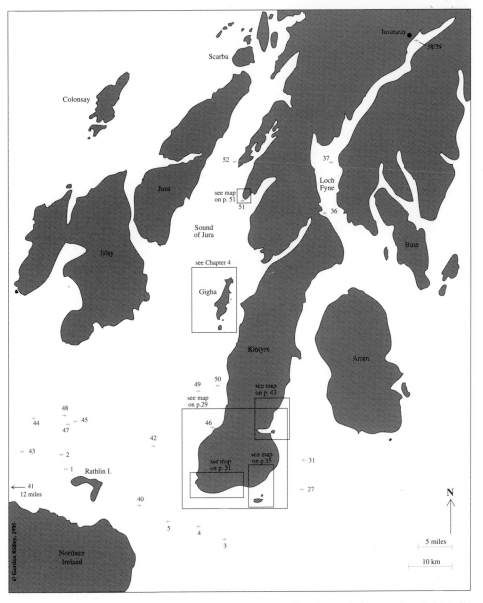

Chart showing the location of wrecks lying off the coast of Kintyre

THE WRECKS

GODETIA

Wreck No : 1	**Date Sunk :** 06 09 1940
Latitude : 55 19 12 N	**Longitude :** 06 05 42 W
Decca Lat : 5519.20 N	**Decca Long :** 0605.70 W
Location : ¾ mile ENE of Rathlin Island	**Area :** N. Channel
Type : Corvette	**Tonnage :** 940 gross.
Length : 205.0 ft. **Beam :** 33.0 ft.	**Draught :** 14.5 ft.
How Sunk : Collision with SS *Marsa*	**Depth :** metres

The Flower Class corvette HMS *Godetia*, built by Smiths Dock, Middlesbrough in 1940, was lost in collision with SS *Marsa*, 3 miles North of Altacarry Head, Ireland at 2300 hours, on 6th September 1940.

ANDANIA

Wreck No : 2	**Date Sunk :** 27 01 1918
Latitude : 55 20 00 N PA	**Longitude :** 06 12 00 W PA
Decca Lat : 5520.00 N	**Decca Long :** 0612.00 W
Location : 2 miles NNE of Rathlin LH.	**Area :** N. Channel

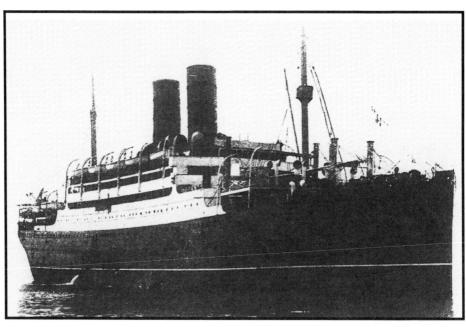

The Andania (Photograph courtesy of John Clarkson, Longton)

Type : Steamship

Length : 520.3 ft.　　Beam : 64.0 ft.

How Sunk : Torpedoed

Tonnage : 13405 gross.

Draught : 43.1 ft.

Depth :　　　metres

The Cunard liner *Andania*, built in 1913 by Scotts S. B. Co., was torpedoed two miles NNE of Rathlin Island by the U-46 on 27th January 1918 while en route from Liverpool to New York. Seven lives were lost. *Lloyds War Losses* gives the position of attack as 3 to 4 miles NNE of Altacarry Light Vessel.

PARTHENIA

Wreck No : 3

Latitude : 55 10 00 N

Decca Lat : 5510.00 N

Location : 7 miles SW of Sanda Island

Type : Steamship

Length : 399.7 ft.　　Beam : 51.9 ft.

How Sunk : Collision

Date Sunk : 29 11 1940

Longitude : 05 40 30 W

Decca Long : 0540.50 W

Area : S. Kintyre

Tonnage : 4872 gross.

Draught : 26.9 ft.

Depth :　　　metres

The British steamship *Parthenia*, (ex-*Kirkholm*), built in 1917 by Russell & Co. of Port Glasgow, was en route from Montreal to Glasgow with a general cargo when she was sunk in collision with the *Robert F Hand* about seven miles South west of Sanda Island on 29th November 1940.

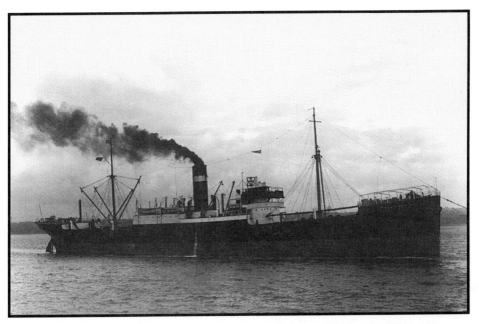

The Parthenia (Photograph courtesy of John Clarkson, Longton)

PERELLE

Wreck No : 4
Latitude : 55 12 00 N PA
Decca Lat : 5512.00 N
Location : 5 miles S of Mull of Kintyre
Type : Steamship
Length : 177.0 ft.   **Beam :** 28.1 ft.
How Sunk :

Date Sunk : 14 03 1942
Longitude : 05 48 00 W PA
Decca Long : 0548.00 W
Area : S. Kintyre
Tonnage : 659 gross.
Draught : 10.9 ft.
Depth :   metres

Perelle, (ex-*Stainburn*), was built in 1922 by Wm. Adam & Co., Larne, engine by Campbell & Calderwood, Paisley. She is not mentioned in Rohwer's *Axis Submarine Successes 1939-45*.

UB-82

Wreck No : 5
Latitude : 55 13 00 N PA
Decca Lat : 5513.00 N
Location : In North Channel
Type : Submarine
Length : 183.2 ft.   **Beam :** 18.9 ft.
How Sunk : Depth-charged

Date Sunk : 17 04 1918
Longitude : 05 55 00 W PA
Decca Long : 0555.00 W
Area : S. Kintyre
Tonnage : 516 gross.
Draught :   ft.
Depth :   metres

Some 516 tons surfaced, 647 tons submerged, *UB-82* (Becker), was depth-charged by HM drifters *Young Fred* and *Pilot Me* in the North Channel.

The latitude and longitude is a Hydrographic Dept. PA, 7 miles South west of the Mull of Kintyre. Another positionrecorded is 5513N 0515W.

BYRON DARNTON

Wreck No : 6
Latitude : 55 16 25 N
Decca Lat : 5516.42 N
Location : SW side of The Ship, Sanda Is.
Type : Steamship
Length : 441.5 ft.   **Beam :** 57.0 ft.
How Sunk : Ran aground

Date Sunk : 17 03 1946
Longitude : 05 35 01 W
Decca Long : 0535.02 W
Area : S. Kintyre
Tonnage : 7176 gross.
Draught : 27.0 ft.
Depth : 5 metres

The *Byron Darnton* was a Liberty Ship built by Bethlehem Fairfield in December 1943, engined by the General Machinery Corporation of Hamilton, Ohio.

She ran aground on 17th March 1946 below the lighthouse at the South west side of the promontory called *The Ship* at the South side of Sanda Island, while outward bound from the Clyde to the United States.

Over a period of 18 hours in terrible conditions, the Campbeltown lifeboat *Duke Of Connaught* rescued all 52 aboard, including seven Norwegian girls, a war bride and a dog. Badly battered by heavy seas, she broke in two just as the lifeboat pulled clear. Despite engine trouble the lifeboat returned safely to Campbeltown.

Until the wreck was scrapped on site in October 1953, but the remains are visible at all states of the tide as a large rusty wreck lying on its side, and very prominent when viewed from East or West. Wreckage extends down to 16 metres.

MYRTLE

Wreck No : 7	**Date Sunk :** 04 08 1854
Latitude : 55 16 30 N PA	**Longitude :** 05 36 00 W PA
Decca Lat : 5516.50 N	**Decca Long :** 0536.00 W
Location : Baron Reef, near Sanda Island	**Area :** S. Kintyre
Type : Paddle steamer	**Tonnage :** 212 gross.
Length : 178.2 ft. **Beam :** 22.6 ft.	**Draught :** 13.1 ft.
How Sunk : Ran aground	**Depth :** metres

Myrtle was a 3-masted iron paddle steamer built in 1853.

CLANSMAN

Wreck No : 8	**Date Sunk :** 07 1869
Latitude : 55 17 00 N PA	**Longitude :** 05 36 00 W PA
Decca Lat : 5517.00 N	**Decca Long :** 0536.00 W
Location : W side of Sanda Island	**Area :** S. Kintyre
Type : Paddle steamer	**Tonnage :** 414 gross.
Length : 192.0 ft. **Beam :** 26.0 ft.	**Draught :** 13.0 ft.
How Sunk : Ran aground	**Depth :** metres

The paddle steamer *Clansman* ran aground in fog on the West side of Sanda Island in July 1869.

DUCHESS OF LANCASTER

Wreck No : 9	**Date Sunk :** 26 01 1863
Latitude : 55 17 00 N PA	**Longitude :** 05 48 00 W PA
Decca Lat : 5517.00 N	**Decca Long :** 0548.00 W
Location : Off Mull of Kintyre	**Area :** S. Kintyre
Type : Schooner	**Tonnage :** gross.
Length : ft. **Beam :** ft.	**Draught :** ft.

How Sunk : Foundered   **Depth :**   metres

The schooner *Duchess of Lancaster* foundered off the Mull of Kintyre on 26th January 1863.

ST. KILDA

Wreck No : 10   **Date Sunk :** 26 01 1863
Latitude : 55 17 00 N PA   **Longitude :** 05 48 00 W PA
Decca Lat : 5517.00 N   **Decca Long :** 0548.00 W
Location : Off Mull of Kintyre   **Area :** S. Kintyre
Type : Steamship   **Tonnage :**   gross.
Length :   ft.   **Beam :**   ft.   **Draught :**   ft.
How Sunk : Foundered   **Depth :**   metres

The steamship *St. Kilda* foundered off the Mull of Kintyre on 26th January 1863.

ADEPT

Wreck No : 11   **Date Sunk :** 17 03 1942
Latitude : 55 17 05 N   **Longitude :** 05 32 26 W
Decca Lat : 5517.08 N   **Decca Long :** 0532.43 W
Location : Paterson's Rock   **Area :** S. Kintyre
Type : Tug   **Tonnage :** 700 gross
Length : 157.0 ft.   **Beam :** 33.5 ft.   **Draught :** 11.0 ft.
How Sunk : Ran aground   **Depth :**   metres

The tug *Adept* was built by Cochranes of Selby in 1941. On 17th March 1942 she ran on to Paterson's Rock at high tide. The tug *Zwart Zee* made an unsuccessful attempt to pull the *Adept* off, and her very smashed remains now lie close in to the West side of Paterson's Rock. Her boiler is standing upright with other wreckage close by.

STEAM DREDGER NO. 285

Wreck No : 12   **Date Sunk :** 29 08 1891
Latitude : 55 17 15 N PA   **Longitude :** 05 34 18 W PA
Decca Lat : 5517.25 N   **Decca Long :** 0534.30 W
Location : Between Sanda and Sheep Island   **Area :** S. Kintyre
Type : Dredger   **Tonnage :** 195 gross.
Length :   ft.   **Beam :**   ft.   **Draught :**   ft.
How Sunk : Ran aground   **Depth :**   metres

The steam dredger *No.285* was lost on a reef between Sanda and Sheep Island on 29th August 1891. She had been en route from Renfrew to Blyth. Her remains may be on the reef which extends northwards from Sanda Island, or on Scart Rocks.

UNKNOWN

Wreck No : 13

Date Sunk :

Latitude : 55 17 21 N

Longitude : 05 33 12 W

Decca Lat : 5517.35 N

Decca Long : 0533.20 W

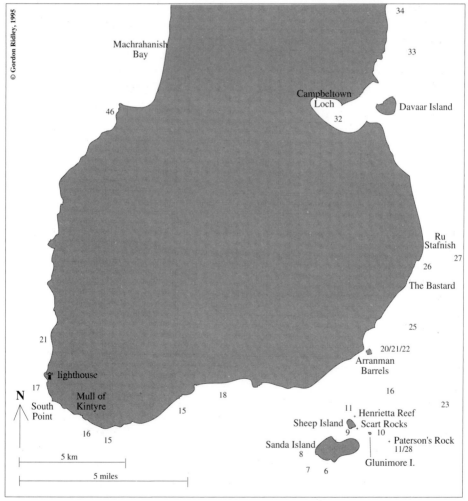

The wrecks of South Kintyre

Location : Glunimore Is., nr Sanda Island **Area :** S. Kintyre
Type : **Tonnage :** gross
Length : ft. **Beam :** ft. **Draught :** ft.
How Sunk : Ran aground **Depth :** metres

Charted off the North east of Glunimore Island, ½ mile North east of Sanda Island, and visible at all states of the tide.

UNKNOWN - STATELY?

Wreck No : 14 **Date Sunk :** 12 09 1927
Latitude : 55 17 42 N **Longitude :** 05 43 24 W
Decca Lat : 5517.70 N **Decca Long :** 0534.40 W
Location : N tip of Sheep Island **Area :** S. Kintyre
Type : Drifter **Tonnage :** gross
Length : ft. **Beam :** ft. **Draught :** ft.
How Sunk : Ran aground **Depth :** metres

Charted at the North tip of Sheep Island, visible at all states of the tide. This may be the steam drifter *Stately* which ran aground here on 12th September 1927.

NEW YORK

Wreck No : 15 **Date Sunk :** 28 09 1895
Latitude : 55 17 24 N **Longitude :** 05 45 24 W
Decca Lat : 5517.40 N **Decca Long :** 0545.40 W
Location : Rubha Clachan, S tip of Kintyre **Area :** S. Kintyre
Type : Steamship **Tonnage :** 2050 gross.
Length : ft. **Beam :** ft. **Draught :** ft.
How Sunk : Ran aground **Depth :** 20 metres

The wreck charted close under the cliffs at Rubha Clachan, about 600 yards East of Sron Uamha, the southernmost point of Kintyre, is the steamship *New York*.

In the late afternoon of 12th June 1858, the *New York* left Greenock, bound for New York with 220 passengers and 80 crew. By the time she passed Sanda Light at 11.00 pm darkness had fallen and there was also a thick fog. In spite of this she was running at 10 knots. An hour later breakers were sighted ahead and, despite altering course and going full astern, she ran on to the reef at Rubha Clachan. She remained perched on the rocks until daybreak when the passengers were landed ashore in the ship's boats. One of the crew members also landed and went to Campbeltown to raise the alarm.

At midday on the 13th the steamer *Celt* arrived on the scene and took off 130 passengers, the remainder travelling overland as the sea was by then becoming too rough to continue transhipping them. Five tugs were unable to pull the *New York* off the rocks, but recovered most of the cargo.

Wreckage, including some quite large sections with portholes, runs from 5 to 20 metres down the slope of the reef.

BUTE

Wreck No : 16	**Date Sunk : 18 12 1890**
Latitude : 55 17 24 N	**Longitude :** 05 45 32 W
Decca Lat : 5517.40 N	**Decca Long :** 0545.53 W
Location : Sron Uamha, S tip of Kintyre	**Area :** S. Kintyre
Type : Steamship	**Tonnage :** gross
Length : 75.9 ft. **Beam :** 19.8 ft.	**Draught :** 10.0 ft.
How Sunk : Ran aground	**Depth :** 20 metres

The steamship *Bute* ran aground under the cliffs at Sron Uamha, the southernmost point of Kintyre, on 18th December 1890.

Her cargo was reportedly either whisky or salt, but perhaps she carried both.

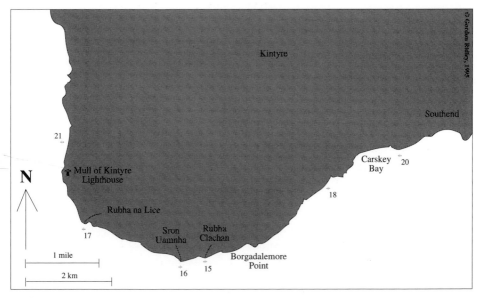

The wrecks of the Mull of Kintyre

SIGNAL

Wreck No : 17	**Date Sunk :** 28 09 1895
Latitude : 55 17 55 N PA	**Longitude :** 05 47 40 W PA
Decca Lat : 5517.92 N	**Decca Long :** 0547.67 W
Location : ¾ mile SSE Mull of Kintyre Lt.	**Area :** S. Kintyre
Type : Paddle steamer	**Tonnage :** 345 gross.
Length : 160.1 ft. **Beam :** 25.1 ft.	**Draught :** 11.6 ft.
How Sunk : Ran aground	**Depth :** metres

The 174 tons net steel paddle steamer *Signal* hit a submerged rock ¾ mile SSE of Mull of Kintyre lighthouse. That suggests she possibly struck the rocks off Rubha na Lice, or below the cliffs in the small bay immediately to the east.

She was built by Caird of Greenock in 1883 for the Commissioners for Northern Lighthouses, and was carrying lighthouse supplies from Islay to Sanda Island.

MOBEKA

Wreck No : 18	**Date Sunk :** 19 01 1942
Latitude : 55 18 18 N	**Longitude :** 05 42 18 W
Decca Lat : 5518.30 N	**Decca Long :** 0542.30 W
Location : 2 miles W of Southend	**Area :** S. Kintyre
Type : Steamship	**Tonnage :** 5277 gross
Length : 426.5 ft. **Beam :** 55.7 ft.	**Draught :** 25.0 ft.
How Sunk : Ran aground	**Depth :** 2 metres

The 6111 tons gross Belgian motor vessel *Mobeka*, built in 1937, ran ashore 2 miles West of Southend on 19th January 1942. The wreck is charted as visible at all states of the tide. The *Mobeka* was one of several ships in an outward bound convoy waiting in the early morning darkness for the arrival of a naval escort to take them through the North Channel.

Before dawn the trawler *Anna Maria* went ashore at Carskiey and fired distress flares; these were mistaken by the *Mobeka*'s captain for the signal that the Navy had arrived. The *Mobeka* set off towards the flares causing the trawler's crew, when they saw her approaching the shore, to fire more flares to warn her that she was heading into danger. When the *Mobeka*'s captain realised the situation he attempted to alter course, but it was too late to prevent his vessel running ashore.

Southend coastguards were already at the scene attempting to rescue the crew of the trawler. Two of the *Mobeka*'s boats were smashed in an attempt to land passengers but, by firing lines ashore, nine men were landed in a third boat. The remaining 44 aboard were taken off later that morning by Campbeltown lifeboat. Most of the cargo was salvaged. The wreck is now very broken up, but some of the cargo of vehicles, tyres, cables and engines are scattered in shallow water close to shore.

UNKNOWN

Wreck No : 19
Latitude : 55 18 00 N
Decca Lat : 5518.00 N
Location : 2 miles NE of Sanda Island
Type :
Length : ft. **Beam :** ft.
How Sunk :

Date Sunk :
Longitude : 05 31 00 W
Decca Long : 0531.00 W
Area : S. Kintyre
Tonnage : gross
Draught : ft.
Depth : 20 metres

ARBUTUS

Wreck No : 20
Latitude : 55 18 00 N PA
Decca Lat : 5518.00 N
Location : Near Southend, Kintyre
Type : Steamship
Length : 179.8 ft. **Beam :** 22.6 ft.
How Sunk : Ran aground

Date Sunk : 06 08 1878
Longitude : 05 40 00 W PA
Decca Long : 0540.00 W
Area : S. Kintyre
Tonnage : 348 gross.
Draught : 12.3 ft.
Depth : metres

The iron steamship *Arbutus* was outward bound from Greenock to Londonderry when she ran on to the rocks near Southend in a fog on 6th August 1878. Some 70 or 80 passengers and crew reached the shore safely before she slipped off the rocks and sank in deep water.

Another report in *Parliamentary Papers* describes her as a 336 ton iron steamship which was lost ¼ mile from Mull of Kintyre light while en route from Londonderry to Glasgow with a general cargo and 55 passengers on 18th April 1878.

Charted as a wreck at 20 metres.

MACEDONIA

Wreck No : 21
Latitude : 55 19 18 N
Decca Lat : 5519.30 N
Location : Mull of Kintyre
Type : Steamship
Length : 315.0 ft. **Beam :** 34.0 ft.
How Sunk : Ran aground

Date Sunk : 30 05 1881
Longitude : 05 48 00 W
Decca Long : 0548.00 W
Area : S. Kintyre
Tonnage : 2273 gross.
Draught : 24.2 ft.
Depth : 14 metres

Macedonia was a British iron steamship wrecked in fog ¾ mile North of the Mull of Kintyre lighthouse while en route from New York to the Clyde with a general cargo including cattle.

For several days the sea remained calm and this allowed most of her cargo to be saved. When the weather eventually blew up the ship was battered about on the rocks and quickly broke up.

Some of the wreck is visible amongst the rocks from depths of 8 to 14 metres, but most of it is buried in sand. Storms move the sand, sometimes uncovering some of the wreckage.

UNKNOWN

Wreck No : 22	**Date Sunk :** Pre - 1943
Latitude : 55 19 01 N	**Longitude :** 05 27 47 W
Decca Lat : 5519.02 N	**Decca Long :** 0527.78 W
Location : 4 miles NE of Sanda Island	**Area :** S. Kintyre
Type :	**Tonnage :** gross
Length : ft. **Beam :** ft.	**Draught :** ft.
How Sunk :	**Depth :** 47 metres

An unknown vessel was first located here in 1943. Least depth charted as 47 metres in a general depth of 50 metres.

ARGO

Wreck No : 23	**Date Sunk :** 27 02 1903
Latitude : 55 19 20 N PA	**Longitude :** 05 33 10 W PA
Decca Lat : 5519.33 N	**Decca Long :** 0533.17 W
Location : Arranman Barrels	**Area :** S. Kintyre
Type : Barque	**Tonnage :** 623 gross.
Length : 154.3 ft. **Beam :** 33.1 ft.	**Draught :** 18.1 ft.
How Sunk : Ran aground	**Depth :** metres

The 584 tons net Norwegian wooden barque *Argo* was dashed on to Arranman Barrels in a Force 10 SSE storm on 27th February 1903. She was en route from Wilmington, North Carolina to London with a cargo of rosin.

SAINT CONON

Wreck No : 24	**Date Sunk :** 30 08 1939
Latitude : 55 19 24 N	**Longitude :** 05 33 12 W
Decca Lat : 5519.40 N	**Decca Long :** 0533.20 W
Location : Arranman Barrels	**Area :** S. Kintyre
Type : Steamship	**Tonnage :** 719 gross

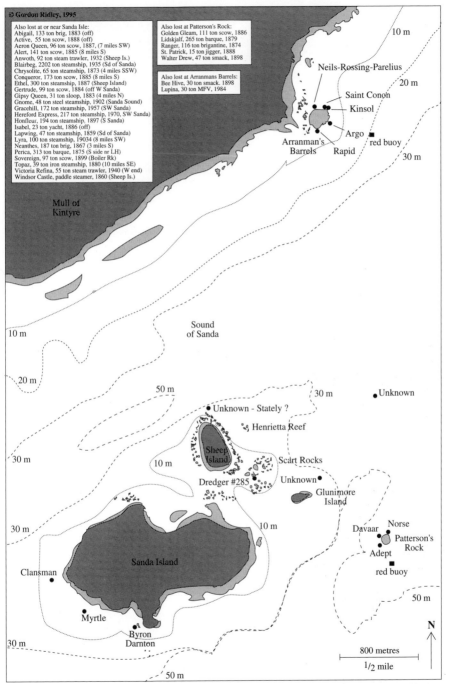

© Gordon Ridley, 1995

Also lost at or near Sanda Isle:
Abigail, 133 ton brig, 1883 (off)
Active, 55 ton scow, 1888 (off)
Aeron Queen, 96 ton scow, 1887, (7 miles SW)
Alert, 141 ton scow, 1885 (8 miles S)
Anworth, 92 ton steam trawler, 1932 (Sheep Is.)
Blairbeg, 2202 ton steamship, 1935 (Sd of Sanda)
Chrysolite, 65 ton steamship, 1873 (4 miles SSW)
Conqueror, 173 ton scow, 1885 (8 miles S)
Ethel, 300 ton steamship, 1887 (Sheep Island)
Gertrude, 99 ton scow, 1884 (off W Sanda)
Gipsy Queen, 31 ton sloop, 1883 (4 miles N)
Gnome, 48 ton steel steamship, 1902 (Sanda Sound)
Gracehill, 172 ton steamship, 1957 (SW Sanda)
Hereford Express, 217 ton steamship, 1970, SW Sanda)
Honfleur, 194 ton steamship, 1897 (S Sanda)
Isabel, 23 ton yacht, 1886 (off)
Lapwing, 47 ton steamship, 1859 (Sd of Sanda)
Lyra, 100 ton steamship, 19034 (8 miles SW)
Neanthes, 187 ton brig, 1867 (3 miles S)
Perica, 313 ton barque, 1875 (S side nr LH)
Sovereign, 97 ton scow, 1899 (Boiler Rk)
Topaz, 39 ton iron steamship, 1880 (10 miles SE)
Victoria Refina, 55 ton steam trawler, 1940 (W end)
Windsor Castle, paddle steamer, 1860 (Sheep Is.)

Also lost at Patterson's Rock:
Golden Gleam, 111 ton scow, 1886
Lidskjalf, 265 ton barque, 1879
Ranger, 116 ton brigantine, 1874
St. Patrick, 15 ton jigger, 1888
Walter Drew, 47 ton smack, 1898

Also lost at Arranmans Barrels:
Bee Hive, 30 ton smack. 1898
Lupina, 30 ton MFV, 1984

Wrecks around Sanda Island and on the reef of Arranman Barrels

Length : 188.5 ft.   **Beam :** 28.7 ft.   **Draught :** 11.1 ft.
How Sunk : Ran aground   **Depth :** 15 metres

The steamship *St. Conon* (ex-*Princetown*), built in 1937, was en route from Ayr to Sligo when she stranded on Arranman Barrels at 2.15 am on 30th August 1939. This reef lies at the South east of Kintyre, and breaks the surface at low water. It is also known as Arranmore Barrels, and is named Otter More on the Ordnance Survey map.

There are two steamship wrecks on the North side of Arranmore Barrels. The smaller wreck is the remains of a steam lighter named *Kinsol* which struck the reef during an attempt to recover the coal from the *St. Conon*.

The depth ranges down to about 15 metres.

NIELS-ROSSING-PARELIUS

Wreck No : 25   **Date Sunk :** 10 05 1894
Latitude : 55 19 24 N   **Longitude :** 05 33 12 W
Decca Lat : 5519.40 N   **Decca Long :** 0533.20 W
Location : Arranman Barrels   **Area :** S. Kintyre
Type : Steamship   **Tonnage :** 450 gross.
Length : 146.3 ft.   **Beam :** 24.6 ft.   **Draught :** 15.3 ft.
How Sunk : Ran aground   **Depth :**   metres

The 354 tons net Norwegian iron steamship *Niels-Rossing-Parelius* (ex-*Dagmar*), was lost on Arranman Barrels in a Force 6 West south westerly on 10th May 1894 while en route from Glasgow to Drontheim (Trondheim?) with a cargo of coal. The vessel was built in Gothenburg in 1882.

RAPID

Wreck No : 26   **Date Sunk :** 11 01 1852
Latitude : 55 19 24 N   **Longitude :** 05 33 12 W
Decca Lat : 5519.40 N   **Decca Long :** 0533.20 W
Location : Arranman Barrels   **Area :** S. Kintyre
Type : Paddle steam tug   **Tonnage :**   gross.
Length :   ft.   **Beam :**   ft.   **Draught :**   ft.
How Sunk : Ran aground   **Depth :**   metres

The steam paddle tug *Rapid* was lost on Arranman Barrels on 11th January 1852.

UNTAMED

Wreck No : 27	**Date Sunk** : 30 05 1943
Latitude : 55 20 00 N PA	**Longitude** : 05 30 00 W PA
Decca Lat : 5520.00 N	**Decca Long** : 0530.00 W
Location : Off Sanda Island	**Area** : S. Kintyre
Type : Submarine	**Tonnage** : 540 gross.
Length : 192.3 ft. **Beam** : 16.1 ft.	**Draught** : 15.0 ft.
How Sunk : Foundered but raised	**Depth** : metres

The British submarine *Untamed* (Lt. G. M. Noll), was built by Vickers-Armstrong, at Newcastle-on-Tyne. She was completed on 14th April 1943, and foundered off Sanda Island during exercises on 30th May 1943. The crew had assembled in the engine room, and were preparing to escape from that compartment when they were overcome by carbon dioxide before they could get out. Although the submarine was subsequently raised, the crew were all lost.

The cause of the disaster was found to be a series of fatal errors resulting from faulty workmanship and lack of training. Like surface ships, submarines also use a patent log to record speed and distance travelled. The log is driven by a small propeller which is rotated by the force of the water flowing through it due to the forward motion of the vessel. The device was located in a tube under the keel of the submarine. During the exercise on 30th May 1943, the log ceased to function, and in order to repair it, the device had to be taken into the submarine. To achieve this, the outside end of the tube had first to be closed to the sea by a valve installed for that purpose, then the inboard end could be opened to give access to the mechanism from within the submarine. Unfortunately, the gear for closing the valve at the outboard end of the tube had been incorrectly fitted, as a result of which the outside valve could not be closed. The crew of the submarine were not aware that this valve remained open, and when the inboard end of the tube was opened, a powerful jet of sea water rushed into the forward torpedo stowage compartment. The crew moved aft to the engine compartment, shutting the watertight bulkhead doors behind them. The weight of water in the flooded forward section forced the submarine to sink to the sea bed. To allow the escape hatch to be opened, it was necessary to equalise the pressure inside the compartment with that on the outside. A special valve to flood the engine compartment was installed for that purpose, but the mechanism for operating this valve had also been wrongly connected, and the valve could not be opened. There were alternative means for flooding the compartment, but only very slowly. A third valve, which should have opened to the sea, was wrongly connected to a small-bore drainpipe leading to the bilges in the after end of the submarine. There was no other means of flooding that section of the boat. During all this time, the oxygen in the air in the compartment was gradually being used up, and before the pressures could be equalised, the air in the compartment had become too contaminated to breathe. The crew had to resort to breathing oxygen from their Davis Submerged Escape Apparatus, and as the submarine was sunk in about 50 metres of water, they probably all died from oxygen poisoning.

The submarine was eventually raised on 5th July 1943, and the log book told the story of the crew's struggle to raise her for seven hours before they finally realised the impossibility of their task. The rising water inside the boat had stopped all their watches at 20.20 hours, 12 hours after the flooding accident.

Untamed was refitted and renamed *Vitality*. She was finally broken up in 1946.

DAVAAR

Wreck No : 28	**Date Sunk :** 10 12 1878
Latitude : 55 17 00 N PA	**Longitude :** 05 32 30 W PA
Decca Lat : 5517.00 N	**Decca Long :** 0532.50 W
Location : Patterson's Rock, nr Sanda Is.	**Area :** E. Kintyre
Type : Steamship	**Tonnage :** 268 gross.
Length : ft. **Beam :** ft.	**Draught :** ft.
How Sunk : Ran aground	**Depth :** metres

The 268 tons net iron steamship *Davaar*, which had been built at Campbeltown only about a month before, ran aground and was wrecked on Patterson's Rock, near Sanda Island on 10th December 1878. She had been bound from Glasgow to Limerick with a general cargo and two passengers.

FANNY

Wreck No : 29	**Date Sunk :** 23 04 1884
Latitude : 55 20 25 N	**Longitude :** 05 30 35 W
Decca Lat : 5520.42 N	**Decca Long :** 0530.58 W
Location : 4 miles NE of Sanda Island	**Area :** E. Kintyre
Type : Smack	**Tonnage :** gross.
Length : ft. **Beam :** ft.	**Draught :** ft.
How Sunk : Ran aground ?	**Depth :** 34 metres

This wreck is about 5 miles South of Davaar Island and one mile offshore. There are strong tidal streams here. This is probably the iron smack *Fanny* which foundered four miles North east of Sanda on 23rd April 1884.

ELISABETH

Wreck No : 30	**Date Sunk :** 02 09 1935
Latitude : 55 21 30 N	**Longitude :** 05 31 12 W
Decca Lat : 5521.50 N	**Decca Long :** 0531.20 W

Location : Johnston's Point, SE Kintyre
Type : Steamship
Length : 224.3 ft. Beam : 33.6 ft.
How Sunk : Ran aground

Area : E. Kintyre
Tonnage : 945 gross.
Draught : 13.5 ft.
Depth : metres

In the early morning of Saturday 2nd September 1935, the Danish steamship *Elisabeth* was driven by a strong South easterly gale on to the sunken reef at Johnston's Point, Kintyre. The vessel, which was en route from Irvine to Wisbech, was holed forward and making water. Her SOS signals were seen from the top of the high cliffs above Johnston's Point. Campbeltown lifeboat and the Southend lifesaving brigade were called out, but when the lifeboat arrived at the scene, she was unable to approach the vessel because of the danger of being dashed to pieces on the rocks. When the lifeboat crew saw that the lifesaving brigade had the situation in hand, she returned to Campbeltown. The Southend brigade brought all 16 of the crew safely ashore with their breeches buoy equipment.

QUESADA

Wreck No : 31
Latitude : 55 22 18 N
Decca Lat : 5522.30 N
Location : 3 miles E of Ru Stafnish
Type : Motor vessel
Length : 58.4 ft. Beam : 12.6 ft.
How Sunk : Foundered

Date Sunk : 23 05 1966
Longitude : 05 27 00 W
Decca Long : 0527.00 W
Area : E. Kintyre
Tonnage : 43 gross.
Draught : 7.1 ft.
Depth : 28 metres

The twin screw motor yacht *Quesada* was built in Southampton in 1938, and was powered by two Dorman engines. She was probably a converted ex-MTB or similar vessel. Eight lives were lost when she sank at 2.00 am after the engine room flooded. Least depth 28 metres in 31 metres.

BREDA

Wreck No : 32
Latitude : 55 24 56 N
Decca Lat : 5524.93 N
Location : Campbeltown Loch
Type : Yacht
Length : 285.0 ft. Beam : 35.2 ft.
How Sunk : Collision

Date Sunk : 18 02 1944
Longitude : 05 34 57 W
Decca Long : 0534.95 W
Area : E. Kintyre
Tonnage : 1207 gross.
Draught : 14.0 ft.
Depth : 9 metres

The wreck lies in 9-15 metres, standing up 4 metres from the seabed, about 200 yds

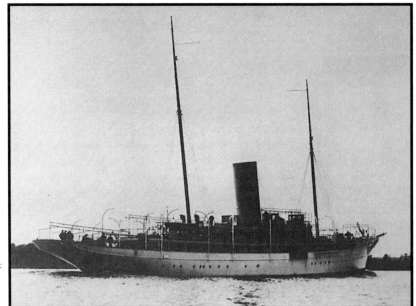

*The yacht
Breda
(Photograph:
Author's
Collection)*

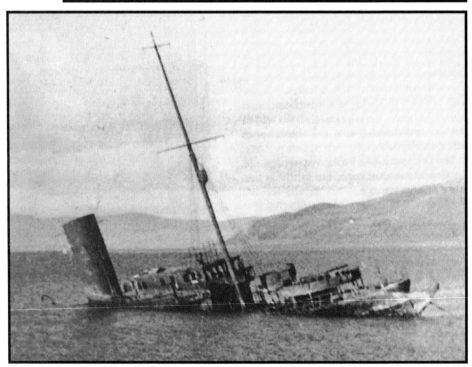

*The Breda sunk in Campbeltown Loch
(Photograph courtesy of Glasgow Museums and Art Galleries)*

offshore, directly out from the burn at Kilkerran on the South side of Campbeltown Loch. Because of the outfall from the burn, visibility underwater can be very poor, especially after heavy rain.

Breda (ex-*Sapphire*) was built in 1912 by John Brown of Clydebank, as a steam yacht for the Duke of Bedford. She was taken over by the Admiralty during the First World War as an auxiliary patrol vessel stationed at Gibraltar, and requisitioned again in the Second World War as a submarine tender.

On 18th February 1944 she was damaged in collision with a submarine, and was being taken to Campbeltown Harbour, but had to be beached before reaching there, and salvage operations were abandoned. Her bows point toward the shore. The forward section of the wreck is fairly broken, but the after section is still intact.

GLENHEAD

Wreck No : 33		**Date Sunk :** 24 03 1890	
Latitude : 55 27 06 N		**Longitude :** 05 31 12 W	
Decca Lat : 5527.10 N		**Decca Long :** 0531.20 W	
Location : Off Peninver		**Area :** E. Kintyre	
Type : Puffer		**Tonnage :**	gross
Length : ft.	**Beam :** ft.	**Draught :** ft.	
How Sunk :		**Depth :** 38 metres	

The steam puffer *Glenhead* was built by Scotts of Bowling in 1887.

On 24th March 1890 she was en route from Glasgow to Campbeltown with a cargo of coal when she foundered in heavy seas near the entrance to Campbeltown Loch. The four crew narrowly escaped in their small boat as the puffer sank under them.

The wreck is intact and sitting upright on a sandy bottom at 38 metres.

COLONIAL

Wreck No : 34		**Date Sunk :** 18 09 1950	
Latitude : 55 29 04 N		**Longitude :** 05 31 01 W	
Decca Lat : 5529.06 N		**Decca Long :** 0531.02 W	
Location : N side of Black Bay		**Area :** E. Kintyre	
Type : Steamship		**Tonnage :** 8371 gross	
Length : 449.8 ft.	**Beam :** 54.9 ft.	**Draught :** 27.8 ft.	
How Sunk : Ran aground		**Depth :** 12 metres	

The Anchor Line steamship *Colonial* (ex-*Assyria*, ex-*Ypiranga*), built in 1908 by Krupp and owned by Cia. Colonial de Navigacao, was sold for scrap to the British Iron and Steel Corporation. The work of breaking her up was given to Arnot Young at Dalmuir.

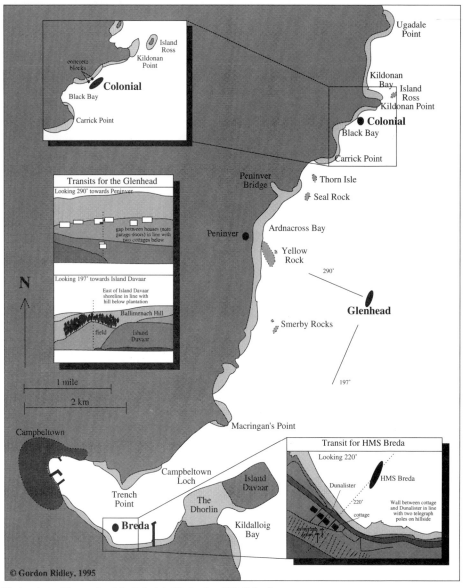

The locations of the wrecks of the Colonial, Glenhead and HMS Breda

While under tow towards that yard by the tug *Turmoil* (which was later to make a famously heroic but unfortunately unsuccessful attempt in January 1953 to tow the American Victory ship *Flying Enterprise* to Falmouth), the towline broke in a hurricane force gale on 18th September 1950. Attempts to attach another towline failed and the *Colonial* was blown towards the Kintyre coast. Campbeltown lifeboat was unable to

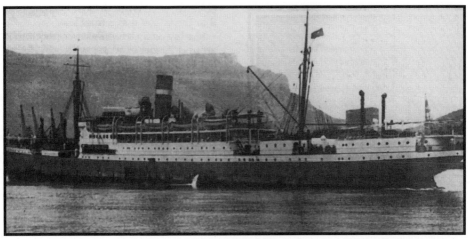

The Colonial (*Photograph courtesy of the World Ship Society*)

approach close enough to take off the towing crew in the prevailing conditions, but kept close by the drifting vessel until the *Colonial* grounded at the North side of Black Bay, three miles North of the Entrance to Campbeltown Loch. Southend Coastguards used breeches buoy equipment to take off the small number of men who were on board for the towing passage.

The *Colonial* was later scrapped on site, a temporary pier being constructed on the reef to enable the salvors to reach the wreck. The concrete pillars of this pier are still visible and quite a lot of wreckage, including non-ferrous items, is strewn around the reef. This reef slopes steeply to about 14 metres and is covered by a thick kelp forest.

VANDAL

Wreck No : 35	**Date Sunk : 24 02 1943**
Latitude : 55 43 48 N	**Longitude : 05 22 24 W**
Decca Lat : 5543.80 N	**Decca Long : 0522.40 W**
Location : Inchmarnock Water, Kilbrannan	**Area :** E. Kintyre
Type : Submarine	**Tonnage : 540 gross.**
Length : 192.3 ft. **Beam : 16.1 ft.**	**Draught : 15.2 ft.**
How Sunk : Foundered	**Depth : 66 metres**

The *Vandal* was a new British submarine built by Vickers-Armstrong. She was completed at their Barrow-in-Furness yard on 20th February 1943.

Only three days later, under the command of Lt. J. S. Bridger, she was undergoing trials in Inchmarnock Water, Kilbrannan Sound, when she failed to surface. She had left Lochranza on the morning of 23rd February 1943 for deep dive exercises in Kilbrannan Sound, and was due back in Holy Loch that night.

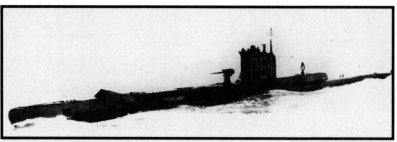

HMS Vandal
(With
acknowledgement
to the Royal
Naval
Submarine
Museum,
Gosport)

She was not located. until June 1994 - 51 years after her disappearance - when the minehunter HMS *Hurworth* made a sonar contact off Arran. A positive identification was made through further sonar and photographic images obtained by the minehunters HMS *Walney* and HMS *Sandown* in December 1994.

Although the *Vandal* and her sister submarine *Untamed*, which was lost three months after the *Vandal*, were both built by Vickers-Armstrong at about the same time, they were not built in the same yard. Both were brand new when lost during trials, or training exercises. The cause of loss of the *Untamed* was established when she was raised about five weeks after sinking (refer to Wreck No. 27: *Untamed* for details.). One cannot help wondering if the loss of the *Vandal* was due to the same, or a similar cause.

As the *Vandal* has only recently been found, and is considered to be a war grave, she is unlikely ever to be disturbed, and the cause of her loss will remain a mystery.

UNKNOWN - PRE-1966

Wreck No : 36	**Date Sunk :** Pre - 1966
Latitude : 55 52 15 N	**Longitude :** 05 24 17 W
Decca Lat : 5552.25 N	**Decca Long :** 0524.28 W
Location : East Loch Tarbert	**Area :** E. Kintyre
Type : Trawler	**Tonnage :** gross
Length : ft. **Beam :** ft.	**Draught :** ft.
How Sunk :	**Depth :** metres

This is reported to be a steam trawler broken into several pieces, first located in 1966. In 1967, an unknown vessel was reported at 555213N, 052417W. This is almost certainly the same trawler.

TARBERT CASTLE

Wreck No : 37	**Date Sunk :** 16 01 1839
Latitude : 55 58 00 N PA	**Longitude :** 05 20 30 W PA
Decca Lat : 5558.00 N	**Decca Long :** 0520.50 W
Location : Silver Rocks, Kilfinnan Bay	**Area :** E. Kintyre

Type : Paddle steamer		**Tonnage :** 100 gross.	
Length : 122.2 ft.	**Beam :** 18.9 ft.	**Draught :** 10.0 ft.	
How Sunk : Ran aground		**Depth :**	metres

The wooden paddle steamer *Tarbert Castle* was built in 1836 by Wood & Mills for the Loch Fyne service, and was wrecked on the Silver Rocks, Kilfinnan Bay on 6th January 1839. Her engines were subsequently salved and fitted to the third *Inveraray Castle*.

LCP 578

Wreck No : 38		**Date Sunk :** 13 12 1942	
Latitude : 56 12 00 N PA		**Longitude :** 05 10 00 W PA	
Decca Lat : 5612.00 N		**Decca Long :** 0510.00 W	
Location : At Inveraray, Loch Fyne		**Area :** E. Kintyre	
Type : Landing Craft Personnel		**Tonnage :** 11 gross.	
Length : ft.	**Beam :** ft.	**Draught :** ft.	
How Sunk :		**Depth :**	metres

Landing Craft Personnel (Ramped) *No. 578* of 9-11 tons was lost at Inveraray. The approximate position given is only a rough estimate in the general area.

About 420 LCPs of 3.75-5.5 tons were built in Britain between 1941-43, and 1200 of 10.75 tons were US-built between 1940-43.

LCV 579

Wreck No : 39		**Date Sunk :** 13 12 1942	
Latitude : 56 12 00 N PA		**Longitude :** 05 10 00 W PA	
Decca Lat : 5612.00 N		**Decca Long :** 0510.00 W	
Location : At Inveraray, Loch Fyne		**Area :** E. Kintyre	
Type : Landing Craft Vehicle		**Tonnage :** 11 gross.	
Length : 36.0 ft.	**Beam :** ft.	**Draught :** ft.	
How Sunk :		**Depth :**	metres

Landing Craft Vehicle *No. 579* of 10-11 tons was lost at Inveraray. The approximate position given is only a rough estimate in the general area.

About 700 LCVs of 11.0 - 11.5 tons were built in the United States between 1942-43. They were able to carry 36 troops or a 3 ton vehicle.

UNKNOWN U-BOAT

Wreck No : 40	**Date Sunk :** 12 1945
Latitude : 55 16 48 N	**Longitude :** 05 59 27 W
Decca Lat : 5516.80 N	**Decca Long :** 0559.45 W

Location : 7 miles W of Mull of Kintyre
Area : W. Kintyre
Type : Submarine
Tonnage : gross
Length : ft. **Beam :** ft.
Draught : ft.
How Sunk : Foundered / *Deadlight*
Depth : metres

This is reported to be a U-Boat which foundered under tow in *Operation Deadlight*. It was located in 1953 in the North Channel, 7 miles East of Rathlin and 7 miles West of the Mull of Kintyre.

U-1014

Wreck No : 41
Date Sunk : 04 02 1945
Latitude : 55 17 00 N PA
Longitude : 06 44 00 W PA
Decca Lat : 5517.00 N
Decca Long : 0644.00 W
Location : In the North Channel
Area : W. Kintyre
Type : Submarine
Tonnage : 769 gross
Length : 221.4 ft. **Beam :** 20.5 ft.
Draught : 15.8 ft.
How Sunk : Depth-charged
Depth : metres

U-1014 (KL Glaser), was depth-charged in the North Channel on 4th February 1945 by HM ships *Loch Scavaig*, *Nyasaland*, *Papua* and *Loch Shin*. The first attack was at 552100N, 065100W, and the U-Boat finally sank at 551700N, 064400W, leaving a German sailor's cap floating in a two square mile slick of light oil. There were no survivors.

DUCHESS

Wreck No : 42
Date Sunk : 12 12 1939
Latitude : 55 22 00 N PA
Longitude : 06 02 00 W PA
Decca Lat : 5522.00 N
Decca Long : 0602.00 W
Location : North Channel, 6 miles NE of Rathlin
Area : W. Kintyre
Type : Destroyer
Tonnage : 1375 gross.
Length : 326.0 ft. **Beam :** 33.0 ft.
Draught : 8.5 ft.
How Sunk : Collision with HMS *Barham*
Depth : metres

The British destroyer *Duchess*, built in 1932 by Palmer & Co., sank in collision in fog, with the battleship *Barham* in the North Channel on 12th December 1939. 129 lives were lost. There were only 23 survivors.

According to *Warship Losses of WW2*, the collision took place 293° 8.6 miles off the Mull of Kintyre at 5519N, 0606W, but the position has also been given as 552200N, 060200W.

UNKNOWN U-BOAT

Wreck No : 43   **Date Sunk** : 30 12 1945
Latitude : 55 24 12 N   **Longitude** : 06 29 40 W
Decca Lat : 5524.20 N   **Decca Long** : 0629.67 W
Location : 18 miles S of Rinns Pt., Islay   **Area** : W. Kintyre
Type : Submarine   **Tonnage** :   gross
Length :   ft.   **Beam** :   ft.   **Draught** : ft.
How Sunk : Foundered / *Deadlight*   **Depth** :   metres

The position given for this wreck is 18 miles South of Rinns Point, Islay, and about 10 miles North of Benbane Head, Northern Ireland. This is one of the surrendered U-Boats which foundered while under tow to the intended scuttling position.

Loch Ryan and Lough Foyle were the two main marshalling points for the 153 U-Boats surrendered at the end of WW2. Scuttling was the chosen means of disposing of the majority of these U-Boats. During November/December 1945 and January 1946, in *Operation Deadlight*, 110 surrendered U-Boats were taken out to sea and sunk in deep water North west of Malin Head. The planned scuttling position was 5600N, 1005W, but almost half of them foundered in tow while en route to that position. One report suggests that some of them may have been chained together in groups of five or six before being scuttled. This method of disposal would today no doubt be regarded as very wasteful, but at that time their value as scrap metal was obviously not considered worth the time and effort of breaking them up, and there were also fairly strong emotions after the war which probably made sinking an attractive option.

At 1.34 am on 5th May 1945, the code word *Regenbogen* - (Rainbow), was transmitted by U-Boat HQ. This was the signal to all the U-Boats then at sea to scuttle themselves rather than surrender. Despite another signal sent eight minutes later, countermanding that order, 215 U-Boats were scuttled by their own crews to avoid the ignominy of surrendering them. Twenty U-Boats were retained by the Royal Navy for a short time for evaluation purposes before being transferred to Russia, Norway, France and the United States.

U-1105 had been entirely covered by the Germans with a synthetic rubber coating in an experiment to find a method of absorbing Asdic pings to reduce the chances of detection while submerged. This boat, nicknamed *The Black Panther*, was evaluated by the Royal Navy in late 1945 before being transferred to the United States. After further trials there, the U. S. Navy scuttled her. (The rubber material proved unsuitable for the purpose, but became today's neoprene). The Germans had also experimented with another U-Boat which had a sponge rubber coating on the snorkel, painted with an aluminium paint in a similar attempt to foil detection on the surface by radar. This boat was nicknamed *The White Puma*.

U-1407 was powered by a German experimental Walter hydrogen peroxide engine. This gave a very much higher submerged speed than was possible with diesel electric engines because it did not require an external supply of air. Therefore the main engines could be used underwater, rather than the less powerful electric motors. The Russians and the Americans both gave up in their attempts to develop submarines powered by this revolutionary engine, but the Royal Navy persisted until a degree of success was achieved. This method of propulsion was finally abandoned, no doubt to the relief of many, when it was overtaken by nuclear power. Some idea of the magnitude of the problems may be deduced from the nicknames *Excruciator* and *Exploder* by which the two experimental hydrogen peroxide submarines *Excaliber* and *Explorer* were generally known!

UNKNOWN U-BOAT

Wreck No : 44	**Date Sunk :** 12 1945
Latitude : 55 25 00 N	**Longitude :** 06 25 51 W
Decca Lat : 5525.00 N	**Decca Long :** 0625.85 W
Location : 12 miles SSW of Mull of Oa	**Area :** W. Kintyre
Type : Submarine	**Tonnage :** gross
Length : ft. **Beam :** ft.	**Draught :** ft.
How Sunk : Foundered / *Deadlight*	**Depth :** metres

This is one of the U-Boats surrendered at the end of WW2, which foundered while under tow from Loch Ryan towards the intended scuttling position at 5600N, 1005W in *Operation Deadlight*.

This U-Boat was relocated in 1953, in the North Channel, 10 miles North of Benbane Head, Northern Ireland, and 18 miles South of Rinns Point, Islay.

UNKNOWN U-BOAT

Wreck No : 45	**Date Sunk :** 12 1945
Latitude : 55 25 00 N	**Longitude :** 06 19 10 W
Decca Lat : 5525.00 N	**Decca Long :** 0619.17 W
Location : North Channel	**Area :** W. Kintyre
Type : Submarine	**Tonnage :** gross
Length : ft. **Beam :** ft.	**Draught :** ft.
How Sunk : Foundered / *Deadlight*	**Depth :** metres

This is one of the U-Boats which foundered in *Operation Deadlight*, while under tow from Loch Ryan in December 1945.

FAIRY QUEEN

Wreck No : 46	**Date Sunk :** 19 07 1876
Latitude : 55 25 00 N PA	**Longitude :** 05 46 00 W PA

Decca Lat : 5525.00 N
Location : Near Macrihanish
Type : Steamship
Length : 175.3 ft.   Beam : 23.0 ft.
How Sunk : Ran aground?

Decca Long : 0546.00 W
Area : W. Kintyre
Tonnage : 317 gross.
Draught : 12.6 ft.
Depth :   metres

An iron steamship built in 1860, lost near Macrihanish (Ran aground?).

CALGARIAN

Wreck No : 47
Latitude : 55 25 00 N PA
Decca Lat : 5525.00 N
Location : North Channel
Type : Cruiser
Length : 568.8 ft.   Beam : 70.3 ft.
How Sunk : Torpedoed by U-19

Date Sunk : 01 03 1918
Longitude : 06 15 00 W PA
Decca Long : 0615.00 W
Area : W. Kintyre
Tonnage : 17515 gross.
Draught : 41.6 ft.
Depth :   metres

The armed merchant cruiser HMS *Calgarian*, built in 1914 by Fairfields, was torpedoed and sunk by the *U-19* on 1st March 1918, while escorting a convoy of 30 merchant ships in the North Channel off Rathlin Island, between Ireland and Kintyre. She was hit by four torpedoes and sank very quickly with the loss of 49 lives.

U-296 ?

Wreck No : 48
Latitude : 55 25 48 N
Decca Lat : 5525.80 N
Location : In North Channel
Type : Submarine
Length : 221.4 ft.   Beam : 20.5 ft.
How Sunk : Depth-charged

Date Sunk : 22 03 1945
Longitude : 06 19 48 W
Decca Long : 0619.80 W
Area : W. Kintyre
Tonnage : 769 gross.
Draught : 15.8 ft.
Depth : 120 metres

U-296 was a type VIIC/41 Atlantic U-Boat, 769 tons surfaced, 871 tons submerged. She was depth-charged by RAF aircraft in the North Channel on 22nd March 1945.
   The wreck in this position is given as a U-Boat sunk 1945/6, and as this is not one of the positions recorded for the foundering of a U-Boat in *Operation Deadlight*, I have assumed it to possibly be the *U-296*. The nearest U-Boat sunk in *Operation Deadlight* is not far away at 552500N, 061910W. This does, however, look suspiciously like a PA, and the actual position for the *Deadlight* boat might be as given above. If that is the case where is the *U-296*?

U-482

Wreck No : 49	**Date Sunk :** 15 01 1945
Latitude : 55 30 00 N PA	**Longitude :** 05 53 00 W PA
Decca Lat : 5530.00 N	**Decca Long :** 0553.00 W
Location : 10 miles SSW Gigha, 6 miles W of Kintyre	**Area :** W. Kintyre
Type : Submarine	**Tonnage :** 769 gross.
Length : 221.4 ft. **Beam :** 20.5 ft.	**Draught :** 15.7 ft.
How Sunk : Depth-charged	**Depth :** 63 metres

On 15th January 1945, the Type VIIC U-Boat, *U-482* (KL Graf von Matuschka), 769 tons surfaced, 871 tons submerged, was depth-charged by five ships in the North Channel, 6 miles North west of Macrihanish.(RN sloops *Amethyst, Hart, Peacock*, and *Starling*, and frigate *Loch Craggie*). There were no survivors.

On his first patrol in U-482, Matuschka had sunk the American tanker *Jacksonville* on 30th August 1944. The following day, 1st September 1944, he sank the RN corvette *Hurst Castle*, and a week later, on 8th September, the motor ship *Pinto* and the British steamship *Empire Heritage*.

OSPREY

Wreck No : 50	**Date Sunk :** 06 04 1935
Latitude : 55 31 00 N PA	**Longitude :** 05 45 00 W PA
Decca Lat : 5531.00 N	**Decca Long :** 0545.00 W
Location : 1 mile offshore, W. Kintyre	**Area :** W. Kintyre
Type : Trawler	**Tonnage :** 295 gross.
Length : 130.0 ft. **Beam :** 23.0 ft.	**Draught :** 13.0 ft.
How Sunk : Collision with *Caldew*	**Depth :** 18 metres

The steam trawler *Osprey*, built in 1911 by Smiths Dock, Middlesbrough, was sunk in collision with a vessel named *Caldew* 8 miles SE by E of Otter Rock.

This position is about 13 miles N of Mull of Kintyre, 1 mile offshore, in about 24 metres of water.

CHRISTINE ROSE

Wreck No : 51	**Date Sunk :** 10 09 1941
Latitude : 55 53 04 N	**Longitude :** 05 41 27 W
Decca Lat : 5553.07 N	**Decca Long :** 0541.45 W
Location : Knap Rock, Sound of Jura	**Area :** W. Kintyre
Type : Drifter	**Tonnage :** gross
Length : ft. **Beam :** ft.	**Draught :** ft.

How Sunk : Ran aground **Depth :** metres

Christine Rose was a French drifter in Admiralty service as an examination vessel at the time of her loss by running aground on Knap Rock.

There is a group of dangerous rocks very close to the surface about ½ mile off Knap Point, at the North of the entrance to Loch Caolisport, West Kintyre. Knap Rock is not named on the chart, but is presumably Bow of Knap, which is the most prominent of that group, and has a beacon on it. Back Bow is the only other named rock in the group. The wreck lies about 100 yards ESE of the beacon.

UNKNOWN

Wreck No : 52 **Date Sunk :**
Latitude : 55 57 52 N **Longitude :** 05 42 14 W
Decca Lat : 5557.87 N **Decca Long :** 0542.23 W
Location : Rubha Riabhaig, nr. Knap Point **Area :** W. Kintyre
Type : **Tonnage :** gross
Length : ft. **Beam :** ft. **Draught :** ft.
How Sunk : Ran aground? **Depth :** metres

In the bay at Rubha Riabhaig, between Kilmory Bay and Knap Point, i.e. between Loch Sween and Carsaig Bay, there is the wreck of a small steel vessel.

© Gordon Ridley, 1995

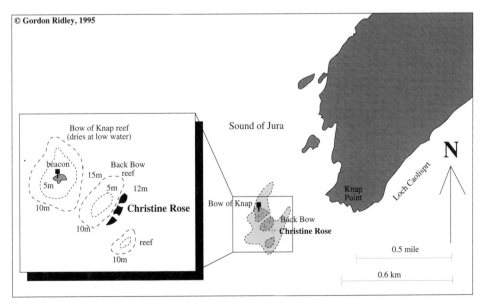

Location of the Christine Rose

CHAPTER 3

THE WRECKS OF ISLAY

INTRODUCTION

Islay measures 25 miles North to South, and 20 miles East to West. It lies 14 miles West of Kintyre, and a mile South west of Jura.

The West coast of the Rinns is rocky, with sandy beaches. Further North, there are high cliffs, and a short distance inland from these cliffs is Loch Gorm, the largest expanse of fresh water on Islay, which attracts enormous numbers of geese every winter. The eastern part of Islay is mountainous, giving way to flatter, low-lying land towards the sandy shores of Loch Indaal.

The Oa peninsula, the most southerly part of Islay, has a rocky coastline with high, sheer cliffs, penetrated by many caves. At the top of the cliffs on the Mull of Oa stands the Memorial, built by the American Red Cross, to commemorate U.S. servicemen lost when the *Tuscania* was torpedoed in February 1918, and the *Otranto* was wrecked in October that same year. Many of the bodies were washed ashore here.

The south eastern area of Islay, with many off-lying rocky islets is perhaps the most attractive part of the island. Many of Islay's distilleries are located in this area.

Port Ellen is the largest centre of population on the island, and one of the two ferry terminals. The other is Port Askaig on the Sound of Jura.

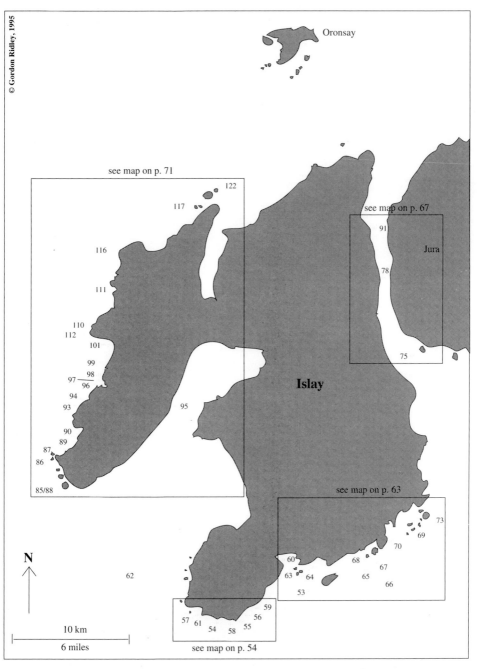

© Gordon Ridley, 1995

Oronsay

see map on p. 71

122

117

116

111

110
112

101

99
97 98
96

94
93

90
89

87
86

85/88

see map on p. 67

91

Jura

78

75

Islay

95

N

62

see map on p. 63

73
69
70
60
68
67
63 64 65
66
53

59
56
57 61 54 58 55

see map on p. 54

10 km

6 miles

Chart showing the location of wrecks lying off the coast of Islay

THE WRECKS

ST. TUDWAL

Wreck No : 53	Date Sunk : 12 08 1934
Latitude : 55 34 00 N PA	Longitude : 06 15 00 W PA
Decca Lat : 5534.00 N	Decca Long : 0615.00 W
Location : 4 miles SW by W of Texa Island	Area : SE Islay
Type : Steamship	Tonnage : 207 gross.
Length : 115.0 ft. Beam : 20.5 ft.	Draught : 8.8 ft.
How Sunk :	Depth : metres

The Yarmouth-registered steel steamship *St. Tudwal*, built in 1895 by Swan Hunter of Newcastle, engine by J. P. Rennoldson of South Shields, sank after being abandoned 4 miles SW by W of Texa Island, Islay on 12th August 1934. That would place it off Rubha nan Leacan, the most southerly point of Islay.

EILEEN M

Wreck No : 54	Date Sunk : 12 01 1966
Latitude : 55 34 46 N	Longitude : 06 17 37 W
Decca Lat : 5534.77 N	Decca Long : 0617.62 W
Location : Mull of Oa	Area : SE Islay
Type : Motor tanker	Tonnage : 323 gross.
Length : 136.0 ft. Beam : 25.0 ft.	Draught : 10.0 ft.
How Sunk : Ran aground	Depth : 12 metres

The British motor tanker *Eileen M* ran aground with a cargo of oil under the 400 ft cliffs of the Mull of Oa. She lies North/South, to the East of a small islet, wedged into rocky gullies. Depth at the stern is 12 metres, but some of the wreckage is at only 3 metres.

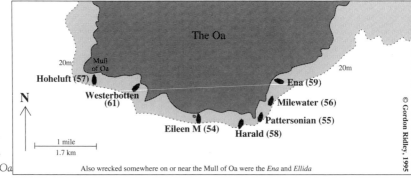

Location of wrecks near the Mull of Oa

Also wrecked somewhere on or near the Mull of Oa were the *Ena* and *Ellida*

© Gordon Ridley, 1995

PATTERSONIAN

Wreck No : 55	**Date Sunk :** 11 09 1945
Latitude : 55 34 43 N	**Longitude :** 06 16 44 W
Decca Lat : 5534.72 N	**Decca Long :** 0616.73 W
Location : Mull of Oa	**Area :** SE Islay
Type : Steamship	**Tonnage :** 300 gross.
Length : 135.3 ft. **Beam :** 23.6 ft.	**Draught :** 9.1 ft.
How Sunk : Ran aground	**Depth :** metres

The *Pattersonian* was wrecked on the Mull of Oa while carrying RAF stores to Port Ellen. It has also been suggested that the date of loss may have been 30th January 1946.

MILEWATER

Wreck No : 56	**Date Sunk :** 10 05 1931
Latitude : 55 34 44 N	**Longitude :** 06 16 21 W
Decca Lat : 5534.73 N	**Decca Long :** 0616.35 W
Location : Strennish, Mull of Oa	**Area :** SE Islay
Type : Steam tug	**Tonnage :** gross
Length : ft. **Beam :** ft.	**Draught :** ft.

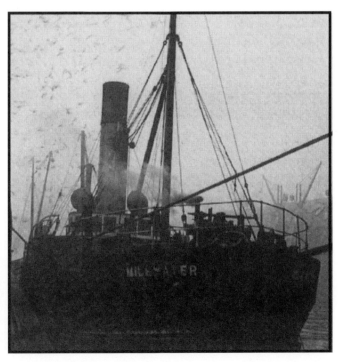

The steam tug Milewater *(Photograph courtesy of Glasgow Museums and Art Galleries).*

How Sunk : Ran aground   Depth :   metres

Milewater was a steam tug with twin propellers, wrecked at Strennish, near the Mull of Oa on 10th May 1931. Her crew were saved and her machinery was salvaged. In 1975 it was reported that the boiler remained intact, but the rest of the vessel had broken up.

HOHELUFT

Wreck No : 57	Date Sunk : 25 12 1924
Latitude : 55 35 00 N PA	Longitude : 06 20 00 W PA
Decca Lat : 5535.00 N	Decca Long : 0620.00 W
Location : Wrecked on Mull of Oa	Area : SE Islay
Type : Steam trawler	Tonnage : gross
Length : 125.3 ft. Beam : 22.6 ft.	Draught : 9.2 ft.
How Sunk : Ran aground	Depth : metres

All but one of the eleven crew were lost when the German steam trawler *Hoheluft* was wrecked on Mull of Oa on 25th December 1924.

HARALD

Wreck No : 58	Date Sunk : 15 08 1909
Latitude : 55 354 43 N	Longitude : 06 16 22 W
Decca Lat : 5534.72 N	Decca Long : 0616.37 W
Location : Mull of Oa	Area : SE Islay
Type : Sailing ship	Tonnage : 1435 gross.
Length : 233.7 ft. Beam : 37.9 ft.	Draught : 22.9 ft.
How Sunk : Ran aground	Depth : 10 metres

The 1435 tons net Norwegian iron ship *Harald* (ex-*Hornby Castle*, ex-*Duncan Coupland*) ran on to the Mull of Oa on 15th August 1909 while en route from Cardiff to Sandefiord, Norway with a cargo of coal.

She hit the rocks at the foot of the cliffs 200 yards West of Rubha nan Leacan, the southernmost point of Islay. Her crew of 19 were all saved.

ENA

Wreck No : 59	Date Sunk : 20 10 1911
Latitude : 55 35 00 N PA	Longitude : 06 20 00 W PA
Decca Lat : 5535.00 N	Decca Long : 0620.00 W
Location : Mull of Oa	Area : SE Islay
Type : Steamship	Tonnage : 1071 gross.

Length : 228.6 ft. **Beam :** 36.2 ft. **Draught :** 14.4 ft.
How Sunk : Ran aground **Depth :** metres

The 632 tons net Norwegian steel steamship *Ena* was built in Frederikstadt in 1908. En route from Liverpool to Krageroe with a cargo of salt, she ran on to the Mull of Oa on 20th October 1911.

ELLIDA ?

Wreck No : 60 **Date Sunk :** 11 12 1890
Latitude : 55 35 10 N **Longitude :** 06 18 55 W
Decca Lat : 5535.17 N **Decca Long :** 0618.92 W
Location : Near Mull of Oa **Area :** SE Islay
Type : Brig **Tonnage :** 267 gross.
Length : ft. **Beam :** ft. **Draught :** ft.
How Sunk : **Depth :** metres

A wreck is recorded by the Navy in this position, and it is thought to be a sailing vessel. This may be the 267 tons net Norwegian brig *Ellida* which was lost on the Mull of Oa on 11th December 1890 while en route from Belfast to Drammen.

WESTERBOTTEN

Wreck No : 61 **Date Sunk :** 11 12 1890
Latitude : 55 35 10 N **Longitude :** 06 18 55 W
Decca Lat : 5535.17 N **Decca Long :** 0618.92 W
Location : Mull of Oa **Area :** SE Islay
Type : Barque **Tonnage :** 376 gross.
Length : ft. **Beam :** ft. **Draught :** ft.
How Sunk : Ran aground **Depth :** metres

The Norwegian barque *Westerbotten* ran on to rocks at the Mull of Oa on 11th December 1890, on the same day, and in the same place, as the *Ellida*. The *Westerbotten* had been en route from Liverpool to Christiania, (Oslo), with a cargo of coke. The wind at the time was SSE Force 5.

TUSCANIA

Wreck No : 62 **Date Sunk :** 05 02 1918
Latitude : 55 36 30 N **Longitude :** 06 26 24 W
Decca Lat : 5536.50 N **Decca Long :** 0626.40 W
Location : 4 miles W of Mull of Oa **Area :** SE Islay
Type : Steamship **Tonnage :** 14348 gross.

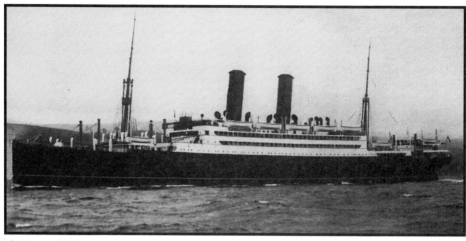

The Tuscania (Photograph courtesy of the World Ship Society)

Length : 549.3 ft. **Beam :** 66.5 ft. **Draught :** 41.7 ft.
How Sunk : Torpedoed by UB-77 **Depth :** 60 metres

The Anchor liner *Tuscania* was built by A. Stephen & Sons in 1914 and was requisitioned as an Armed Merchant Cruiser during the First World War.

Some 166 lives were lost when she was torpedoed by *UB-77* (Meyer), 7 miles north of Rathlin Island.

Lloyds *War Losses* gives the position of attack as 13 miles North west of Rathlin Island, Ireland. She now lies in deep water 4 miles West of Mull of Oa, and is one of the many wrecks around Islay owned by Tim Epps of Port Charlotte.

LIMELIGHT

Wreck No : 63 **Date Sunk :** 10 10 1966
Latitude : 55 37 04 N **Longitude :** 06 11 40 W
Decca Lat : 5537.07 N **Decca Long :** 0611.67 W
Location : 1 mile SSW of Port Ellen **Area :** SE Islay
Type : Motor Vessel **Tonnage :** 143 gross.
Length : 89.0 ft. **Beam :** 19.1 ft. **Draught :** ft.
How Sunk : Ran aground **Depth :** 9 metres

The motor vessel *Limelight*, (ex-*Cristo*), built 1916 by Rennie Forrest S. B. Co., powered by a Bristol oil engine, ran aground en route from Irwin to Port Ellen with a cargo of bricks and cement. She lies on the North west side of Sgeir Thraghaidh.

The vessel has now broken up, the stern section from the engine room bulkhead aft lodged on the rocks at a 45° angle, while the aft section has fallen off the rock and is lying about 30 yards away in 9 metres of water.

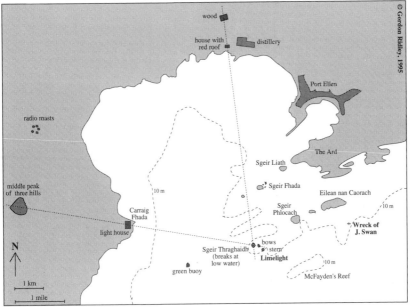

© Gordon Ridley, 1995

Chart showing the location of and transits for the Limelight

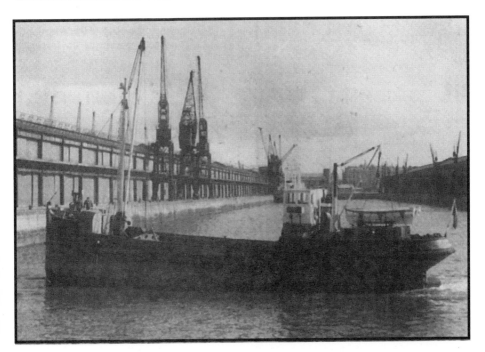

The Limelight
(Photograph courtesy of Glasgow Museums and Art Galleries).

ISLAY

Wreck No : 64
Latitude : 55 37 16 N
Decca Lat : 5537.27 N
Location : SE of Port Ellen
Type : Paddle Steamer
Length : 211.4 ft.   **Beam : 24.1 ft.**
How Sunk : Ran aground

Date Sunk : 15 07 1902
Longitude : 06 11 08 W
Decca Long : 0611.13 W
Area : SE Islay
Tonnage : 497 gross.
Draught : 12.4 ft.
Depth : 13 metres

An iron paddle steamer built in 1872 by Tod & McGregor as the *Princess Louise*. Bought by David MacBrayne and renamed *Islay*, she ran aground in fog and lies on the South side of Sheep Island, to the South east of Port Ellen.

The boiler lies about 40 metres North of the main part of the wreck. Gordon Ridley gives position 553716N, 061008W, while the Navy records the position as 553712N, 061052W. The vessel had been bound from Glasgow to Port Ellen with 76 passengers.

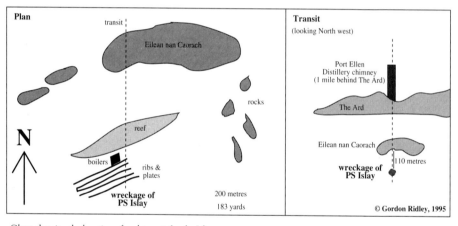

Chart showing the location of and transit for the Islay

LUNEDA

Wreck No : 65
Latitude : 55 37 30 N
Decca Lat : 5537.50 N
Location : SE of Ardbeg
Type : Trawler
Length : 130.0 ft.   **Beam : 23.0 ft.**
How Sunk : Ran aground

Date Sunk : 09 02 1937
Longitude : 06 05 42 W
Decca Long : 0605.70 W
Area : SE Islay
Tonnage : 288 gross.
Draught : 12.7 ft.
Depth : 7 metres

The steel steam trawler *Luneda*, built in 1912 by Cochranes of Selby, engine by C. D.

Holmes, and owned by J. Marr of Fleetwood, ran aground in a blinding snow storm while en route from Fleetwood to the Faröe Islands

The crew of 12 took to the lifeboat as the vessel developed an alarming list and began to fill. Drifting in a cold, biting wind and zero visibility because of the darkness and thickly-falling snow, the men were uncertain of their position until the snowstorm abated at dawn, four hours later, when the lights of Ardbeg became visible, but they dared not approach the shore because of treacherous rocks. Eventually they saw, with relief, the lights of a vessel to which they headed their boat. Their shouts were heard by those aboard the vessel, the *Pibroch*, a steam lighter owned by the Distillers Co. Ltd., and they were taken aboard.

The crew of the *Pibroch* had seen the *Luneda* fast on the rocks, and after checking that there was no-one aboard her, commenced a search for the crew. It was while the *Pibroch* was looking for them that the shipwrecked men saw her lights through the snow.

The *Luneda* sank almost at the same place as the *San Sebastian* had sunk a month previously. The Navy records her position as 553755N, 060519W.

SERB

Wreck No : 66	**Date Sunk :** 05 12 1925
Latitude : 55 37 38 N	**Longitude :** 06 04 42 W
Decca Lat : 5537.63 N	**Decca Long :** 0604.70 W
Location : Iomalloch	**Area :** SE Islay
Type : Steam puffer	**Tonnage :** gross
Length : ft. **Beam :** ft.	**Draught :** ft.
How Sunk : Ran aground	**Depth :** 5 metres

The steam puffer *Serb* sank at the entrance to Lagavullin, Islay in 3 fathoms (5.5 metres), on 5th December 1925. Her crew all safely arrived at Ardbeg. The position of the vessel has also been given as 553739N, 060621W, and there is a further suggestion that she may subsequently have been salved.

SAN SEBASTIAN

Wreck No : 67	**Date Sunk :** 10 01 1937
Latitude : 55 38 03 N	**Longitude :** 06 04 40 W
Decca Lat : 5538.05 N	**Decca Long :** 0604.67 W
Location : SE of Ardbeg	**Area :** SE Islay
Type : Trawler	**Tonnage :** 271 gross.
Length : 125.7 ft. **Beam :** 23.5 ft.	**Draught :** 12.7 ft.
How Sunk : Ran aground	**Depth :** 20 metres

The steam trawler *San Sebastian* was built in 1918 by Collingwood S. B. Co. for the

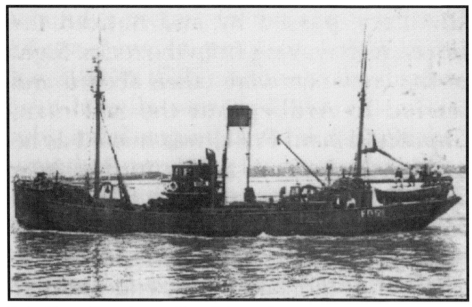

The San Sebastian (Photograph courtesy of the World Ship Society).

Boston Deep Sea Fishing & Ice Co. of Fleetwood.

Weather conditions were bad with a heavy drizzle and strong wind when she sank after striking the submerged reef Corr Sgeir, a mile off Ardbeg at 3.00 o'clock in the morning of 10th January 1937. The *San Sebastian*'s lifeboat was smashed in an attempt to launch it, and the crew, with hastily-donned lifejackets, took to the water. Four of the crew were lost, but nine others succeeded in the darkness in struggling through the icy water to the comparative safety of the rocks where they lay soaked and shivering for five hours before being spotted and rescued by the crew of the *Pibroch*, a steam lighter belonging to Scottish Malt Distillers, a subsidiary of D. C. L.

JOHN STRACHAN

Wreck No : 68 **Date Sunk :** 08 12 1917
Latitude : 55 38 20 N **Longitude :** 06 05 10 W
Decca Lat : 5538.33 N **Decca Long :** 0605.17 W
Location : Eilean Imersay **Area :** SE Islay
Type : Steam puffer **Tonnage :** 82 gross.
Length : ft. **Beam :** ft. **Draught :** ft.
How Sunk : Ran aground **Depth :** 5 metres

The hull of the *John Strachan* is intact, lying on its side in a few feet of water. The machinery has been salvaged. The Navy records the position as 553815N, 060513W.

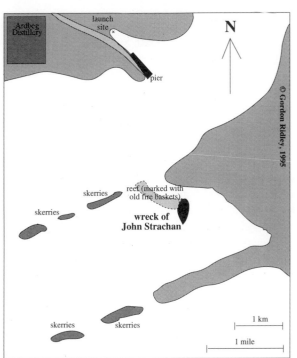

Left: Chart showing the location of the wreck of the John Strachan

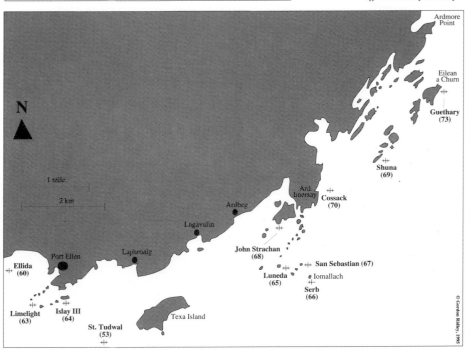

Below: Chart showing the location of wrecks lying off the coast of SE Islay

SHUNA

Wreck No : 69		**Date Sunk :** 17 10 1936	
Latitude : 55 39 05 N		**Longitude :** 06 02 25 W	
Decca Lat : 5539.08 N		**Decca Long :** 0602.42 W	
Location : Eilean Bhride		**Area :** SE Islay	
Type : Steamship		**Tonnage :** 1494 gross.	
Length : 250.0 ft.	**Beam :** 37.3 ft.	**Draught :** 17.2 ft.	
How Sunk : Ran aground		**Depth :** 10 metres	

A certain amount of confusion existed for some time because of apparently conflicting information about the *Shuna*, due to two vessels of that name having been lost, one near Ardmore Point, Mull in 1913, the other near Ardmore Point, Islay in 1936!

On 17th October 1936, the *Shuna* went ashore and became a total wreck at Eilean Bhride, which is two miles East of Ardbeg, South east Islay. In the *Oban Times* of Sat Oct 24, 1936, a report about the *St. Joseph*, which went aground in the Lynn of Lorne on 17th October, mentions that the Islay lifeboat was unable to go to the assistance of the crew of the *St. Joseph* as it was already at sea attending a Glasgow ship off Islay. The vessel referred to was undoubtedly the *Shuna*!

She was built in 1915 by J. Crown & Sons. The Navy has her position as 553858N, 060222W. Her machinery was salvaged. The stern was reported to still be intact in 1975, but the other wreckage is completely broken up and scattered over a wide area.

COSSACK

Wreck No : 70		**Date Sunk :** 13 06 1923	
Latitude : 55 39 10 N PA		**Longitude :** 06 03 50 W PA	
Decca Lat : 5539.17 N		**Decca Long :** 0603.83 W	
Location : Ardmore Sound		**Area :** SE Islay	
Type : Steamship		**Tonnage :** 92 gross.	
Length : 66.0 ft.	**Beam :** 18.0 ft.	**Draught :** 9.0 ft.	
How Sunk : Ran aground		**Depth :** metres	

Cossack struck a submerged rock in Ardmore Sound while en route from Glasgow to Ardbeg. The position 553843N, 060458W given by the Navy plots ashore, but there is no visible sign of wreckage above the water near that position, nor has any wreckage been found in searches of the seabed in the vicinity.

The wreck was reported in 1975 to lie between Ardmore Islands and Ard Imersay. This would suggest a position of about 553910N, 060350W. It has also been reported that the *Cossack* sank ¼ mile from Ardmore Point.

SURPRISE

Wreck No : 71
Latitude : 55 39 18 N
Decca Lat : 5539.30 N
Location : Eilean Bhride
Type : Steam puffer
Length : 121.3 ft.   Beam : 19.5 ft.
How Sunk : Ran aground

Date Sunk : 16 12 1906
Longitude : 06 02 52 W
Decca Long : 0602.87 W
Area : SE Islay
Tonnage : 197 gross.
Draught : 10.3 ft.
Depth : 8 metres

The broken remains of what was thought to be a trawler were reported in 1975 at 553903N, 060235W. I suspect this is the 79 tons net iron steamship *Surprise* (ex-*Sea King*), which was reported lost on a reef about a mile South of Ardmore Point on 16th December 1906. She was en route from Larne to Foyers, Invernesshire with a cargo of coal and aluminium. The vessel was built in 1864 by J. Ash & Co., London, engine by D. Joy & Co. of Middlesbrough.

UNKNOWN

Wreck No : 72
Latitude : 55 39 27 N
Decca Lat : 5539.45 N
Location : Near Rudha Sconash
Type : Yacht
Length :   ft.   Beam :   ft.
How Sunk : Ran aground?

Date Sunk : Pre - 1973
Longitude : 06 04 27 W
Decca Long : 0604.45 W
Area : SE Islay
Tonnage :   gross
Draught : ft.
Depth : 3 metres

Reported in 1973 to be a wooden yacht. Little remains.

GUETHARY

Wreck No : 73
Latitude : 55 40 03 N
Decca Lat : 5540.05 N
Location : Eilean a'Churn, SW Islay
Type : Barque
Length : 277.0 ft.   Beam : 40.4 ft.
How Sunk : Ran aground

Date Sunk : 03 11 1914
Longitude : 06 01 00 W
Decca Long : 0601.00 W
Area : SE Islay
Tonnage : 2178 gross.
Draught : 22.5 ft.
Depth : 8 metres

Eilean a'Churn lies about one mile South of Ardmore Point, the easternmost point of Islay. The wreck lies just off the shore about 100 yards West of the light.
    Guethary was a steel barque built in Nantes, France in 1901. The date of her loss was given in *Parliamentary Papers* as 21st October 1914. The vessel had been bound from New Caledonia to Glasgow with a cargo of mineral nickel.

EARL LENNOX

Wreck No : 74		**Date Sunk :** 23 10 1917	
Latitude :	N	**Longitude :**	W
Decca Lat :	N	**Decca Long :**	W
Location : Off entrance to Sound of Islay		**Area :** E. Islay	
Type : Trawler		**Tonnage :** 226 gross.	
Length : ft.	**Beam :** ft.	**Draught :** ft.	
How Sunk : Mined		**Depth :** metres	

The only positional information I have for the *Earl Lennox* is *off the entrance to the Sound of Islay*, but I do not know whether this refers to the North or the South entrance to the Sound.

CRISCILLA

Wreck No : 75		**Date Sunk :** 03 11 1931	
Latitude : 55 47 37 N		**Longitude :** 06 03 48 W	
Decca Lat : 5547.62 N		**Decca Long :** 0603.80 W	
Location : Black Rock, Sound of Islay		**Area :** E Islay	
Type : Trawler		**Tonnage :** 350 gross.	
Length : 135.4 ft.	**Beam :** 25.0 ft.	**Draught :** 13.4 ft.	
How Sunk : Ran aground		**Depth :** 14 metres	

The *Criscilla* was a trawler built in 1929 by Cochrane & Sons of Selby, engine by Amos & Smith of Hull.

She ran aground on rocks in the Sound of Islay, about 100 yards from the Black Rock buoy. Efforts to pull her off the rocks were unsuccessful, and she finally broke in two and sank leaving only her masts showing at low water, though these are no longer visible.

Tidal streams in the Sound of Islay can run at 5-7 knots, but there is a short period of slack water.

EDITH MORGAN

Wreck No : 76		**Date Sunk :** 16 01 1881	
Latitude : 55 47 44 N		**Longitude :** 06 03 26 W	
Decca Lat : 5547.73 N		**Decca Long :** 0603.43 W	
Location : Black Rock, Sound of Islay		**Area :** E Islay	
Type : Schooner		**Tonnage :** gross	
Length : ft.	**Beam :** ft.	**Draught :** ft.	
How Sunk : Ran aground		**Depth :** metres	

The position of Black Rock in the Sound of Islay 554744N, 060326W. The Navy gives the position of the *Edith Morgan* as 554745N, 060350W.

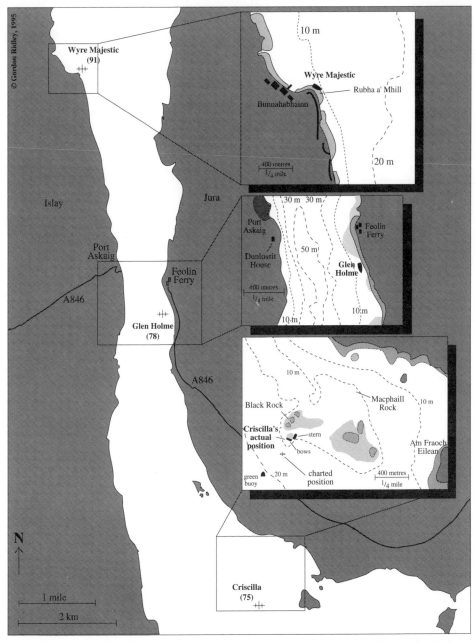

Chart showing the location of wrecks lying in the Sound of Islay

KAY D

Wreck No : 77	**Date Sunk :** 03 04 1982
Latitude : 55 50 00 N PA	**Longitude :** 06 06 00 W PA
Decca Lat : 5550.00 N	**Decca Long :** 0606.00 W
Location : 500 yds from Black Rock buoy	**Area :** E Islay
Type :	**Tonnage :** gross
Length : ft. **Beam :** ft.	**Draught :** ft.
How Sunk : Foundered	**Depth :** metres

Foundered after listing and taking in water 500 yards from the Black Rock buoy in the Sound of Islay.

GLEN HOLME

Wreck No : 78	**Date Sunk :** 28 05 1893
Latitude : 55 50 36 N	**Longitude :** 06 05 20 W
Decca Lat : 5550.60 N	**Decca Long :** 0605.33 W
Location : Feolin Ferry, Sound of Islay	**Area :** E Islay
Type : Steamship	**Tonnage :** 826 gross.
Length : 213.6 ft. **Beam :** 29.2 ft.	**Draught :** 16.2 ft.
How Sunk : Collision	**Depth :** 5 metres

The Maryport-registered iron steamship *Glen Holme*, 532 tons net, was proceeding down the Sound of Islay en route from Windau, Russia, to Ardrossan with a cargo of sleepers, when she was sunk in collision with the Danish steamer *GPA Koch* on 28th May 1893.

The *Glen Holme* (ex-*Margaret Banks*), was built in 1870 by Denton, Gray & Co. of West Hartlepool, engine by Richardsons of Hepple.

LILY MELLING

Wreck No : 79	**Date Sunk :** 02 12 1929
Latitude : 55 52 00 N PA	**Longitude :** 06 06 00 W PA
Decca Lat : 5552.00 N	**Decca Long :** 0606.00 W
Location : Grounded in Sound of Islay	**Area :** E Islay
Type : Steam trawler	**Tonnage :** gross
Length : ft. **Beam :** ft.	**Draught :** ft.
How Sunk : Ran aground	**Depth :** metres

In 1929 the steamship *Lady Anstruther* reported an unknown vessel in this approximate position, which is in the middle of the Sound of Islay, near the lighthouse at Carragh an t-Sruith on Jura. No trace of the wreck was found by HMS *Cook* in 1956.

The steam trawler *Lily Melling* was abandoned after grounding in the Sound of Islay on 2nd December 1929.

It seems possible that this is the vessel reported by the *Lady Anstruther*, in which case she was obviously visible above water for a time after she ran aground, but will have slipped off the rocks, and probably lies close to the more southerly of the outlying rocks off Inver Cottage, just to the North of Whitefarland Bay, Jura. I would suggest 555202N, 054000W may be a more accurate position for the wreck.

MOUNT PARK

Wreck No : 80	**Date Sunk :** 13 06 1887
Latitude : 55 52 00 N PA	**Longitude :** 06 06 00 W PA
Decca Lat : 5552.00 N	**Decca Long :** 0606.00 W
Location : Sound of Islay	**Area :** E Islay
Type : Steamship	**Tonnage :** 302 gross.
Length : ft. **Beam :** ft.	**Draught :** ft.
How Sunk : Ran aground	**Depth :** metres

The 302 tons net iron steamship *Mount Park*, bound from Hamburg to Greenock with a cargo of sugar, was lost by running aground in the Sound of Islay on 13th June 1887.

UNKNOWN - PRE-1922

Wreck No : 81	**Date Sunk :** 1921
Latitude : 55 55 02 N	**Longitude :** 06 04 48 W
Decca Lat : 5555.03 N	**Decca Long :** 0604.80 W
Location : Sgear Traigh, Sound of Islay	**Area :** E Islay
Type : Trawler	**Tonnage :** gross
Length : ft. **Beam :** ft.	**Draught :** ft.
How Sunk :	**Depth :** 6 metres

Sunk in 1921? The position 555500N, 060400W PA has also been given for an unknown trawler, sunk pre-1922.

PORT HOBART

Wreck No : 82	**Date Sunk :** 24 11 1940
Latitude : 55 32 00 N PA	**Longitude :** 06 44 00 W PA
Decca Lat : 5532.00 N	**Decca Long :** 0644.00 W
Location : SW of Islay	**Area :** SW Islay
Type : Steamship	**Tonnage :** 7448 gross.
Length : 466.9 ft. **Beam :** 59.7 ft.	**Draught :** 31.3 ft.
How Sunk : By *Admiral Sheer*	**Depth :** metres

Port Hobart, built by Swan Hunter and Wigham Richardson at Newcastle in 1925, was sunk by the German raider *Admiral Sheer*.

ALMA DAWSON

Wreck No : 83		Date Sunk : 25 11 1940	
Latitude : 55 32 00 N PA		Longitude : 06 44 00 W PA	
Decca Lat : 5532.00 N		Decca Long : 0644.00 W	
Location : SW of Islay		Area : SW Islay	
Type : Steamship		Tonnage : 3985 gross.	
Length : 360.1 ft.	Beam : 51.1 ft.	Draught : 24.3 ft.	
How Sunk : Mined		Depth : metres	

The British steamship *Alma Dawson* was built in 1917 by the Tyne Iron Shipbuilding Co. She sank after striking a British mine while en route from Montreal to Ipswich.

NORMAN

Wreck No : 84		Date Sunk : 25 05 1900	
Latitude : 55 40 00 N PA		Longitude : 06 39 00 W PA	
Decca Lat : 5540.00 N		Decca Long : 0639.00 W	
Location : About 5 miles W of Orsay Light		Area : SW Islay	
Type : Steamship		Tonnage : 524 gross.	
Length : ft.	Beam : ft.	Draught : ft.	
How Sunk : Foundered		Depth : metres	

The 524 tons net steel steamship *Norman* foundered about 5 miles West of Oversay Light in a Force 6 North westerly on 25th May 1900.

THOMAS

Wreck No : 85		Date Sunk : August 1857	
Latitude : 55 40 18 N		Longitude : 06 30 52 W	
Decca Lat : 5540.30 N		Decca Long : 0630.87 W	
Location : Near Orsay Light		Area : SW Islay	
Type : Brig		Tonnage : gross	
Length : ft.	Beam : ft.	Draught : ft.	
How Sunk : Ran aground		Depth : 3 metres	

Reputed to be the sailing brig *Thomas*, bound for Canada with two railway engines as deck cargo.

Part of the wreck site does consist of wreckage which appears to be the remains of at least one steam locomotive and possibly some rolling stock.

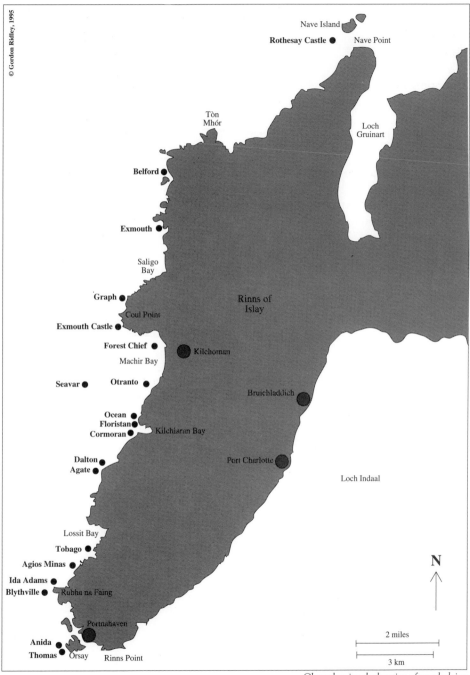

© Gordon Ridley, 1995

Nave Island

Rothesay Castle ●   Nave Point

Tòn
Mhór

Loch
Gruinart

Belford ●

Exmouth ●

Saligo
Bay

Graph ●

Rinns of
Islay

Coul Point

Exmouth Castle ●

Forest Chief ●

Kilchoman

Machir Bay

Seavar ●   Otranto ●

Bruichladdich

Ocean ●
Floristan ●
Cormoran ●

Kilchiaran Bay

Dalton ●
Agate ●

Port Charlotte

Loch Indaal

Lossit Bay

Tobago ●

Agios Minas ●

Ida Adams ●
Blythville ●

Rubha na Faing

N

↑

Portnahaven

2 miles

Anida ●
Thomas ●   Orsay   Rinns Point

3 km

*Chart showing the location of wrecks lying
off the Rinns of Islay*

BLYTHVILLE

Wreck No : 86	**Date Sunk :** 03 06 1908
Latitude : 55 41 36 N	**Longitude :** 06 31 57 W
Decca Lat : 5541.60 N	**Decca Long :** 0631.95 W
Location : Frenchman's Rocks, SW Islay	**Area :** SW Islay
Type : Steamship	**Tonnage :** 1325 gross.
Length : 248.0 ft. **Beam :** 32.1 ft.	**Draught :** 18.4 ft.
How Sunk : Ran aground	**Depth :** 16 metres

The iron steamship *Blythville* was built in 1877 by W. Gray & Co. of West Hartlepool, and owned by the Zapata Steamship Co. En route in ballast from Stornoway to Swansea at reduced speed in fog and darkness, she ran aground on rocks off the Rinns of Islay. According to *Parliamentary Papers* she ran aground about one mile North of Oversay Light. The position recorded by the Navy is 554018N, 063100W PA, which is off the South west of Orsay Island, near the lighthouse, but she floated off and drifted away to sink elsewhere.

The wreck was found amongst the southernmost of Frenchman's Rocks at 554136N, 063157W in 1975.

It was described as a large wreck of about 1000 tons, and wreckage consisting of machinery and steel plating is scattered amongst gullies in the rocks. The bell was recovered in 1983, and is on display at the museum of Islay life at Port Charlotte.

WARNING:
There are very strong tidal streams in this area. These, along with the usual sea state here, only allow diving on this site a few days a year. Take great care!

IDA ADAMS

Wreck No : 87	**Date Sunk :** 21 11 1930
Latitude : 55 42 00 N PA	**Longitude :** 06 32 00 W PA
Decca Lat : 5542.00 N	**Decca Long :** 0632.00 W
Location : Frenchman's Rocks	**Area :** SW Islay
Type : Trawler	**Tonnage :** 275 gross.
Length : 125.0 ft. **Beam :** 22.0 ft.	**Draught :** 11.0 ft.
How Sunk : Ran aground	**Depth :** metres

The Fleetwood trawler *Ida Adams*, owned by the Fleetwood Fishselling Co. was lost on Frenchman's Rocks, Islay on 21st November 1930.

ANIDA

Wreck No : 88
Latitude : 55 41 00 N PA
Decca Lat : 5541.00 N
Location : Oversay Light
Type : Trawler
Length :   ft.   **Beam :**   ft.
How Sunk : Ran aground

Date Sunk : 21 11 1930
Longitude : 06 31 00 W PA
Decca Long : 0631.00 W
Area : SW Islay
Tonnage : 275 gross.
Draught :   ft.
Depth :   metres

The Fleetwood trawler *Anida* was wrecked at Oversay Light on 20th October 1924.

AGIOS MINAS

Wreck No : 89
Latitude : 55 42 06 N
Decca Lat : 5542.10 N
Location : 2 miles N of Portnahaven
Type : Steamship
Length : 322.5 ft.   **Beam :** 43.0 ft.
How Sunk : Ran aground

Date Sunk : 08 09 1968
Longitude : 06 30 36 W
Decca Long : 0630.60 W
Area : SW Islay
Tonnage : 2677 gross.
Draught : 18.2 ft.
Depth : 15 metres

The Liberian freighter *Agios Minas* ran aground on 8th September 1968, about 2 miles North of Portnahaven, West Islay, while en route from Archangel to Bristol with a 15 ft high deck cargo of timber. She was holed in three places, and stuck firmly by the bows, listing to port. The Greek crew of 16 were taken off by Islay lifeboat while awaiting the arrival of the Clyde tug *Cruiser*. Refloating attempts failed, and it was impossible to pull her off the rocks without tearing her bottom. She was declared a total wreck six days after running aground in poor misty weather.

She is now owned by a Mr. Burke of Islay, and lies parallel to the shore, well broken up, with the stern section about 125 yards off the rocks.

TOBAGO

Wreck No : 90
Latitude : 55 42 22 N
Decca Lat : 5542.37 N
Location : S of Lossit Bay
Type : Steamship
Length : 191.0 ft.   **Beam :** 30.6 ft.
How Sunk : Ran aground

Date Sunk : 12 08 1940
Longitude : 06 30 00 W
Decca Long : 0630.00 W
Area : SW Islay
Tonnage : 774 gross.
Draught : 12.3 ft.
Depth : 5 metres

The Latvian steamship *Tobago* (ex-*Latava*, ex-*Sundmar*, ex-*Erica*, ex-*Vinga*), was built in 1900 by Lindholmens of Gothenburg.

She ran aground in bad weather while en route from Reykjavik to Ardrossan with a cargo of dried fish.

WYRE MAJESTIC

Wreck No : 91
Latitude : 55 52 58 N
Decca Lat : 5552.90 N
Location : Rubha a'Mhill, Sound of Islay
Type : Trawler
Length : 132.0 ft.   **Beam :** 27.3 ft.
How Sunk : Ran aground

Date Sunk : 18 10 1974
Longitude : 06 07 12 W
Decca Long : 0607.20 W
Area : W Islay
Tonnage : 338 gross.
Draught : 13.5 ft.
Depth :   metres

The steam trawler *Wyre Majestic* left Oban about 15.10 hours on 18th October, bound for Fleetwood. At about 19.40 hours in the darkness, she ran aground at full speed (10-11 knots), and is now dry on the Islay shore at Rubha a Mhill, four miles North of Port Askaig. All of the crew were saved. Her position is recorded by the Navy as 555258.5N, 060711.5W.

Trawlers are more vulnerable than many cargo vessels in that they do not have double bottom tanks which give some additional protection in the event of stranding.

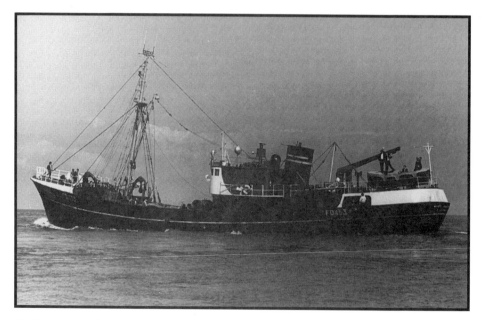

The Wyre Majestic *(Photograph courtesy of Maritime Photo Library)*

JUSTICIA

Wreck No : 92
Latitude : 55 38 00 N PA
Decca Lat : 5538.00 N
Location : W of Islay
Type : Steamship
Length : 776.0 ft.   **Beam :** 86.3 ft.
How Sunk : Torpedoed by *UB-64, UB-124*

Date Sunk : 20 07 1918
Longitude : 07 39 00 W PA
Decca Long : 0739.00 W
Area : W Islay
Tonnage : 32234 gross.
Draught : 43.0 ft.
Depth :   metres

In 1914, the liner *Statendam* was under construction by Harland & Wolff at Belfast for the Holland-Amerika line but, on the outbreak of the First World War, work on her was halted. The unfinished liner was requisitioned by the Admiralty and completed in 1917 as the troopship *Justicia*, managed by the White Star line.

On 19th July 1918, she was torpedoed by the *UB-64* 20 miles W by N¾ N of Skerryvore. The first torpedo struck at 13.50 hours, and this was followed by two more at 16.00 hours. She was taken in tow towards Lough Swilly, but was torpedoed again by the *UB-64* at 19.18 hours. The *UB-64* then had to break off the attack, as she was damaged herself.

At 09.10 hours the next day the *Justicia* was torpedoed by *UB-124*. Three hours later she sank stern first with the loss of 10 lives. *Lloyds War Losses* gives the position as 5538N 0739W.

The *Justicia* was one of the largest ships to be sunk in WW1. At 32234 tons, her gross weight was some 2000 tons greater than that of the *Lusitania* (30296 tons).

Depth-charging forced the *UB-124* to the surface where she was then sunk by gunfire from several ships including the destroyers *Marne*, *Millbrook* and *Pigeon*. The wreck of the *UB-124* must, therefore, be somewhere in the vicinity of the wreck of the *Justicia*.

AGATE

Wreck No : 93
Latitude : 55 43 11 N
Decca Lat : 5543.18 N
Location : Under Cnoc Breac South, Islay
Type : Steamship
Length : 199.4 ft.   **Beam :** 30.1 ft.
How Sunk : Ran aground

Date Sunk : 30 12 1940
Longitude : 06 30 10 W
Decca Long : 0630.17 W
Area : W Islay
Tonnage : 482 gross.
Draught : 11.9 ft.
Depth : 10 metres

The British steam collier *Agate*, built in 1917 by Scott & Sons, was wrecked 4 miles North of Orsay lighthouse, Islay on 30th December 1940. This position is under the southern edge of the cliffs at Rubha Glamraidh on the West coast of Rinns of Islay. Her cargo was 800 tons of coal.

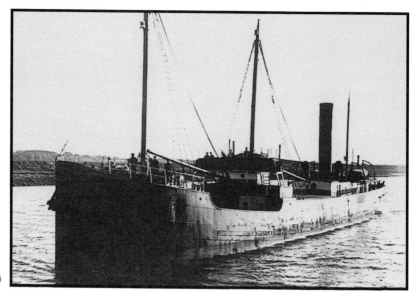

The Agate (Photograph courtesy of the World Ship Society)

DALTON

Wreck No : 94
Latitude : 55 44 08 N
Decca Lat : 5544.13 N
Location : Under Cnoc Breac North, Islay
Type : Steamship
Length : 315.4 ft.   **Beam :** 34.9 ft.
How Sunk : Ran aground

Date Sunk : 28 09 1895
Longitude : 06 29 54 W
Decca Long : 0629.90 W
Area : W Islay
Tonnage : 2030 gross.
Draught : 24.9 ft.
Depth : 15 metres

The British steamship *Dalton*, built in 1881 by A. Leslie & Co. for Lamport & Holt, was wrecked South of Kilchiaran Bay on the West coast of Islay while en route from New York to the Clyde with a cargo of grain, oil and wood. She broke in two and became a total loss under Cnoc Breac North, where a break in the cliffs forms a tiny inlet half a mile West of Tormisdale, and just to the North of Rubha Glamraidh.

The position has also been recorded as 554224N, 062912W.

HENRY CLAY

Wreck No : 95
Latitude : 55 44 30 N PA
Decca Lat : 5544.50 N
Location : At Port Charlotte, Loch Indaal
Type : Sailing Ship

Date Sunk : 28 09 1861
Longitude : 06 22 30 W PA
Decca Long : 0622.50 W
Area : W Islay
Tonnage : 1250 gross.

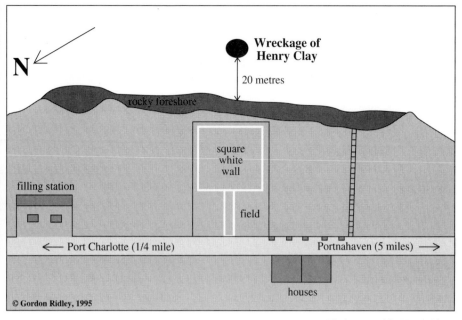

The location of the Henry Clay

Length : ft.   **Beam :** ft.   **Draught :** ft.
How Sunk : Ran aground   **Depth :** 6 metres

Henry Clay was an American sailing vessel which struck a reef off Laggan Bay while en route from Liverpool to New York. She was not in immediate danger of sinking, and made for the shelter of the nearest land to anchor and carry out repairs. Instead of calming, the weather worsened to a storm. Her anchor ropes parted and she was driven on to rocks on the northern side of the loch near Port Charlotte.

The crew were all saved but, despite an attempt by another sailing ship, the *Lady Franklin*, to pull the *Henry Clay* off the rocks, she broke up, and now lies partially buried in sand, in 6 metres of water only 20 yards off the shore.

CORMORAN

Wreck No : 96   **Date Sunk :** 12 01 1926
Latitude : 55 44 42 N   **Longitude :** 06 29 06 W
Decca Lat : 5544.70 N   **Decca Long :** 0629.10 W
Location : Kilchiaran Bay   **Area :** W Islay
Type : Trawler   **Tonnage :** 228 gross.
Length : 120.8 ft.   **Beam :** 21.5 ft.   **Draught :** 11.6 ft.
How Sunk : Ran aground   **Depth :** 5 metres

The Fleetwood trawler *Cormoran* went ashore on rocks between Kilchiaran and Tormisdale in the early hours of 12th January 1926. Five of the crew reached the shore, but a boat with six others was missing until they landed safely on Tiree, 60 miles away, four days later. Rough weather had prevailed in the area for several days.

The *Cormoran* was built in 1909 by Mackie & Thompson, and was owned by Taylor & Co. of Fleetwood.

The boiler is high and dry on the rocks just to the South of Kilchiaran Bay, with the rest of the wreckage broken up and scattered amongst the rocks very close to the shore.

FLORISTAN

Wreck No : 97	**Date Sunk :** 20 01 1942
Latitude : 55 45 06 N	**Longitude :** 06 28 07 W
Decca Lat : 5545.10 N	**Decca Long :** 0628.12 W
Location : Kilchiaran Bay	**Area :** W Islay
Type : Steamship	**Tonnage :** 5478 gross.
Length : 415.3 ft. **Beam :** 54.2 ft.	**Draught :** 27.6 ft.
How Sunk : Ran aground	**Depth :** 12 metres

The steamship *Floristan* was built in 1928 by J. Redhead & Sons, S. Shields. She sank after running aground in fog while en route to the Persian Gulf with a cargo of tanks, jeeps and *DUKWS*, rolling stock, tin coins and gold bullion.

Many coins have been found, along with a great quantity of copper wire. She lies close to the shore in shallow water, very broken up, about 6 miles North of Orsay light, on the North side of the entrance to Kilchiaran Bay. The boilers are the highest part of the wreckage, and are within 1 metre of the surface at low water.

The wreck is owned by Tim Epps, and is charted at 554509N, 062830W.

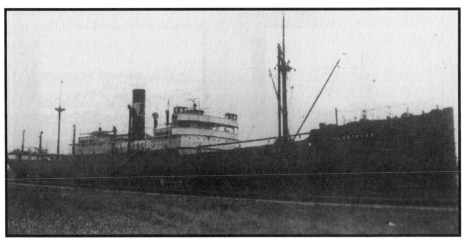

The Floristan *(Photograph courtesy of the World Ship Society)*

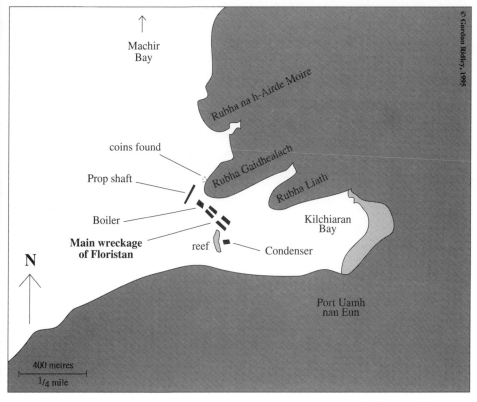

The location of the
Floristan

OCEAN

Wreck No : 98
Latitude : 55 45 18 N
Decca Lat : 5545.30 N
Location : Rubha na h-Airde Moire
Type : Barque
Length : 231.1 ft.   **Beam :** 37.1 ft.
How Sunk : Ran aground

Date Sunk : 03 11 1911
Longitude : 06 28 28 W
Decca Long : 0628.47 W
Area : W Islay
Tonnage : 1324 gross.
Draught : 23.4 ft.
Depth : 5 metres

The 1239 tons net iron barque *Ocean*, built by J. Reid of Port Glasgow in 1873, and registered in Mariehamn, Finland, left Dublin in ballast for Norway. En route, she experienced the full force of a gale off the West of Islay. Her sails were blown away, and the vessel drifted towards the rocky coast at Rubha na h-airde Moire, to the North of Kilchiaran Bay. The crew of sixteen men were seen clustered in the bow which first struck the rocks. The ship instantly slewed round, the stern striking the rocks, and before the men could leave their shelter, suddenly parted in the middle.

Tremendous seas broke over the ship, which with the rising tide was pounding on the rocks within 70 yards of the shore in a wild full gale on the beam. The captain, A. Christophen, dived into the water to swim ashore, and reached the rocks, only to be dashed against them and instantly killed. His body was then washed away. The stern mast then fell landwards, and one by one the crew attempted to crawl along the mast and throw themselves into the boiling surf. Two of them were drowned, but twelve succeeded in reaching the shore.

OTRANTO

Wreck No : 99
Latitude : 55 45 46 N
Decca Lat : 5545.77 N
Location : At S of Machir Bay
Type : Steamship
Length : 535.3 ft.   **Beam :** 64.0 ft.
How Sunk : Collision with *Kashmir*

Date Sunk : 06 10 1918
Longitude : 06 28 40 W
Decca Long : 0628.67 W
Area : W Islay
Tonnage : 12124 gross.
Draught : 38.6 ft.
Depth : 18 metres

The 12124 tons gross liner *Otranto* was built by Workman Clark & Co., Belfast, for the Orient Steam Navigation Company in 1909. Measuring 535.3 x 64 x 38.6 ft. she was launched on 21st March, and completed on 30th June. Her six boilers were coal fired, and her top speed was 18 knots. Her maiden voyage commenced on 1st October 1909 on the Australian mail run.

On the outbreak of the First World War she was taken over by the Admiralty for

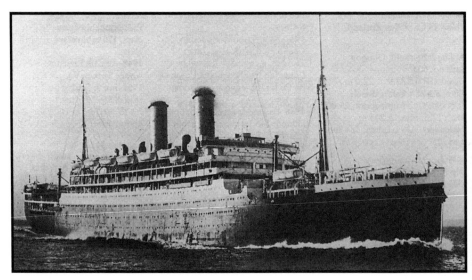

The Otranto (Photograph courtesy of John Clarkson, Longton)

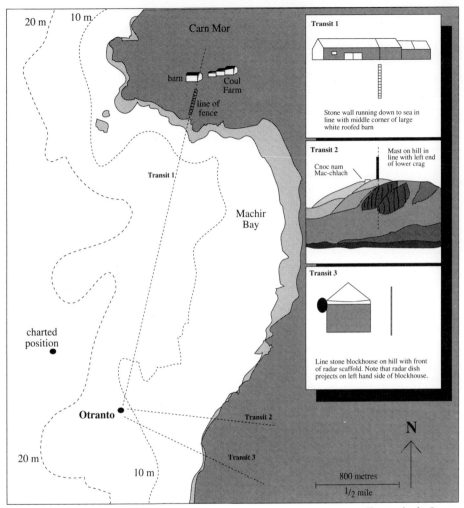

Transits for the Otranto

service as an auxiliary cruiser, and armed with eight 4.7" guns. In February 1916 she was refitted at Sydney, Australia, her 4.7" guns being replaced with 6" guns, and in 1917, one additional 6" gun was fitted.

The *Otranto* sailed from New York on 24th September 1918 as part of Convoy HX50, which consisted of 13 ships - 12 British and one French - escorted by two US cruisers, the *Louisiana* and the *St. Louis*, and the US destroyer *Dorsey*. The convoy was bringing over 20000 American troops via Liverpool and Glasgow to the battlefields of Flanders.

One of the columns of ships in the convoy was led by the *Otranto*, and to the left of her, the 8841 tons gross P&O liner *Kashmir* led another. Soon after the convoy left, a radio message was received that two U-boats were operating in the area of the

Nantucket lightship, and the convoy altered course to the North to avoid them.

On the 26th, two days after setting out, the first of many deaths occurred on the ships from Spanish influenza. The total number of deaths from this disease is not known, but 20 died on the *Kashmir* alone.

Steaming without lights in mid Atlantic on the night of 1st October, in cold and foggy weather, the convoy crossed the path of a fleet of 22 French fishing vessels which were also sailing without lights. This, of course, was standard practice during the War, to avoid advertising their presence to any U-boats which might be waiting to attack.

One of the French fishing vessels, *Barquentine Croisine*, was hit in the side by the *Otranto* as she came steaming through the fog. The French ship was rendered immobile with broken spars, and was taking in water. The *Otranto* stopped, and Captain Davidson sent one of his officers, F.R.O'Sullivan, in a small boat to rescue the French fishermen. He returned top the *Otranto* with the French crew of 36, including her captain Jules Le Hoerff and his pet dog.

The abandoned French vessel was still afloat, and to prevent her falling into enemy hands, Captain Davidson ordered her to be sunk, to the delight of the *Otranto*'s gun crews. The *Otranto* then set off to catch up with the rest of the convoy, which had continued to steam on ahead.

On 5th October, about 200 miles West of Ireland, the American escorts left the convoy, their duties being taken over by a British escort which had come out to meet them. The following morning, 6th October, in worsening weather with waves up to 40ft high, a light, which was assumed to be Tory Island Light was seen. In the deteriorating weather and huge seas, the convoy was spread out over a wide area. One of the British destroyers was seen in the distance.

During the day, the mist and fog cleared, and some ships sighted land ahead and to the left. Mistaking this for the Scottish mainland, many of the ships turned southward. Because of the bad weather, the convoy had actually been blown some 20 miles North of their intended course, and the land they saw was in fact Islay. The *Otranto*, half a mile to the right, mistook the land for Northern Ireland, and turned northwards. After turning North and battling through heavy seas for a hour or so in poor visibility, the *Kashmir*, which was having difficulty steering due to the sea conditions, suddenly appeared out of one of the great waves, heading directly for the port side of the *Otranto*.

To Captain Davidson's horror, the *Kashmir* was carried up the side of a huge wave, and smashed down almost at right angles into the *Otranto*, tearing a massive hole in her amidships. The *Kashmir* then regained some control of her steering and headed for the Scottish coast, not realising the extent of the damage she had inflicted on the *Otranto*, which at first seemed to suffer no ill effect from the collision. The *Otranto* continued steaming for a further hour or so, but by that time she had taken in so much water that her engines finally stopped, and the liner was left drifting helplessly toward the cliffs of Machir Bay on the West coast of Islay.

Despite dropping her anchors, the *Otranto* continued to drift toward the Islay shore in the heavy weather prevailing, and sent out SOS messages. These were answered by the torpedo boat destroyer HMS *Mounsey*, commanded by Lt.F.W.Craven. The

Mounsey was in sight of the *Otranto* by about 10.00 am that morning, and Captain Davidson advised the *Mounsey* not to come alongside in the heavy seas, Lt. Craven realised that he had to attempt just that if anyone aboard the *Otranto* was to survive.

In such terrible sea conditions, a normal approach to lie alongside the liner was impossible. By steaming head into the wind until she was parallel with the *Otranto*, Lt. Craven let the wind carry the *Mounsey* toward the stricken liner. Captain Davidson understood Lt. Craven's intention, and lowered the *Otranto's* starboard lifeboats to act as fenders to cushion the inevitable impact between the two ships as the gap closed. The men on board were lined up on deck without their heavy coats and boots, and as the *Mounsey* smashed into her side, the first line of men were ordered to jump. Many of the men made it to the deck, but many others did not. Some of the men were terribly injured as they landed on the heaving deck of the *Mounsey*, and others landed on the deck only to be swept overboard by the huge waves washing over the decks. Lt. Craven repeated his excellent feat of seamanship a further three times, and each time she smashed alongside, men jumped for the comparative safety of the *Mounsey's* decks. By the fourth and last time, the *Otranto's* lifeboats had been smashed to matchwood, and it was every man for himself, each man jumping when his chance came. One wave washed about a dozen men over the side, and another who jumped for the tossing deck below landed on a wire stay, and was neatly cut in two.

By mid-day, the *Mounsey*, with survivors lashed to anything which a rope could be got around, headed for the Irish shore. Captain Davidson was last seen standing on his bridge, and was never seen alive again. He had ordered *Abandon Ship*, but of the 400 or so still aboard the *Otranto*, only 16 made the long hard swim to the Islay shore. The following morning, over 150 bodies had been recovered from the shore line and placed in the church on Islay. The loss of life was very heavy. 431 persons had been drowned, including 351 US soldiers, but there were 367 survivors according to one report, 596 according to another.

Meanwhile, the *Otranto* drifted ashore on the West of Islay and became a total wreck. Her wrecked remains lie scattered over a wide area about ¼ mile off the cliffs at the South of Machir Bay, below a radar installation. Large portions of the wreck remain reasonably intact, and the 6" guns and shells are still there. The broken wreckage lies across a reef in depths of 8-18 metres of water. The boilers lie in three pairs side by side in a gully near the edge of the reef in about 8-9 metres of water.

Two large pieces of cast iron pipe are visible about 15 metres above sea level under the cliffs. These are actually part of a stepping piece for one of *Otranto's* masts.

The wreck was eventually bought by Tim Epps of Port Charlotte, and some of the artefacts recovered by divers, including the ship's telegraph and steam whistle, have been renovated and are on display in the bar of the Port Charlotte Hotel.

The *Otranto* was not the only troop ship to be sunk off Islay. On 5th February 1918, the Anchor liner *Tuscania*, bringing over 2000 American soldiers to Britain, was torpedoed off the south of Islay by the *UB-77* (commanded by KL Wilhelm Meyer), with the loss of 166 lives, A monument to those lost on the *Tuscania* and the *Otranto* was erected on the Mull of Oa in the South east of Islay.

SEAVAR

Wreck No : 100
Latitude : 55 46 00 N PA
Decca Lat : 5546.00 N
Location : 4 miles W of Machir Bay
Type : Trawler
Length :   ft.   **Beam :**   ft.
How Sunk :

Date Sunk : 18 05 1950
Longitude : 06 35 00 W PA
Decca Long : 0635.00 W
Area : W Islay
Tonnage :   gross
Draught : ft.
Depth : 5 metres

Seavar was a steam trawler.

FOREST CHIEF

Wreck No : 101
Latitude : 55 46 30 N PA
Decca Lat : 5546.50 N
Location : Kilchoman, NW Islay
Type :
Length :   ft.   **Beam :**   ft.
How Sunk : Ran aground

Date Sunk : 06 11 1872
Longitude : 06 28 00 W PA
Decca Long : 0628.00 W
Area : W Islay
Tonnage : 1054 gross.
Draught : ft.
Depth :   metres

The 1054 tons net ship *Forest Chief*, en route from New York to Londonderry with a cargo of Indian corn, was blown ashore in a WSW hurricane, Force 11, at Kilchoman, on the North west of Islay, on 6th November 1872. One member of the crew was lost.

Kilchoman is not actually on the coast, but is a small settlement about ½ mile inland from the beach at Machir Bay. *Forest Chief* was presumably blown ashore on this beach.

LA PLATA

Wreck No : 102
Latitude : 55 46 30 W PA
Decca Lat : 5546.50 N
Location : Macharie Bay
Type : Barque
Length :   ft.   **Beam :**   ft.
How Sunk : Ran aground

Date Sunk : 16 11 1888
Longitude : 06 28 00 W PA
Decca Long : 0628.00 W
Area : W Islay
Tonnage : 596 gross.
Draught : ft.
Depth :   metres

The 596 tons net Norwegian barque *La Plata*, en route from Newcastle to Buenos Aires with a cargo of coke and coal was blown ashore and wrecked in a WSW storm, Force 10, at Macharie Bay, Islay, on 16th November 1888.

UNKNOWN - PRE-1957

Wreck No : 103   **Date Sunk :** Pre - 1957
Latitude : 55 46 37 N   **Longitude :** 06 16 18 W
Decca Lat : 5546.62 N   **Decca Long :** 0616.30 W
Location : Dries at Bowmore, Loch Indaal   **Area :** W Islay
Type :   **Tonnage :**   gross
Length : ft.   **Beam :** ft.   **Draught :** ft.
How Sunk :   **Depth :**   metres

A drying wreck was reported here in 1957.

UNKNOWN

Wreck No : 104   **Date Sunk :**
Latitude : 55 46 58 N   **Longitude :** 06 27 30 W
Decca Lat : 5546.97 N   **Decca Long :** 0627.50 W
Location : Machir Bay   **Area :** W Islay
Type : Paddle steamer   **Tonnage :**   gross
Length : ft.   **Beam :** ft.   **Draught :** ft.
How Sunk :   **Depth :** 2 metres

The drying wreck of a paddle steamer was reported here.

COLONIAL EMPIRE

Wreck No : 105   **Date Sunk :** 01 02 1880
Latitude : 55 47 00 N PA   **Longitude :** 06 28 00 W PA
Decca Lat : 5547.00 N   **Decca Long :** 0628.00 W
Location : N of Machrie Bay   **Area :** W Islay
Type : Barque   **Tonnage :** 1269 gross.
Length : ft.   **Beam :** ft.   **Draught :** ft.
How Sunk : Ran aground   **Depth :**   metres

The Aberdeen barque *Colonial Empire* ran aground North of Machir Bay in a Force 10 SW storm on 1st February 1880. She had been en route from Liverpool to Pensacola, Florida.

NILS GORTHON

Wreck No : 106	**Date Sunk :** 13 08 1940
Latitude : 55 47 00 N PA	**Longitude :** 07 00 00 W PA
Decca Lat : 5547.00 N	**Decca Long :** 0700.00 W
Location : 25 miles NNE of Malin Head	**Area :** W Islay
Type : Steamship	**Tonnage :** 1809 gross.
Length : 260.9 ft. **Beam :** 40.9 ft.	**Draught :** 17.5 ft.
How Sunk : Torpedoed by U-60	**Depth :** 43 metres

The Swedish steamship *Nils Gorthon*, built in 1921 by Howaldtswerke, torpedoed by *U-60* (Schnee), 25 miles NNE of Malin Head, when she straggled from a convoy bound from St. Johns, Newfoundland, to Ridham dock.

The trawler *St. Kenan* picked up nine survivors two days later, and a *Sunderland* aircraft spotted a raft with another eight survivors who were picked up by HMS *Anthony*.

LEXINGTON?

Wreck No : 107	**Date Sunk :** 13 08 1940
Latitude : 55 47 26 N	**Longitude :** 06 59 50 W
Decca Lat : 5547.43 N	**Decca Long :** 0659.83 W
Location : 16 miles W of Islay	**Area :** W Islay
Type : Sailing ship	**Tonnage :** 344 gross.
Length : ft. **Beam :** ft.	**Draught :** ft.
How Sunk : Foundered	**Depth :** 43 metres

The 344 ton barque *Lexington* foundered off Coul, Islay on 25th December 1865. She had a cargo of coal and three passengers. One life was lost.

The wreck was first located in 1967 and was thought to be the Swedish steamship *Nils Gorthon* but, in 1983, and again in 1986, the wreck was identified as a large sailing vessel lying on her port side, oriented 040/220 degrees, standing 10 metres high in about 46 metres.

JACKSONVILLE

Wreck No : 108	**Date Sunk :** 30 08 1944
Latitude : 55 47 37 N	**Longitude :** 06 54 04 W
Decca Lat : 5547.62 N	**Decca Long :** 0654.07 W
Location : 15 miles W of Coul Point	**Area :** W Islay
Type : Tanker	**Tonnage :** 10448 gross.
Length : 504.0 ft. **Beam :** 68.2 ft.	**Draught :** 39.2 ft.
How Sunk : Torpedoed by U-482	**Depth :** 26 metres

The *Jacksonville* was an American tanker built in 1944 by the Kaiser Corporation. She was torpedoed by *U-482* (KL Graf von Matuschka) 200 miles North of Ireland while en route from New York to Shellhaven with a cargo of 14300 tons of petrol.

The ship broke in two, the forepart sinking immediately. The stern section remained afloat, on fire, and only three of the 78 crew were saved, although badly injured. Least depth of 84 ft (25 metres), in a general depth of 145 ft (44 metres).

CHEVALIER

Wreck No : 109	**Date Sunk** : 20 01 1883
Latitude : 55 48 00 N PA	**Longitude** : 06 30 00 W PA
Decca Lat : 5548.00 N	**Decca Long** : 0630.00 W
Location : Coul	**Area** : W Islay
Type : Barque	**Tonnage** : 829 gross.
Length : ft. **Beam** : ft.	**Draught** : ft.
How Sunk : Ran aground	**Depth** : metres

The wooden barque *Chevalier*, with a cargo of coal from Troon to Matanzas, was blown ashore by a North westerly severe gale, Force 9, at Coul, Islay on 20th January 1883.

GRAPH

Wreck No : 110	**Date Sunk** : 20 03 1944
Latitude : 55 48 48 N	**Longitude** : 06 27 38 W
Decca Lat : 5548.80 N	**Decca Long** : 0627.63 W
Location : ¾ mile N of Coul Point	**Area** : W Islay
Type : U-Boat	**Tonnage** : 880 gross.
Length : 220.2 ft. **Beam** : 20.3 ft.	**Draught** : 15.7 ft.
How Sunk : Ran aground under tow	**Depth** : 5 metres

HMS *Graph* (ex-German Type VIIC U-Boat *U-570*) ran aground under tow on the West coast of Islay. The conning tower and aft section are reported intact but little remains of the forward section. The position is also recorded as 554808N, 062832W.

Type VIIC U-Boats displaced 749 tons surfaced, and 871 tons submerged. They were powered by two diesel engines and two electric motors, and were armed with 5 torpedo tubes (4 bow and 1 stern), 1 x 88 mm and 1 x 20 mm guns. Maximum diving depth was 309 ft. (94 metres).

Although she was reportedly scrapped in situ in 1947, the conning tower and after section were still intact in 1970, but by 1981 the wreck was reported to be broken up. The bronze torpedo tubes were recovered by Keith Jessup of HMS *Edinburgh* fame. A large winch used during the salvage operations overlooks the site.

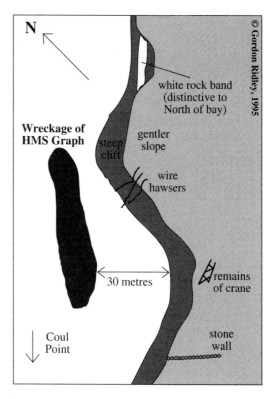

The location of the wreck of HMS Graph.

Only two U-Boats were captured and taken in tow during the war: *U-110* (Lemp), which sank on 11th May 1941 while under tow South of Iceland after being captured by HMS *Bulldog* (Cdr. John Baker-Cresswell). This was not officially disclosed until 1966 for security reasons. (A complete *Enigma* coding machine and code books were captured intact from her before she sank), and *U-570*, (HMS *Graph*), captured in the North Atlantic on 28th August 1941 by HMS *Burwell* and HMT *Northern Chief*, after being depth-charged by RAF aircraft of *269 Squadron* the previous day. She was used by the Royal Navy for a time, and ran aground on Islay when the tow broke while en route from Chatham to the Clyde.

EXMOUTH

Wreck No : 111
Latitude : 55 49 50 N
Decca Lat : 5549.83 N
Location : Rubha Lamanais
Type : Trawler
Length : 120.0 ft.   **Beam :** 21.1 ft.

Date Sunk : 09 03 1938
Longitude : 06 27 30 W
Decca Long : 0627.50 W
Area : W Islay
Tonnage : 236 gross
Draught : 11.7 ft.

How Sunk : Ran aground   **Depth :**   metres

The 236 ton Fleetwood trawler *Exmouth*, built in 1912, ran aground in fog on rocks off Smaull Point, which must either be another name for Rubha Lamanais, or the headland immediately to the North.

Three of the crew were washed away by waves breaking over their vessel, but the eight others did succeed in reaching the shore in their small boat. The *Exmouth* was soon pounded to pieces by the waves.

EXMOUTH CASTLE

Wreck No : 112   **Date Sunk :** 28 04 1847
Latitude : 55 51 10 N PA   **Longitude :** 06 27 20 W PA
Decca Lat : 5551.17 N   **Decca Long :** 0627.33 W
Location : An Clachan   **Area :** W Islay
Type : Sailing ship   **Tonnage :** 322 gross.
Length :   ft.   **Beam :**   ft.   **Draught :** ft.
How Sunk : Ran aground   **Depth :** 5 metres

A sailing vessel built in1818, the *Exmouth Castle* left Londonderry for Quebec on 25th April 1847, with a crew of 11 and 243 emigrants. Three days out, she encountered very bad weather, and ran for shelter. A light, which had been assumed to be Tory Island light, was, in fact, Orsay light on the point of the Rinns of Islay. By the time this mistake had been realised, it was too late to prevent the vessel driving ashore. Three of the crew survived, but all 251 others aboard were drowned.

After climbing a hill at dawn the next day, the survivors spotted a lone farmhouse about a mile away, and made for it to seek help. They were taken in and given dry clothes and the farmer set out for the wreck site to look for any more survivors, but there were none.

A total of 108 bodies were washed up and recovered in the days following the wrecking.

A clue to the position of the disaster is given in a poem written by William Roach, one of the three survivors. One verse reads:

"Next day about eleven o'clock, we got a dreadful shock,
the vessel came with all her might, against the Sanaig rock.
The mainmast fell overboard; and three of us got ashore,
and the rest of us to the bottom went, who never see no more."

Sanaig Rock is a name which could readily apply to An Clachan, the rocky headland about one mile West of the isolated farmhouse at Sanaigmore.

UNKNOWN

Wreck No : 113		**Date Sunk :** Pre - 1967
Latitude : 55 49 18 N		**Longitude :** 06 36 26 W
Decca Lat : 5549.30 N		**Decca Long :** 0636.43 W
Location : 5 miles W of Rubha Lamanais		**Area :** W Islay
Type :		**Tonnage :** gross
Length : ft.	**Beam :** ft.	**Draught :** ft.
How Sunk :		**Depth :** 35 metres

This is an unknown vessel, first located in 1967. Least depth to the wreck is 35 metres in a general depth of 45 metres, hence this appears to be a large wreck.

The *Atos* was lost on in this vicinity 3rd August 1940. Some 800 ft. (240 metres) WNW of the above position there is either another piece of the same wreck, or a different, smaller wreck. The depths are charted as 35 and 31 metres in general depths of 45 metres.

UNKNOWN

Wreck No : 114		**Date Sunk :** Pre - 1967
Latitude : 55 49 23 N		**Longitude :** 06 36 37 W
Decca Lat : 5549.38 N		**Decca Long :** 0636.62 W
Location : W of Saligo Bay		**Area :** W Islay
Type :		**Tonnage :** gross
Length : ft.	**Beam :** ft.	**Draught :** ft.
How Sunk :		**Depth :** 32 metres

Unknown vessel first located in 1967. Least depth of 104 ft. (31 metres), in a general depth of 130 ft. (39 metres). This is probably part of the wreck at 554918N, 063626W.

BRITTANY

Wreck No : 115		**Date Sunk :** 05 02 1918
Latitude : 55 50 00 N PA		**Longitude :** 08 03 00 W PA
Decca Lat : 5550.00 N		**Decca Long :** 0803.00 W
Location : W of Islay		**Area :** W Islay
Type : Steamship		**Tonnage :** 2926 gross.
Length : 330.0 ft.	**Beam :** 43.0 ft.	**Draught :** 16.6 ft.
How Sunk : Collision		**Depth :** metres

The 1890 tons net steel steamship *Brittany* was built in 1898 by Richardson & Duck of Stockton, engine by Blair & Co.

En route from Liverpool to Montevideo with a cargo which included coal and livestock, she was sunk in a collision off Islay on 5th February 1918. Six lives were lost.

BELFORD

Wreck No : 116
Latitude : 55 50 06 N
Decca Lat : 5550.10 N
Location : At Smaull, N of Rubha Lamanais
Type : Steamship
Length : 325.0 ft.   **Beam :** 47.0 ft.
How Sunk : Ran aground

Date Sunk : 09 02 1916
Longitude : 06 27 26 W
Decca Long : 0627.43 W
Area : W Islay
Tonnage : 3216 gross.
Draught : 24.3 ft.
Depth : 5 metres

The *Belford* was a steel steamship of 2076 tons net, built in 1901 by J. Priestman & Co., and registered in Sunderland.

A wild north-westerly gale was blowing on 9th February 1916 when a coast watcher saw a drifting steamer in the early morning, but did not suspect her to be in distress. About 2.00 pm he observed a mast above the rocks, and hurrying to the place, found the steamer *Belford* close up to a high rock. The coast near Smaull is the wildest in Islay, with high rocks towering above the land - one of the worst places at which a vessel could strike. Her papers showed that she was bound from Barry to New York in ballast. When off the coast of Ireland her propeller struck some wreckage, breaking the blades, and the vessel had drifted helplessly in the storm since January 30th. The log recorded the constant sending up of distress signals, and it is surprising how the steamer could have drifted such a length of time without being observed. The boats were gone, and it is probable that the 13 crew saw their vessel nearing the huge rocks, took to the boats

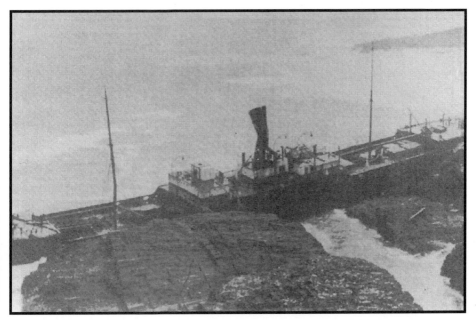

The Belford *ashore (Photograph courtesy of the World Ship Society)*

and were lost. The body of the 29 year old second mate was washed ashore near Ballinaby about the time of the wreck. He had evidently died only a short time before, and his body was interred at Kilchoman churchyard. A broken boat was also washed ashore. The very wild weather continued, and by the evening only half of the ship remained visible, with huge seas dashing her to pieces.

The wreck is now very broken up. The position has also been given as 554924N, 062742W.

ROTHESAY CASTLE

Wreck No : 117	**Date Sunk :** 05 01 1940
Latitude : 55 53 36 N	**Longitude :** 06 21 48 W
Decca Lat : 5553.60 N	**Decca Long :** 0621.80 W
Location : Eilean Beag	**Area :** NW Islay
Type : Steamship	**Tonnage :** 7016 gross.
Length : 443.5 ft. **Beam :** 61.3 ft.	**Draught :** 32.0 ft.
How Sunk : Ran aground	**Depth :** 10 metres

The Union Castle Line vessel *Rothesay Castle* was en route from New York to Glasgow when she ran aground a few minutes before midnight on 4th January 1940. Her SOS was heard just before 1.00 am on the 5th, and the Islay lifeboat *Charlotte Elizabeth* went out from Port Askaig in the darkness to her aid. The *Rothesay Castle's* position had not been given accurately, and it was not until dawn that the lifeboat saw her aground on a reef on the North side of Eilean Beag, to the South west of Nave Island. A tug was called, but was unable to pull her off the rocks. Fourteen of the crew were taken off by the lifeboat on the 6th, and the next day, the remaining crew members were taken off by the tug.

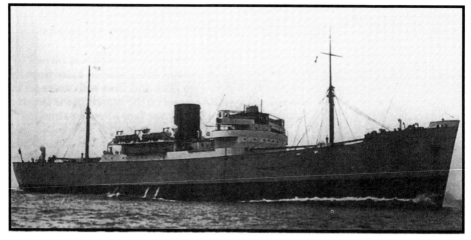

The Rothesay Castle
(Photograph courtesy of the World Ship Society).

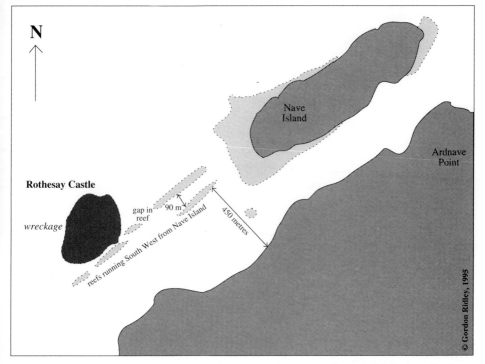

N

Nave
Island

Ardnave
Point

Rothesay Castle

gap in '90 m
reef

wreckage

450 metres

reefs running South West from Nave Island

© Gordon Ridley, 1995

Location of the Rothesay Castle

A few days later the ship started to break up in a storm, and now lies completely broken up and scattered over a fairly wide area. Some of the wreckage is only 10 ft below the surface and covered in kelp. Tidal streams in this area are very strong with considerable turbulence in the water.

The position was given by the Admiralty as 555345N, 062100W, and has also been recorded (by Gordon Ridley) as 555306N, 062148W or 555309N, 062142W.

BOKA

Wreck No : 118
Latitude : 55 54 00 N PA
Decca Lat : 5554.00 N
Location : NW of Islay
Type : Steamship
Length : 400.3 ft.　　**Beam :** 52.4 ft.
How Sunk : Torpedoed by *U-138*

Date Sunk : 20 04 1940
Longitude : 07 24 00 W PA
Decca Long : 0724.00 W
Area : NW Islay
Tonnage : 5399 gross.
Draught : 28.0 ft.
Depth :　　　metres

The Panamanian steamship *Boka (ex-Canadian Planter)*, built in 1920, was torpedoed at 555400N, 072400W at 21.23 hours on 20th September 1940 by the *U-138* (Luth).

NEW SEVILLA

Wreck No : 119		**Date Sunk** : 21 09 1940
Latitude : 55 54 05 N		**Longitude** : 07 29 54 W
Decca Lat : 5554.08 N		**Decca Long** : 0729.90 W
Location : NW of Islay		**Area** : NW Islay
Type : Steamship		**Tonnage** : 13801 gross.
Length : 550.2 ft.	**Beam** : 63.3 ft.	**Draught** : 47.9 ft.
How Sunk : Torpedoed by *U-138*		**Depth** : metres

The 13801 ton British steamship *New Sevilla* (ex-*Runic II*), formerly a whaling factory ship, built by Harland and Wolff in 1900, was torpedoed by *U-138* (Luth), at 554800N, 072200W at 21.20 hours on the 20th September 1940. She had been en route from Liverpool to Aruba and South Georgia.

She was taken in tow by the tug *Salvonia* at 21.40 hours on the 21st, but sank two hours later with the loss of two of the crew.

One report says she sank 9 miles West of the Mull of Kintyre, but the Hydrographic Department has recorded her position of sinking as 555405N, 072954W.

EMPIRE ADVENTURE

Wreck No : 120		**Date Sunk** : 20 09 1940
Latitude : 55 55 00 N PA		**Longitude** : 07 25 00 W PA
Decca Lat : 5555.00 N		**Decca Long** : 0725.00 W
Location : NW of Islay		**Area** : NW Islay
Type : Steamship		**Tonnage** : 5145 gross.
Length : ft.	**Beam** : ft.	**Draught** : ft.
How Sunk : Torpedoed by *U-138*		**Depth** : metres

Empire Adventure was in convoy OB216 with the *New Sevilla*, *Boka* and the *City of Simla*. All four ships were torpedoed by the *U-138*. *Empire Adventure* had been outward bound from the Tyne to Wabana, Newfoundland; 21 of her 39 crew were lost.

The tug *Superman* took the *Empire Adventure* in tow, but she sank en route to the Clyde.

CITY OF SIMLA

Wreck No : 121		**Date Sunk** : 21 09 1940
Latitude : 55 55 00 N PA		**Longitude** : 08 20 00 W PA
Decca Lat : 5555.00 N		**Decca Long** : 0820.00 W
Location : NW of Islay		**Area** : NW Islay
Type : Steamship		**Tonnage** : 10138 gross.
Length : 476.7 ft.	**Beam** : 58.2 ft.	**Draught** : 39.8 ft.
How Sunk : Torpedoed by *U-138*		**Depth** : metres

The 10138 tons British steamship *City of Simla*, built by W. Gray of West Hartlepool in 1921, was torpedoed by *U-138* (Luth), at 0227 hours on 21st September 1940 in position 555500N, 082000W, and sank by the stern within 20 minutes. Two passengers and one crewman died. 32 survivors were picked up by the trawler *Van Dyck*, and a further 142 were rescued by the SS *Guinean* and landed at Gourock.

VENI

Wreck No : 122	**Date Sunk :** 11 01 1948
Latitude : 55 55 18 N	**Longitude :** 06 17 30 W
Decca Lat : 5555.30 N	**Decca Long :** 0617.50 W
Location : Balach Rocks, NE of Ard Noamh	**Area :** NW Islay
Type : Steamship	**Tonnage :** 2982 gross.
Length : 324.1 ft. **Beam :** 47.1 ft.	**Draught :** 21.8 ft.
How Sunk : Ran aground	**Depth :** metres

The *Veni* (ex-*Tonbridge*), was built in 1901 by W. Pickersgill of Sunderland, and was registered in Stavanger, Norway.

   She ran aground on Balach Rocks, which are three rocks that break the surface at all states of the tide, 3 miles North east of Ardnave Point.

   The *Veni* lies on her port side in 18 metres of water, standing up 8-10 metres from the bottom, about 150 yards East of the northernmost rock.

ATLANTIC SUN

Wreck No : 123	**Date Sunk :** 18 03 1918
Latitude : 55 55 55 N	**Longitude :** 06 54 50 W
Decca Lat : 5555.92 N	**Decca Long :** 0654.83 W
Location : W of Islay	**Area :** NW Islay
Type : Steamship	**Tonnage :** 2333 gross.
Length : 297.0 ft. **Beam :** 39.6 ft.	**Draught :** 26.4 ft.
How Sunk : Torpedoed	**Depth :** 55 metres

A wreck was reported at 555600N, 065600W PA in 1939. 555555N, 065450W is presumably the accurate position for that wreck.

   The 2333 tons gross American steel steamship *Atlantic Sun* (ex-*Iris*), was torpedoed off the North west of Islay on 18th March 1918 at 555500N, 070900W PA.

Chapter 4

The Wrecks of Gigha, Jura, Colonsay and Oronsay

Introduction

The West Coast of Scotland can be one of the most beautiful places in the world but, in inclement weather, its shores and seas are unforgiving. Tides race through the Dorus Mor between Craignish Point and Garbh Reisa at 8 knots at spring tides, and up to 10 knots through the Gulf of Corryvreckan, (the cauldron of Breachan), between Jura and Scarba. A pinnacle of rock rising from the seabed causes violent overfalls and breakers, with whirlpools on the Scarba side. This is a good place to avoid in bad weather, when conditions can be so awful that it used to be considered by the Royal Navy to be unnavigable!

According to legend, Breachan, a Scandinavian prince, fell in love with the daughter of an island chief. The chief would consent to their marriage only if Breachan would anchor for three days and nights in the eye of the whirlpool. To hold his anchor, he obtained three ropes, one of wool, one of hemp, and one woven from virgins' hair which was considered to be infallible. The wool rope failed on the first night, the hemp on the second. The rope of virgins' hair lasted until the final hour, when it also failed, apparently because some of the hair did not meet the specification. (Virgin's hair was obviously a very scarce commodity, even in those days!) Breachan was drowned, and his body was washed ashore in Bagh Glean nam Muc, and buried in Uamh Breachan - Breachan's cave.

More recently, in the 1950s and 1960s, a farmer kept his sheep on Scarba. One day, his dog fell in the rough water and was lost. That night the farmer dreamed he saw his dog on a particular rock. The next morning he returned to Scarba and found his dog on the rock of his dream.

In addition to the Dorus Mor and the Corryvreckan, the north-going tidal stream in the Sound of Jura is very strong.

Oronsay is Norse for *Ebb Tide Island*, and Jura is Norse for *Deer Island*. Jura is 28 miles

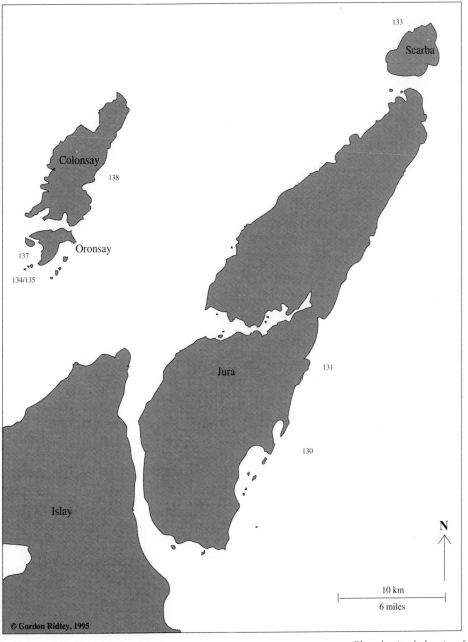

Chart showing the location of wrecks lying off the coast of Jura, Colonsay and Oronsay

long by 8 miles wide. Most of the island is inaccessible, and uninhabited by humans, but there is a large population of red deer, goats and adders. The human population, which numbers only about 250, all live on the East coast, most of them in the village of Craighouse, in the South of Small Isles Bay. It was while living in the remote farmhouse at Barnhill in the North of the island, that George Orwell wrote his novel Nineteen Eighty Four.

The most prominent features of the island are the three conical shaped hills known as the Paps of Jura, and they are visible for many miles.

THE WRECKS

ASKA

Wreck No : 124	**Date Sunk :** 16 09 1940
Latitude : 55 38 18 N	**Longitude :** 05 45 19 W
Decca Lat : 5538.30 N	**Decca Long :** 0545.32 W
Location : Cara Island, S of Gigha	**Area :** Gigha
Type : Steamship	**Tonnage :** 8323 gross.
Length : 444.6 ft. **Beam :** 61.2 ft.	**Draught :** 25.2 ft.
How Sunk : Bombed, drifted ashore	**Depth :** metres

The British steam liner *Aska* left Bathurst, Gambia, West Africa on 7th September 1940 with 350 French troops aboard, some of whom were landed in France.

At 02.50 hours on 16th September, at 551500N, 055500W, between Rathlin Island and Maidens Rock, the *Aska* was attacked by a German aircraft and hit by three bombs. Twelve of the crew were killed; 75 survivors, including 65 French Colonial troops, were picked up by trawlers and transferred to a Naval ship which landed them in Greenock. Meanwhile, the *Aska* drifted ashore, on fire, just below Cara House on Cara Island,

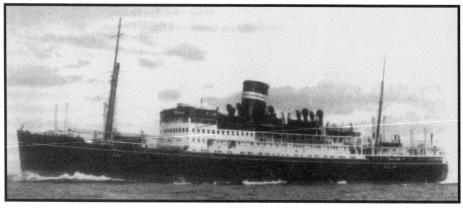

The Aska (Photograph courtesy of the World Ship Society).

South of the island of Gigha, off the West coast of Kintyre.
Parts of her machinery now show above the surface at low water springs. The
Hydrographic Department gives her position as 553742 N 054519W PA, but this is a
little too far South of her true position, and she is actually on the off-lying Cara Rocks,
rather than immediately ashore.

UDEA

Wreck No : 125
Latitude : 55 39 42 N
Decca Lat : 5539.70 N
Location : Cath Sgeir, W side of Gigha
Type : Steamship
Length : 110.5 ft.   **Beam :** 18.1 ft.
How Sunk : Ran aground

Date Sunk : 08 04 1894
Longitude : 05 47 12 W
Decca Long : 0547.20 W
Area : Gigha
Tonnage : 157 gross.
Draught : 10.1 ft.
Depth :   metres

The wreck of a small 19th century steamship is reported to lie on the East side of Cath
Sgeir where the rock slopes steeply down to 36 metres.
      The iron steamship *Udea*, belonging to David MacBrayne, was lost on Cara Rocks
(Cath Sgeir), on 8th April 1894. She had been en route from Glasgow to Portness, Butt
of Lewis with a cargo of coal and iron.
      The *Udea* was built in Newcastle in 1873.

STAFFA

Wreck No : 126
Latitude : 55 39 42 N
Decca Lat : 5539.70 N
Location : Cathskeir Rocks, Gigha
Type : Steamship
Length : 148.3 ft.   **Beam :** 23.1 ft.
How Sunk : Ran aground

Date Sunk : 24 08 1886
Longitude : 05 47 12 W
Decca Long : 0547.20 W
Area : Gigha
Tonnage : 128 gross.
Draught : 11.2 ft.
Depth :   metres

The 128 tons net iron steamship *Staffa* was en route from Greenock to Inverness with a
general cargo and 21 passengers when she ran on to Cathskeir Rock, South of Gigha on
24th August 1886. Fortunately the sea was calm that night and the vessel remained
perched on top of the reef until morning, when the MacBrayne steamer *Fingal* spotted
her as she passed by on her usual route from West Loch Tarbert to Islay. Some of the
passengers were taken off by the *Fingal* and others by several small vessels from Gigha.
      The *Staffa* broke up in storms the following day and wreckage now extends from the
top of the reef to 15 metres down the East side.

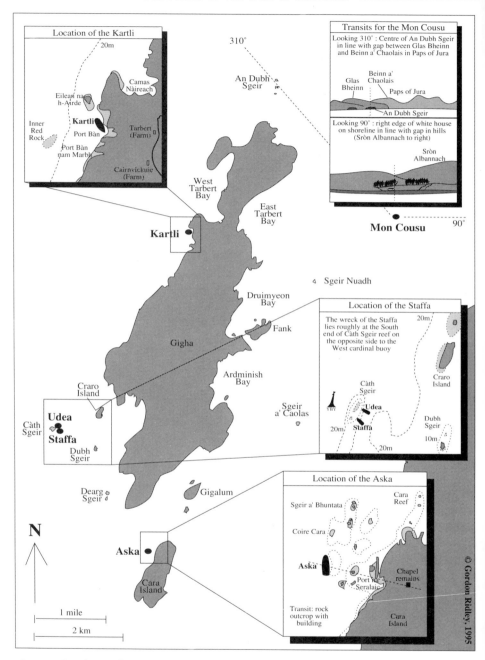

Location of wrecks around the island of Gigha

KARTLI

Wreck No : 127
Latitude : 55 42 10 N
Decca Lat : 5542.17 N
Location : Port Ban, W coast of Gigha
Type : Motor vessel
Length : 263.4 ft.   **Beam :** 43.7 ft.
How Sunk : Ran aground

Date Sunk : 18 12 1991
Longitude : 05 44 45 W
Decca Long : 0544.75 W
Area : Gigha
Tonnage : 1920 gross.
Draught : 17.2 ft.
Depth :   metres

The Russian fish factory ship *Kartli*, which was built in 1966, was hit by two gigantic freak waves while off Islay on Wednesday 18th December 1991. Forty seven of the crew were airlifted to safety by two RAF helicopters. Four others were killed in the accident, two of the bodies being recovered from the ship by helicopter after she drifted ashore on the sandy beach at Port Ban on the West coast of Gigha the day after being abandoned. The *Kartli* had been on her way from Shetland to Bulgaria, and was carrying 180 tons of marine diesel oil in her fuel tanks.

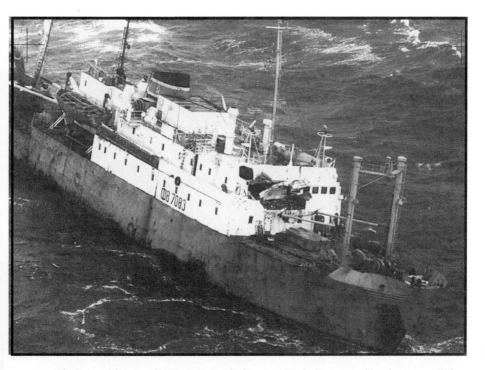

The Russian fish factory ship Kartli showing the damage to the wheelhouse caused by a huge wave off Islay on 18 th December 1991. The hammer and sickle emblem is visible on the funnel, and the cyrillic letters on the side of the ship are the Russian characters for FV 7083 (i.e. Fishing Vessel 7083). This picture of the Kartli was taken from a Nimrod aircraft of RAF Kinloss who kindly supplied the photograph.

MON COUSU

Wreck No : 128
Latitude : 55 42 38 N
Decca Lat : 5542.63 N
Location : N end of Sound of Gigha
Type : Steamship
Length : 235.2 ft.   **Beam : 36.0 ft.**
How Sunk : Scuttled

Date Sunk : 05 01 1944
Longitude : 05 39 49 W
Decca Long : 0539.82 W
Area : Gigha
Tonnage : 1345 gross.
Draught : 16.3 ft.
Depth : 8 metres

The ex-French vessel *Mon Cousu* (ex-*Nestor*), was built in 1912 by Mackay Bros. of Alloa. She was sunk as a bombing target on 5th January 1944, but is no longer used for that purpose.

The wreck lies in a North/South direction, with a least depth of 18 ft in a general depth of 26 ft to a sandy seabed. The position has also been given as 554233N, 053949W

Little remains of the Mon Cousu today and those pieces of tangled wreckage that are left are covered in soft coral.

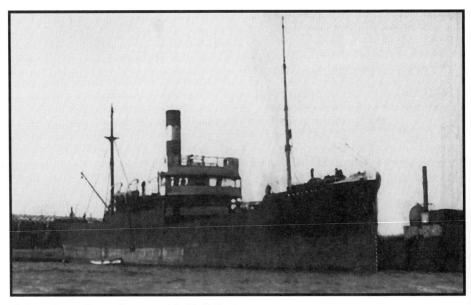

The Mon Cousu. *Photograph courtesy of the World Ship Society.*

STORMLIGHT

Wreck No : 129
Latitude : 55 50 01 N
Decca Lat : 5550.02 N
Location : Rubha Bhride, Sound of Jura
Type : Motor vessel
Length : 88.0 ft.　　**Beam :** 21.0 ft.
How Sunk : Ran aground

Date Sunk : 15 12 1973
Longitude : 05 56 09 W
Decca Long : 0556.15 W
Area : Jura
Tonnage : 158 gross.
Draught : 9.0 ft.
Depth : 5 metres

The motor vessel *Stormlight* ran aground in the Sound of Jura, about 4 miles ENE of Craighouse, South east Jura, while en route in ballast from Campbeltown to Oban.

The bow lies on its port side at the southern tip of Eilean nan Gabhar, about 120 ft from the light, and is visible above water at all states of the tide. The stern portion has broken off and lies in a gully nearby.

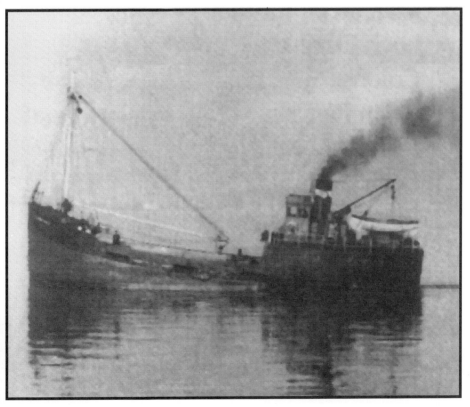

The Stormlight. *(Photograph courtesy of the World Ship Society.*

CHEVALIER

Wreck No : 130

Latitude : 55 53 00 N PA

Decca Lat : 5553.00 N

Location : Iron Rock, Sound of Jura

Type : Paddle steamer

Length : 176.8 ft.   **Beam** : 22.0 ft.

How Sunk : Ran aground

Date Sunk : 24 11 1854

Longitude : 05 50 00 W PA

Decca Long : 0550.00 W

Area : Jura

Tonnage : 229 gross.

Draught : 10.8 ft.

Depth :   metres

The paddle steamer *Chevalier*, built in 1853 by J & G Thomson of Govan, ran on to Iron Rock in the Sound of Jura and foundered. Apparently her decks were only covered at high water, and her engines may have been salvaged.

Iron Rock is not named on present day charts or maps. Where is it? According to Peter Moir and Ian Crawford, it is Skervuile (Sgeir Maoile), about two miles off Lowlandman's Bay, and wreckage which might very well be the remains of the *Chevalier* has been found in 4-12 metres, just off the North west of Skervuile, between the permanently exposed rock and a reef which only shows at low water.

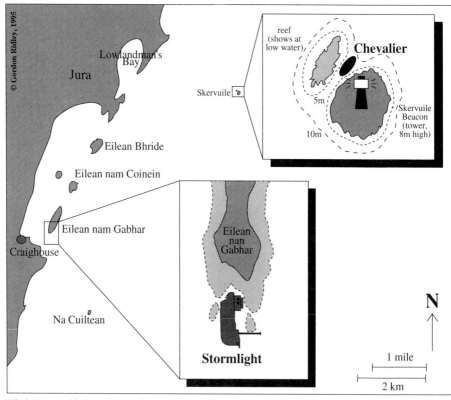

The locations of the Stormlight & the Chevalier.

While Moir/Crawford's argument is pretty convincing, I should also point out that in the Sound of Jura, off Loch Crinan, there is another rock named Sgeir na Maoile at 560700N 053740W, and a rocky island named Eilean na h Eairne at 560636N 053730W. To the uninitiated, this latter name might be anglicised as Iron Island or Iron Rock.

CULZEAN

Wreck No : 131
Latitude : 55 56 20 N PA
Decca Lat : 5556.33 N
Location : SW of ferry slip at Lagg Bay
Type : Sailing ship
Length : 250.8 ft.   **Beam :** 39.6 ft.
How Sunk : Ran aground

Date Sunk : 21 11 1881
Longitude : 05 50 45 W PA
Decca Long : 0550.75 W
Area : Jura
Tonnage : 1572 gross.
Draught : 23.1 ft.
Depth :   metres

The iron sailing ship *Culzean* (built in 1871 by J. Reid & Co.) with a crew of 17 was being towed from Dundee to Greenock for repairs when the towline parted during a furious gale while passing down the Sound of Jura. As far as I am aware, the wreck has never been found, but it lies in Lowlandman's Bay on the East of Jura.

The master of the tug *Conqueror* was in command of both vessels during the tow, and before leaving Dundee, signals had been agreed between the master of the tug and Captain Pirnie of the *Culzean*. En route, a towline was lost in bad weather, and the vessels made for Stornoway to shelter for a time. While there, the loan of another tow rope was offered, but this was declined, and the tow was continued with the tug's one remaining tow rope. After passing Crinan, in a gradually increasing gale, that towline parted, and the *Culzean* was driven ashore and wrecked with the loss of all on board.

The heavily salvaged wreck lies a short distance South east of the ferry slip in Lagg Bay.

COMET

Wreck No : 132
Latitude : 56 07 44 N
Decca Lat : 5607.73 N
Location : Wrecked in Dorus-Mhor
Type : Paddle steamer
Length : 43.5 ft.   **Beam :** 11.2 ft.
How Sunk : Ran aground

Date Sunk : 13 12 1820
Longitude : 05 36 24 W
Decca Long : 0536.40 W
Area : Jura
Tonnage : 24 gross.
Draught : 5.6 ft.
Depth :   metres

The wooden paddle steamer *Comet* was the first passenger steamship, invented by Henry Bell in 1812.

She was wrecked off Crinan in Dorus Mhor channel between Craignish Point and Garbh Reisa when her engines could not cope with the tidal race, and the vessel broke in two. The after section was swept away towards Corryvreckan, but the forward part remained firmly on the rocks. All the passengers and crew were on this section, and were able to reach the shore.

Her engine was later salved, and is now on display in the National Maritime Museum, London.

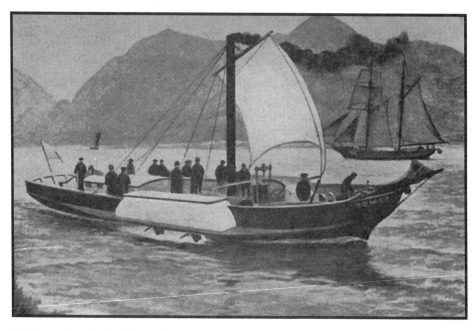

The Comet. *(Photograph: Author's collection).*

WILHELM ABERG

Wreck No : 133
Latitude : 56 12 00 N PA
Decca Lat : 5612.00 N
Location : Scarba
Type : Barque
Length :   ft.   **Beam :**   ft.
How Sunk : Ran aground

Date Sunk : 03 04 1874
Longitude : 05 41 00 W PA
Decca Long : 0541.00 W
Area : Jura
Tonnage : 856 gross.
Draught :   ft.
Depth :   metres

Fifteen lives were lost when the 856 tons net Russian barque *Wilhelm Aberg* ran aground on Scarba in a north-westerly severe gale on 3rd April 1874.
    The barque had been en route from St. Ubes to Borga with a cargo of salt.

MONA

Wreck No : 134
Latitude : 55 59 48 N PA
Decca Lat : 5559.70 N
Location : Chubaidth Rock, Oronsay
Type : Steamship
Length : 160.0 ft.   **Beam :** 24.2 ft.
How Sunk : Ran aground

Date Sunk : 17 08 1908
Longitude : 06 18 00 W PA
Decca Long : 0618.00 W
Area : Oronsay
Tonnage : 413 gross.
Draught : 14.0 ft.
Depth :   metres

The iron steamship *Mona*, (ex-*Margaret*), of 204 tons net, owned by the Ayr Steamship Company, was built in 1878 by Barrow S. B. Co., and registered in Glasgow.
    At Bunessan, she took aboard a cargo of livestock for a farm in Wigtownshire, and nine passengers, bound for Stranraer. About midday on 17th August 1908, a grating sound was heard and the ship stopped. She had stuck fast on Chubaidth (Quebec) Rock, about ¼ mile South west of Oronsay. The passengers and cattlemen landed at Oronsay and raised the alarm.
    Meanwhile, the captain and his crew remained aboard the grounded vessel until it started to fill with water. Shortly after abandoning her, and landing on a small rock between the ship and Oronsay, the *Mona* heeled over, drowning 1000 sheep and 65 bullocks. The steamer *Fern* rescued the captain and his crew from their rocky refuge, and the *Mona* sank completely soon afterwards.

QUEBEC

Wreck No : 135
Latitude : 55 59 48 N PA
Decca Lat : 5559.80 N
Location : Bogha Chubaidth (Quebec Rock)
Type : Steam puffer
Length : ft.   **Beam :** ft.
How Sunk : Ran aground

Date Sunk :
Longitude : 06 18 00 W PA
Decca Long : 0618.00 W
Area : Oronsay
Tonnage : gross
Draught : ft.
Depth : 10 metres

Bogha Chubaidth lies 1 mile SW of Eilean nan Ron, at the south-western tip of Oronsay. A puffer named *Quebec* supposedly ran aground and sank while transporting a farmer's possessions from Mull to Islay. The position has also been estimated as 555913N, 061742W.

I have been unable to find any record of this puffer, but am struck by the similarity of the circumstances of its alleged loss, and that of the *Mona*. I suspect they are one and the same. It might be assumed that the rock took its name from the puffer, but another theory is that the rock was so named after an emigrant vessel bound for Quebec was lost on it. It was already named Bogha Chubaidth when the *Mona* struck it in 1908.

ATOS

Wreck No : 136
Latitude : 56 00 00 N PA
Decca Lat : 5600.00 N
Location : W of Oronsay
Type : Steamship
Length : 291.6 ft.   **Beam :** 42.6 ft.
How Sunk : Torpedoed by U-57

Date Sunk : 03 08 1940
Longitude : 07 30 00 W PA
Decca Long : 0730.00 W
Area : Oronsay
Tonnage : 2161 gross.
Draught : 19.1 ft.
Depth : metres

The Swedish steamship *Atos*, built in 1902 by Helsingors Jernsk, was torpedoed by the *U-57* (Topp) at 08.10 hours on 3rd August 1940, at AM5364 in the German grid system, which would seem to equate to about 570000N, 080000W. According to *DODAS*, she sank some time after having been torpedoed.

Another report gives the position of torpedoing as 40 miles West of Colonsay.

BELFAST

Wreck No : 137	**Date Sunk :** 23 03 1895
Latitude : 56 02 00 N PA	**Longitude :** 06 18 00 W PA
Decca Lat : 5602.00 N	**Decca Long :** 0618.00 W
Location : W coast of Oronsay	**Area :** Oronsay
Type : Steamship	**Tonnage :** 1638 gross.
Length : 265.6 ft. **Beam :** 33.2 ft.	**Draught :** 24.3 ft.
How Sunk : Ran aground	**Depth :** metres

The British iron steamship *Belfast*, built in 1870 by Palmers Co. was wrecked while en route from Sapelo to Belfast with a cargo of timber. The mate and three other crewmen were picked up from a lifeboat by the steamship *Durham City* which took them to Greenock. The rescued men thought they had struck rocks off Iona.

The captain of the *Durham City* reported that he had been in company with the *Belfast* to west of Iona, but as it was a very dark night, he was not absolutely certain of his exact position, and did not know what had become of the other 16 members of the *Belfast*'s crew. He reported that the *Belfast* had struck West Rock of Iona, which is the western outlier of the Torran Rocks, at 561418N, 062739W, and was likely to become a total wreck.

It was later discovered that other crewmen had landed at Colonsay. On the 26th March, the Colonsay sailing packet arrived at Port Askaig and reported that the *Belfast* had struck rocks 1.5 cables West of Oronsay at 10.00 pm on Saturday night and became a total wreck. Nineteen of the crew landed in Colonsay, but the chief officer and three men had left the vessel in a small boat. On the 28th, it was reported that the Colonsay shore was strewn with logs and deals from the *Belfast*.

UNKNOWN - PRE-1919

Wreck No : 138	**Date Sunk :** Pre - 1919
Latitude : 56 04 00 N PA	**Longitude :** 06 10 00 W PA
Decca Lat : 5604.00 N	**Decca Long :** 0610.00 W
Location : Port an Obain, E Colonsay	**Area :** Colonsay
Type :	**Tonnage :** gross
Length : ft. **Beam :** ft.	**Draught :** ft.
How Sunk : Towed here on fire	**Depth :** 6 metres

During the First World War, a small wooden American vessel was towed in here on fire. She was subsequently salvaged, but her kelp-covered remains just break the surface. As a result, she looks like a continuation of the rocks. The position has also been estimated as 560717N, 061036W.

Chapter 5

The Wrecks of Oban

Introduction

Oban is the largest town in the West Highlands, and the main ferry port for the Islands. It is set in magnificent scenery, and offers all the facilities required by the diver and his family for a marvellous holiday. As a touring centre it is unrivalled.

McCaig's Folly, which dominates the skyline over the town, was built between 1897 and 1902 by John Stuart McCaig, banker, gas works owner and philanthropist. Modelled on the Colosseum, and constructed in Bonawe granite, at a cost of £5000, he had it built to provide employment during the winter months, and as a family memorial. It had been McCaig's intention to erect 12 bronze statues of members of his family within the edifice, but he died before ordering the statues.

The Sea Life Centre at Barcaldine, a few miles north of Oban, is well worth a visit.

In 1523, Lachlan Maclean of Duart rowed his wife Elizabeth, the daughter of Archibald Campbell, 2nd Earl of Argyll, out to Liath Sgeir, the rock between Duart Point and Lismore, which covers at high tide, and left her chained on this rock to drown because he wanted to marry the daughter of Maclean of Treshnish. Just in time, however, she was rescued by men from Tayvallich, and Maclean was murdered by her brother, Campbell of Cawdor. To this day, the rock is known as Lady's Rock.

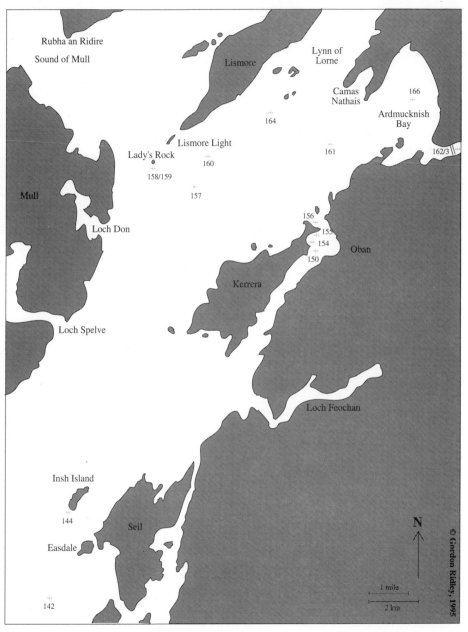

Rubha an Ridire

Sound of Mull

Lismore

Lynn of
Lorne

Camas
Nathais

166

Ardmucknish
Bay

164

Lismore Light

161

162/3

Lady's Rock

160

158/159

157

Mull

Loch Don

156

155

154

150

Oban

Kerrera

Loch Spelve

Loch Feochan

Insh Island

144

Seil

Easdale

N

142

1 mile

2 km

© Gordon Ridley, 1995

*Chart showing the location
of wrecks lying off the
coasts near Oban*

THE WRECKS

BENGHAZI

Wreck No : 139	**Date Sunk :** 23 03 1947
Latitude : 56 14 58 N	**Longitude :** 05 40 56 W
Decca Lat : 5614.97 N	**Decca Long :** 0540.93 W
Location : W of Fladda, nr. Isle of Luing	**Area :** Oban
Type : Trawler	**Tonnage :** 257 gross.
Length : 125.0 ft. **Beam :** ft.	**Draught :** ft.
How Sunk : Ran aground	**Depth :** 40 metres

The steam trawler *Benghazi* (ex-*Flying Admiral*, ex-*John Bullock*), was a Castle class trawler built at South Shields in 1917 for the Admiralty. When released for commercial service she came into the ownership of Hull Merchants Amalgamated Trawlers, and was managed by the Boston Deep Sea Fishing & Ice Co. Ltd.

On 23rd April 1947, while returning from the Icelandic fishing grounds with a crew of 16, she called into Oban for stores, and left there at 10.45 pm that night. About an hour later, in heavy rain and a 70 mph gale, she was swept on to a reef near Fladda lighthouse. One member of the crew was washed away and never seen again, while a second member later died of exposure, having lain in the bottom of their lifeboat for some time, plugging a drain hole with his hand, as the bung for the drain hole could not be found in the darkness.

The wreck has been reported to lie in about 12 metres, well broken up in a strong tidal stream, but a 1971 report stated that the wreck was still intact in 40 metres, and in 1993 divers who recovered several portholes confirmed that she is still intact.

UNKNOWN - MELDON?

Wreck No : 140	**Date Sunk :**
Latitude : 56 15 12 N	**Longitude :** 05 45 15 W
Decca Lat : 5615.20 N	**Decca Long :** 0545.25 W
Location : ¼ mile N of Garvellach Islands	**Area :** Oban
Type :	**Tonnage :** gross.
Length : ft. **Beam :** ft.	**Draught :** ft.
How Sunk :	**Depth :** 47 metres

A wreck with at least 47 metres over it in a total depth of about 58 metres is charted ¼ mile North of the gap between Garbh Eilach, the main island in the Garvellachs, and Dun Chonnuill, the most northerly islet of the group. This is the position of mining of the *Meldon*, ½ mile North of the Gavellachs and ½ mile West of the Isles of the Sea.

The *Meldon*, of course, did not sink here, and it is surprising that a wreck is marked here, apparently with an accurate position rather than PA. I do not believe there is any wreck here at all!

HELENA FAULBAUMS

Wreck No : 141

Latitude : 56 15 15 N

Decca Lat : 5615.25 N

Location : Close off NW Belnahua

Type : Steamship

Length : 280.1 ft.   **Beam :** 41.9 ft.

How Sunk : Ran aground

Date Sunk : 26 10 1936

Longitude : 05 41 42 W

Decca Long : 0541.70 W

Area : Oban

Tonnage : 1951 gross.

Draught : 18.9 ft.

Depth : 55 metres

The *Helena Faulbaums*, (ex- *Firpark*), was built by Grangemouth Dockyard Co. in 1920.

She left the Mersey in ballast on the 26th October 1936, en route for Blyth. In the late afternoon the weather deteriorated quickly, and by early evening she was heading for shelter in the Firth of Lorne. The rough weather and her light load meant that her propeller spent much of the time thrashing uselessly above water. At about 7.00 pm she was struck by a violent gale. Her steering gear failed and the vessel drifted helplessly in the stormy seas. Captain Cughaus gave the order to cast out the anchors, but they did not hold in the deep water channels of the Firth. At 10.00 pm she struck the treacherous rocks at the North west end of Belnahua, broadside on. Within 10 minutes she had sunk in deep water.

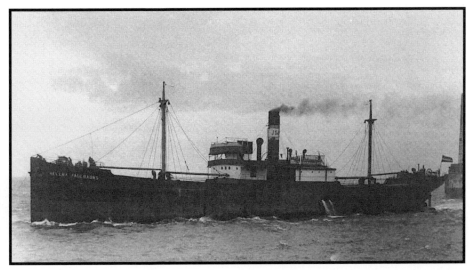

The Helena Faulbaums (*Photograph courtesy of the World Ship Society*)

Four of the crew members managed to drag themselves ashore, but the other 15, including Captain Cughaus and two 18 year old boys perished. The wireless operator, Albert Sultcs, sat frantically sending out SOS messages right up until the ship sank. The storm had wreaked havoc with communications ashore, and the coastguards receiving the SOS were unable to contact the nearest lifeboat at Port Askaig, Islay. Finally, in desperation, the Admiralty was contacted, and a message was broadcast by the BBC in the hope that someone at Port Askaig might receive it. The lifeboat was duly launched and spent most of the night searching the Firth of Lorne for the ship, or survivors from her. The four survivors, meanwhile spent the night in derelict slate-mining cottages on Belnahua. They were rescued the next day. The bodies of the less lucky crew members were recovered from amongst the wreckage which littered the shore of the neighbouring island of Luing.

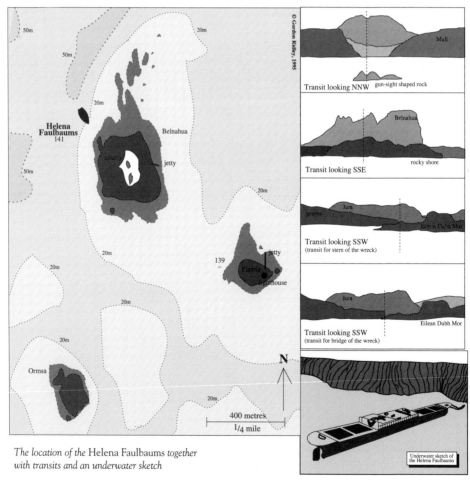

The location of the Helena Faulbaums together
with transits and an underwater sketch

The wreck is sitting upright. Depth to the deck is 55 metres, and to the bottom is 60 metres. It is very dark down there. The front of the bridge has fallen forwards and lies on the deck, projecting over the forward hold. Some portholes and the ship's Walker log have been recovered. As there are very strong tidal streams in this area, the wreck can only be dived at slack water. Launch from Cuan ferry slip.

APOLLO

Wreck No : 142	**Date Sunk :** 15 08 1900
Latitude : 56 16 18 N	**Longitude :** 05 41 00 W
Decca Lat : 5616.30 N	**Decca Long :** 0541.00 W
Location : On Bono Reef, Luing	**Area :** Oban
Type : Steamship	**Tonnage :** 495 gross.
Length : 182.0 ft. **Beam :** 24.0 ft.	**Draught :** 12.0 ft.
How Sunk : Ran aground	**Depth :** 5 metres

The 305 tons net iron steamship *Apollo* was built by Barrow S.B. Co in 1874. En route from Aberdeen to Newport, Mon. with a cargo of granite cobble stones, she ran on to Bono Reef, near Luing on 15th August 1900.

Bono Rock is part of a reef which comes to within a metre of the surface at low water, and is marked with a red can buoy at 561612N, 064036W, about 1.5 miles North of Fladda, and 1.5 miles West of Cuan Point at the North tip of the island of Luing. The top of the reef is about 100 yards North west of the red buoy. It can be found even without an echo sounder as the kelp-covered rock is visible from the surface as a dark area in the water.

Depths adjacent to the rock slope down to 17 metres, but the bulk of the very broken wreckage of the Apollo, and her cargo of hundreds of granite blocks, lies in a gully near the top of the reef in 5-11 metres beneath a thick kelp forest.

HAFTON

Wreck No : 143	**Date Sunk :** 02 1933
Latitude : 56 17 00 N PA	**Longitude :** 05 40 00 W PA
Decca Lat : 5617.00 N	**Decca Long :** 0540.00 W
Location : In the Firth of Lorne	**Area :** Oban
Type : Steamship	**Tonnage :** gross
Length : 66.0 ft. **Beam :** ft.	**Draught :** ft.
How Sunk : Foundered	**Depth :** metres

The *Hafton* was a Clyde puffer, with a 2-cylinder compound engine.

Early puffers had no condensers and the exhaust steam from the engines was routed

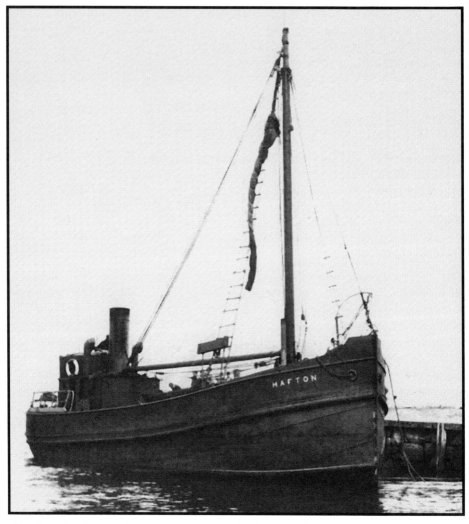

The puffer Hafton *(Photograph courtesy of the executors of P. Ransome-Wallis)*

through the funnel, giving rise to a puffing noise like a steam locomotive. Although later-built vessels were fitted with condensers which eliminated the distinctive sound of the early vessels, they were still generally referred to as puffers.

She must have been about 100 tons gross and had left Toberonochy on the island of Luing, bound for Mull. Nine miles into the journey, the vessel sprang a leak and rapidly filled with water. The crew of five took to their small boat and got ashore at daybreak at Ellanbeich on the island of Seil.

NORVAL

Wreck No : 144	**Date Sunk :**
Latitude : 56 18 27 N	**Longitude :** 05 40 26 W
Decca Lat : 5618.45 N	**Decca Long :** 0540.43 W
Location : Off S of Insch Island	**Area :** Oban
Type : Sailing ship	**Tonnage :** 631 gross.
Length : 161.8 ft. **Beam :** 30.8 ft.	**Draught :** 19.5 ft.
How Sunk : Ran aground	**Depth :** 10 metres

On 20th December 1870 the wooden sailing ship Norval ran aground in fog just to the West of Rubha Sasunaich, the South tip of Insch Island (formerly known as Sheep Island). The remaining wreckage, which includes sections of copper hull sheathing, is well broken up amongst gullies and clefts in the boulders.

UNKNOWN

Wreck No : 145	**Date Sunk :**
Latitude : 56 19 16 N	**Longitude :** 05 35 29 W
Decca Lat : 5619.27 N	**Decca Long :** 0535.48 W
Location : Off N of Seil Island	**Area :** Oban
Type :	**Tonnage :** gross
Length : ft. **Beam :** ft.	**Draught :** ft.
How Sunk :	**Depth :** metres

A wreck has been recorded by the Hydrographic Dept. in this position, ⅓ mile East of Rubha Garbh Airde, the northernmost point of Seil Island.

UNKNOWN

Wreck No : 146	**Date Sunk :** Pre - 1953
Latitude : 56 23 33 N	**Longitude :** 05 30 47 W
Decca Lat : 5623.55 N	**Decca Long :** 0530.78 W
Location : Charted ashore at Gallanach	**Area :** Oban
Type :	**Tonnage :** gross
Length : ft. **Beam :** ft.	**Draught :** ft.
How Sunk :	**Depth :** metres

CATALINA AIRCRAFT

Wreck No : 147
Latitude : 56 23 57 N
Decca Lat : 5623.95 N
Location : Sound of Kerrera
Type : Aircraft
Length :   ft.   **Beam :**   ft.
How Sunk :

Date Sunk :
Longitude : 05 30 51 W
Decca Long : 0530.85 W
Area : Oban
Tonnage :   gross
Draught : ft.
Depth : 25 metres

The position has also been recorded as 562357N, 053031W.

UNKNOWN - AIRCRAFT?

Wreck No : 148
Latitude : 56 24 25 N
Decca Lat : 5624.42 N
Location : Off SE of Heather Island
Type : Aircraft
Length :   ft.   **Beam :**   ft.
How Sunk :

Date Sunk : Pre - 1967
Longitude : 05 30 10 W
Decca Long : 0530.17 W
Area : Oban
Tonnage :   gross
Draught : ft.
Depth : 35 metres

There is reputed to be the wreck of a flying boat, possibly a *Catalina*, fairly close off the South east of Heather Island, in the Sound of Kerrera. An obstruction was reported in the above position in 1967.

UNKNOWN

Wreck No : 149
Latitude : 56 24 30 N
Decca Lat : 5624.50 N
Location : 200 yds E of Heather Island
Type :
Length :   ft.   **Beam :**   ft.
How Sunk :

Date Sunk : Pre - 1967
Longitude : 05 29 50 W
Decca Long : 0529.83 W
Area : Oban
Tonnage :   gross
Draught : ft.
Depth : 40 metres

An unknown wreck was reported here in 1967. This position is in the middle of the Sound of Kerrera, off the North east of Heather Island. Could this be the *Young Fisherman*?

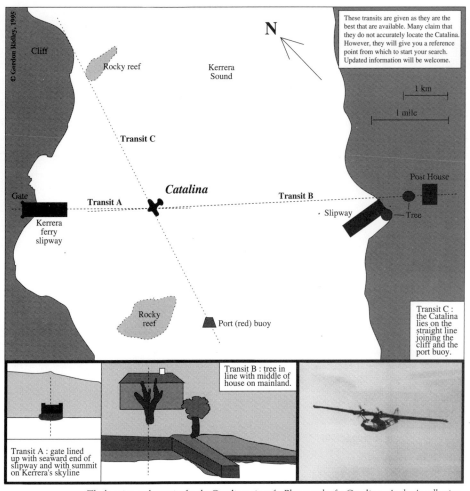

The location and transits for the Catalina aircraft. Photograph of a Catalina, Author's collection.

HELEN WILSON ?

Wreck No : 150
Latitude : 56 25 00 N
Decca Lat : 5625.00 N
Location : Off Ardantrive Bay, Kerrera
Type : Drifter
Length : ft. **Beam :** ft.
How Sunk : Destroyed by fire

Date Sunk : 05 12 1917
Longitude : 05 29 34 W
Decca Long : 0529.57 W
Area : Oban
Tonnage : 44 gross.
Draught : ft.
Depth : 34 metres

According to *British Vessels Lost at Sea 1914-18*, the steam drifter *Helen Wilson* was destroyed by fire at Oban on 5th December 1917.

The remains of a steel wheelhouse and engine lying on a muddy slope at 34 metres, off the South of Ardantrive Bay at the North end of the Sound of Kerrera, were found by Mike Tye of Oban Divers. There is no sign of any part of the hull, which had presumably been wooden.

It is easy to imagine that the remains on the bottom are what is left after a wooden hull has burned away, and as a result, Mike Tye assumed this to be the *Helen Wilson*. Unknown to Mike, however, an advert for the sale, by public auction within the offices of West Highland Auction Mart, of the hull of the *Helen Wilson*, lying at the North Pier, Oban appeared on page 1 of the *Oban Times* of Saturday February 21, 1920.

This was more than two years after she had been reported as destroyed by fire. Thus, what doers the hull lying at Oban North Pier consist of, wasr the engine and wheelhouse still there at that time, who bought the remains, and what happened to them?

An aged local whom I met in *Aulay's Bar* in Oban in 1990, (visit for the many old photographs of ships on the walls of the bar), claimed to remember the *Helen Wilson*, and was of the opinion that her loss had been due to sabotage for her insurance value.

Perhaps the remains of the unknown wooden hull lying on the North shore of Ardantrive Bay at 562515N, 052937W is the *Helen Wilson*. The engine and wheelhouse remains found by Mike Tye are considerably larger than one would expect in a vessel of only 44 tons gross, and I would suggest that they may have come from the *Hyacinth*. The type of engine was not particularly significant to me when I dived this wreck in 1984/1985, but my vague recollection is that it was a diesel engine, whereas the *Helen Wilson* had a steam engine.

GOLDEN GIFT

Wreck No : 151	**Date Sunk :** 06 04 1943
Latitude : 56 25 00 N	**Longitude :** 05 28 32 W
Decca Lat : 5625.00 N	**Decca Long :** 0528.53 W
Location : Off the Esplanade, Oban Bay	**Area :** Oban
Type : Drifter	**Tonnage :** 89 gross.
Length : 120.0 ft. **Beam :** ft.	**Draught :** ft.
How Sunk : Collision with *Lochinvar*	**Depth :** 10 metres

The wooden drifter *Golden Gift* of Lowestoft, on Admiralty service, sank in collision with the MacBrayne ferry *Lochinvar* on 6th April 1943.

She lies about 50 yards out from the shore, directly opposite the Park Hotel on the Esplanade, Oban. The main frames, engine and boiler are there, but the wooden hull is rotting away.

For many years she was erroneously known as *The Puffer*, and was a popular dive until diving was prohibited within the Oban harbour limits, within which she lies.

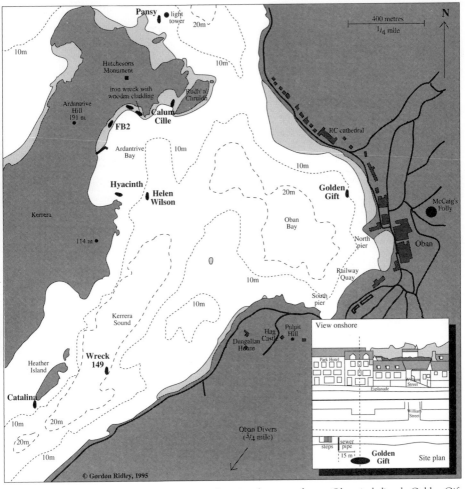

Location of some wrecks near Oban, including the Golden Gift.

YOUNG FISHERMAN

Wreck No : 152
Latitude : 56 25 00 N PA
Decca Lat : 5625.00 N
Location : Oban
Type : Drifter
Length :   ft.   **Beam :**   ft.
How Sunk : Ran aground

Date Sunk : 29 11 1940
Longitude : 05 30 00 W PA
Decca Long : 0530.00 W
Area : Oban
Tonnage : 95 gross.
Draught : ft.
Depth :   metres

The 95 ton drifter *Young Fisherman*, built in 1914, was requisitioned for Admiralty use in June 1940.

The unknown wreck first located in 1967 at 562430N, 052950W may be the *Young Fisherman*, but that position, 200 yards East of Heather Island, in deep water in the middle of the Sound of Kerrera does not seem to accord with running aground, which was the reported cause of loss of the *Young Fisherman*. Perhaps she got off the rocks on which she ran aground and may have been making for the safety of Oban harbour when she sank, but this is only speculation.

KINGFISHER

Wreck No : 153	**Date Sunk :** 01 04 1924
Latitude : 56 25 00 N PA	**Longitude :** 05 30 00 W PA
Decca Lat : 5625.00 N	**Decca Long :** 0530.00 W
Location : Foundered in Oban Bay	**Area :** Oban
Type : Drifter	**Tonnage :** 76 gross.
Length : ft. **Beam :** ft.	**Draught :** ft.
How Sunk : Foundered	**Depth :** metres

The wooden fishing vessel *Kingfisher*, built in 1882 by Hawthorns of Granton, foundered in Oban Bay on 1st April 1924.

HYACINTH

Wreck No : 154	**Date Sunk :** 29 04 1920
Latitude : 56 25 02 N	**Longitude :** 05 29 42 W
Decca Lat : 5625.03 N	**Decca Long :** 0529.70 W
Location : S shore of Ardantrive Bay	**Area :** Oban
Type : Fishing boat	**Tonnage :** gross
Length : ft. **Beam :** ft.	**Draught :** ft.
How Sunk : Towed here after fire	**Depth :** metres

A 1922 report stated that two masts of a wreck were showing at low water springs, 178°, 595 yds from Hutcheson's monument. The wreck is of an iron-hulled vessel, visible above water at all states of the tide, on the South shore of Ardantrive Bay. The bows stand about three metres above water at low tide, and a vertical boiler protrudes above the fo'c'sle. The stern is level with the water surface, while the keel at the stern is in about three metres of water.

On 29th April 1920, the Fraserburgh fishing boat *Hyacinth* caught fire off Maiden Island and within a couple of hours, became a total wreck. The fire, which started in the engine at the stern of the boat, spread rapidly, and the crew were about to launch a small boat when they were taken aboard a drifter which was passing on its way into Oban.

Later, the hull of the *Hyacinth* was towed to the Kerrera side of Oban Bay, where it now lies.

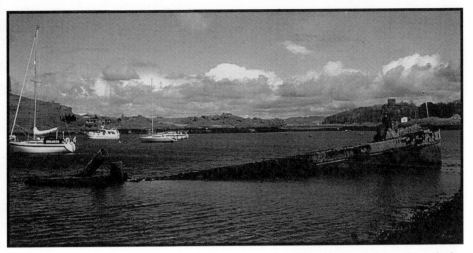

The anchorage in Ardantrive Bay with what are possibly the remains of the Hyacinth. (Photograph: Bob Baird)

CALUM CILLE

Wreck No : 155
Latitude : 56 25 15 N
Decca Lat : 5625.25 N
Location : N shore of Ardantrive Bay
Type : Fishing boat
Length :   ft.   **Beam :**   ft.
How Sunk :

Date Sunk :
Longitude : 05 29 37 W
Decca Long : 0529.62 W
Area : Oban
Tonnage :   gross
Draught : ft.
Depth :   metres

There are three wrecks on the shore on the North side of Ardantrive Bay, two of them are wooden fishing vessels, one with the registration OB151, and the name Calum Cille still visible on the starboard bow. Another is gradually disappearing as someone seems to be sawing it up for firewood. The third wreck is the keel and ribs of what appears to be a very old iron-hulled vessel with wooden cladding on the hull.

On the western shore lies a fourth wreck, that of a barge constructed of ferro-concrete, probably dating from WW2. The faded lettering of the name FB2 is still discernible on both sides of the bows, and there is a large hole in the starboard side of the hull.

There are also two or three small iron barges sunk in the southern part of the Bay. Is one of the wooden vessels perhaps the hull of the Helen Wilson?

PANSY

Wreck No : 156
Latitude : 56 25 30 N
Decca Lat : 5625.50 N
Location : Red Lady Beacon, N Kerrera
Type : MFV
Length :   ft.   **Beam :**   ft.
How Sunk : Ran aground

Date Sunk : 02 11 1958
Longitude : 05 29 32 W
Decca Long : 0529.53 W
Area : Oban
Tonnage :   gross
Draught : ft.
Depth :   metres

The Stornoway-registered line fishing vessel *Pansy* was on her way to Oban from Tobermory, and misjudged the entrance to Oban Bay on Sunday night, 2nd November 1958. She went firmly on the rocks at the North end of Kerrera, close to the warning light of the Red Lady beacon. Fortunately the sea was fairly calm, and the crew were taken off safely in darkness by the Lossiemouth seine-netter *Valkyrie*. The first attempt to pump the *Pansy* off the rocks at high tide next morning was unsuccessful. A second attempt was to be made by the *Valkyrie*, assisted by the *Alert*, but this was abandoned.

SOLWAY FIRTH

Wreck No : 157
Latitude : 56 26 30 N PA
Decca Lat : 5626.50 N
Location : Firth of Lorne
Type : Trawler
Length : 53.0 ft.   **Beam :**   ft.
How Sunk :

Date Sunk : 08 02 1977
Longitude : 05 34 00 W PA
Decca Long : 0534.00 W
Area : Oban
Tonnage : 53 gross.
Draught : ft.
Depth : 36 metres

The *Solway Firth* was an MFV. I have 53 ft as the length and 53 as the tonnage. Which is correct? The PA is 1.75 miles ESE of Lady's Rock.

MOUNTAINEER

Wreck No : 158
Latitude : 56 26 40 N
Decca Lat : 5626.67 N
Location : Off SW tip of Lady's Rock
Type : Paddle steamer
Length : 195.7 ft.   **Beam :** 17.6 ft.
How Sunk : Ran aground

Date Sunk : 27 09 1889
Longitude : 05 37 00 W
Decca Long : 0537.00 W
Area : Oban
Tonnage : 188 gross.
Draught : 8.0 ft.
Depth :   metres

The MacBrayne paddle steamer *Mountaineer*, built in 1852 by J & G Thomson of Clydebank, lived up to its name when it ran on to Lady's Rock on 27th September

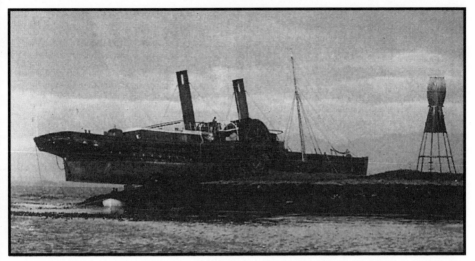

The Mountaineer perched on Lady's Rock at low tide
(Photograph courtesy of Mitchell Library, Glasgow City Libraries)

1889, and remained perched there, high and dry, until 7th October when she broke in two and slipped off the rock. The weather during this period had been too bad to allow any salvage to be carried out.

Pieces of the wreckage still lie off the South west of Lady's Rock, and the rock itself has a groove gouged out by the keel of the *Mountaineer* where she went aground. The light on Lady's Rock was first put there in September 1907. Prior to that, a tall, unlit tower was erected on the rock.

CLYDESDALE

Wreck No : 159

Latitude : 56 26 40 N

Decca Lat : 5626.76 N

Location : Lady's Rock, Lynne of Lorne

Type : Steamship

Length : 196.7 ft.   **Beam :** 24.1 ft.

How Sunk : Ran aground

Date Sunk : 13 01 1905

Longitude : 05 37 00 W

Decca Long : 0537.00 W

Area : Oban

Tonnage : 468 gross.

Draught : 13.5 ft.

Depth :   metres

On Friday 13th January 1905, MacBrayne's iron steamship *Clydesdale* was on her outward voyage with the mails and 17 passengers from Oban to Barra. Heavy sleet driven by a Force 6 North westerly obscured Lismore Light, and shortly after 7.00 am she went on to Lady's Rock in the Lynne of Lorne. The passengers were taken off by the *Carabineer* on her inward run from Tobermory, and landed at Oban.

Clydesdale was built in 1862 by J&G Thompson.

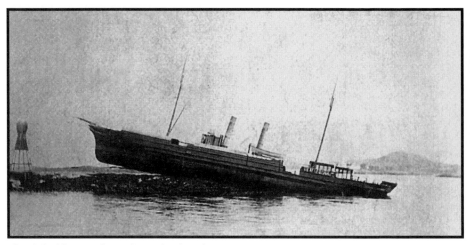

The Clydesdale *aground on Lady's Rock at low tide*
(Photograph: Author's collection)

APPLETREE

Wreck No : 160

Latitude : 56 27 10 N

Decca Lat : 5627.17 N

Location : E of Lismore Light

Type : Drifter

Length : ft. **Beam :** ft.

How Sunk : Collision/RAF pinnace

Date Sunk : 15 10 1940

Longitude : 05 33 40 W

Decca Long : 0533.67 W

Area : Oban

Tonnage : 84 gross.

Draught : ft.

Depth : 42 metres

The drifter *Appletree* was hired by the Admiralty in January 1940 as a harbour defence patrol craft, and was sunk in a collision with RAF pinnace No. 50, 1.5 miles ESE of Lismore Light in the Lynne of Lorne at 20.15 hours on 15th October 1940, in rain and bad visibility. According to one report, two of the crew were lost. Another report says the crew were all saved, but the confidential books were lost.

She supposedly lies in a deep muddy trench. I have two positions recorded: 552710N, 053340W and 552710N, 053318W.

MADAM ALICE

Wreck No : 161

Latitude : 56 27 22 N

Decca Lat : 5627.37 N

Location : 1.1 miles NW of Ganavan

Type : Steamship

Date Sunk : 16 02 1918

Longitude : 05 29 14 W

Decca Long : 0529.23 W

Area : Oban

Tonnage : 478 gross.

Length : 168.7 ft. **Beam :** 25.8 ft. **Draught :** 10.4 ft.

How Sunk : Collision with *Iolaire* **Depth :** 42 metres

Madam Alice, (ex-*Bay Fisher*), was a 3-masted steel screw steamer built in 1904 by Dublin Dockyard, for J. Fisher & Sons of Barrow. She had a welldeck with machinery aft - engine by Renfrew Bros, of Irvine.

While en route from Oban to Stornoway on 16th February 1918 with a cargo of empty barrels (presumably for the herring fishing industry), she was struck on the port side at the boiler room by the Admiralty vessel *Iolaire*, and went down by the stern in a very short time. All 17 of the crew were saved.

After several years of searching, the wreck was finally found in May 1985 by the author and Campbell McKellar. (The last year of the search was so intense that our wives were almost convinced we were having an affair with a lady named Alice! I suppose, in a way, we were - and it was wonderful!)

The collision damage on the port side is obvious, and the wreck lies with a bow-up

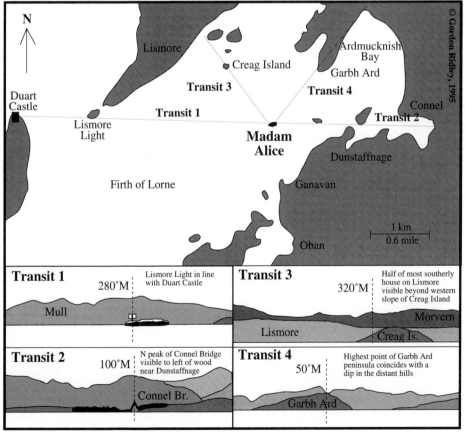

Location and transits for the Madam Alice

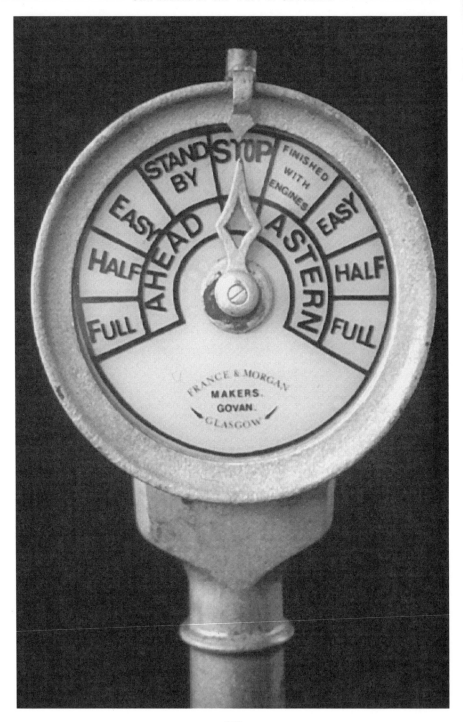

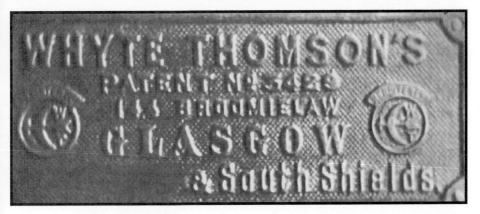

Above: The plate off the binnacle of the Madam Alice (a photograph of the author with the binnacle itself appears on page 5).
Opposite: The bridge telegraph of the Madam Alice after restoration.
Photographs : Bob Baird.

attitude, partially embedded in a silty bottom, listing about 45° to port. Lost fishing nets covered in tube worms are festooned over her bow, with more net snagged on the gun mounted on the stern deck housing. The bows themselves rise about 4 metres up from the mud, while the nets extend upward for about another 5 metres, held in suspension by the spherical floats attached to them.

The wheelhouse has largely collapsed inwards, and two compass binnacles, the bridge telegraph (which was still reading *Easy Astern*), several portholes, the steam whistle, engine room gauges and various other items have been recovered.

The wreck lies directly on the route of the Oban to Lismore ferry, in a very exposed position, subject to almost instantaneous weather and sea state changes.

EARL OF CARRICK

Wreck No : 162	**Date Sunk :** 29 09 1878
Latitude : 56 27 36 N	**Longitude :** 05 17 30 W
Decca Lat : 5627.60 N	**Decca Long :** 0517.50 W
Location : Above Connel Bridge, L. Etive	**Area :** Oban
Type : Steamship	**Tonnage :** 161 gross.
Length : ft. **Beam :** ft.	**Draught :** ft.
How Sunk : Ran aground	**Depth :** metres

The 161 ton net iron steamship *Earl Of Carrick* ran aground off Connel on 29th September 1878 while carrying a cargo of rails from Workington to Bonawe for the Callander to Oban railway.

This is the wreck above the Falls of Lora, mentioned in Oban Divers Guide, and has been reported to lie 80 ft East of Connel Bridge. A report at the time said that the after part of the vessel was lying upside down on a rock 45 yards from the south shore, while the fore part, also upside down, lay about 80 yards north of this. Because of the extremely strong tidal streams, there was no hope of salvage.

EXIT

Wreck No : 163		**Date Sunk** : 28 06 1892	
Latitude : 56 27 36 N PA		**Longitude** : 05 17 30 W PA	
Decca Lat : 5627.60 N		**Decca Long** : 0517.50 W	
Location : Falls of Lora, Loch Etive		**Area** : Oban	
Type : Schooner		**Tonnage** : 84 gross.	
Length : ft.	**Beam** : ft.	**Draught** : ft.	
How Sunk : Ran aground		**Depth** : metres	

The *Exit* of Campbeltown, from Glasgow to Ardchattan with coal, struck the reef on the North side of the channel, (Great Connel Rock), while attempting passage of the rapids of Lora, and stuck fast there, broadside to the tide, lying on her beam ends. The crew stood by her in their boat, and she floated off two hours later, but a large part of her keel was wrenched off. The crew immediately boarded her and tried to run her ashore, but after being hauled up at *Little Connel*, they got a rope ashore and had the forepart aground when she keeled over and sank in deep water. As the tide receded, the main mast again became visible above the surface at the place where she went down. According to the *Oban Times* of 9 July, 1892, the wreck then drifted into Ardchattan Bay - a distance of 3 miles! - and the foremast was visible above water at all states of the tide.

She was sold as she lay to a Mr. William Black of Black Crofts, on the North shore of Loch Etive, and it was reported that he intended to raise her, but there is no further report in the *Oban Times* to tell of the success, or otherwise, of his efforts. I am more than a little sceptical about the reported drift of some three miles after she sank to the bottom, and suspect she still lies where she originally sank, a short distance into Loch Etive from the Connel bridge.

Is *Little Connel* what is now called North Connel? I think a search around 552730N, 052306W, off the jetty in the bay to the North east of Connel Bridge, or just above the Falls of Lora, is more likely to bear fruit than a search of Ardchattan Bay.

This may be the wreck mentioned in *Oban Divers Guide* just above the Falls of Lora at about 562724N, 052233W, half a mile above the Connel Bridge.

THALIA

Wreck No : 164
Latitude : 56 28 09 N
Decca Lat : 5628.15 N
Location : 0.43 miles SW of Creag Island
Type : Steam yacht
Length : 108.8 ft.   **Beam :** 21.1 ft.
How Sunk : Collision

Date Sunk : 11 10 1942
Longitude : 05 31 24 W
Decca Long : 0531.40 W
Area : Oban
Tonnage : 161 gross.
Draught : 9.4 ft.
Depth : 54 metres

The *Thalia*, (ex-*Protector*), built in 1904, was purchased by the Admiralty as a dan layer in March 1940, and was *reportedly* used as a water carrier, supplying the ships at anchor in the Firth of Lorne, assembling for convoys. Her skipper was the father of Norman Budge, the harbourmaster at Oban, who refutes the suggestion that the *Thalia* was used as a water carrier, as she was not equipped with tanks suitable for that purpose.

According to Norman Budge, his father and the mate took the *Thalia* out on alternate days, and the *Thalia* was sunk in collision with a Norwegian tanker while under the command of the mate on 11th October 1942. She now lies at 562809N, 053124W, 0.43 miles South west of Creag Island in the Lynne of Lorne.

Some years ago, Norman Budge asked a group of Navy clearance divers to recover the bell of the *Thalia* for him. They apparently got a line around the bell bracket after fighting their way through layers of fishing net, but had to abandon the attempt and were unwilling to try again.

A local prawn fisherman got his creels entangled in the nets on the wreck in 1985, and in attempting to free them with his hydraulic line hauler, pulled the nets all the way to the surface but had to cut the line as his boat, the *New Venture*, was listing so severely under the strain of the pull that he was in danger of capsizing his vessel! The other end of the nets remained firmly attached to the *Thalia*, 54 metres below.

There is just enough room to trawl between the wreck and Creag Island, but tidal streams in the area make this a very tricky operation - hence the nets on the *Thalia*.

ST. JOSEPH

Wreck No : 165
Latitude : 56 28 30 N
Decca Lat : 5628.50 N
Location : Off Liath Sgeir, Lynn of Morven
Type : Steamship
Length : 258.0 ft.   **Beam :** 39.7 ft.
How Sunk : Ran aground

Date Sunk : 17 10 1936
Longitude : 05 36 45 W
Decca Long : 0536.75 W
Area : Oban
Tonnage : 1749 gross.
Draught : 16.3 ft.
Depth : 25 metres

The charted depth at this position is about 25 metres to a sand and shingle bottom at the North west of Liath Sgeir, which is Gaelic for Grey Rock.

The Norwegian steamer *St. Joseph*, en route from Tonsberg to Manchester with a cargo of iron ore, struck the Grey Rock during a south-westerly gale on 17th October 1936. Rockets were fired and an SOS sent out, which was picked up by the Coast Line vessel *Northern Coast*. There was no lifeboat based in Oban at that time, and Islay lifeboat was already at sea attending to another distressed vessel off Islay, (the *Shuna*), and was therefore not able to respond to the needs of the *St. Joseph*, but the Barra boat left for the Sound of Mull, 75 stormy miles away. Meantime, a Granton trawler lying at Oban had noticed the distress rockets and immediately put to sea, but when she arrived at the Grey Rock, the sea was so rough that there was no possibility of her effecting a rescue. She stood by the stricken vessel until the *Northern Coast* appeared. The Barra lifeboat arrived during the afternoon of the following day, but at first the crew of the Norwegian steamer would not leave their ship. Later, the *Northern Coast* took off 17 members of the crew. The next morning, Barra lifeboat took off the captain and the three remaining crew from the *St. Joseph* and brought them into Oban. By jettisoning her cargo during salvage efforts over the following two weeks, the Leith tug *Bullger* was finally able to get the *St. Joseph* off the rocks.

Wreckage remaining is therefore only cargo and steel plates.

BREDA

Wreck No : 166		**Date Sunk :** 24 12 1940	
Latitude : 56 28 33 N		**Longitude :** 05 25 00 W	
Decca Lat : 5628.55 N		**Decca Long :** 0525.00 W	
Location : Ardmucknish Bay		**Area :** Oban	
Type : Steamship		**Tonnage :** 6941 gross.	
Length : 418.6 ft.	**Beam :** 58.3 ft.	**Draught :** 34.7 ft.	
How Sunk : Bombed		**Depth :** 9 metres	

On 23rd December 1940, the Dutch vessel *Breda* was bombed during a German air raid on Oban roads. She was anchored there with several other ships marshalling for a convoy awaiting a Naval escort to continue her voyage from London to Mombasa and Bombay. The attacking aircraft were five *Heinkel 111*s from Stavanger, Norway. These aircraft made the attack at very low level, flying from South to North, and hit several vessels. One of the other vessels attacked, the 4652 tons gross Dutch motor vessel *Tuva*, on which seven of the crew were killed, was en route from Hull to Buenos Aires with a cargo of coal. She was beached first of all on Bogha Garbh Ard on the 23rd, but was floated off this rock pinnacle to be re-beached on the sand in Camas Nathais Bay. An unexploded bomb was found in her No. 3 hold. She was again refloated after being patched up sufficiently well to enable her to proceed to a repair port.

The 2092 ton Danish steamship *Flynderborg* was hit by two bombs and strafed, but was not seriously damaged, although her radio operator was badly injured. A bomb which entered the foc'sle of the 5117 ton *Dan Y Bryn*, failed to explode. The harbour

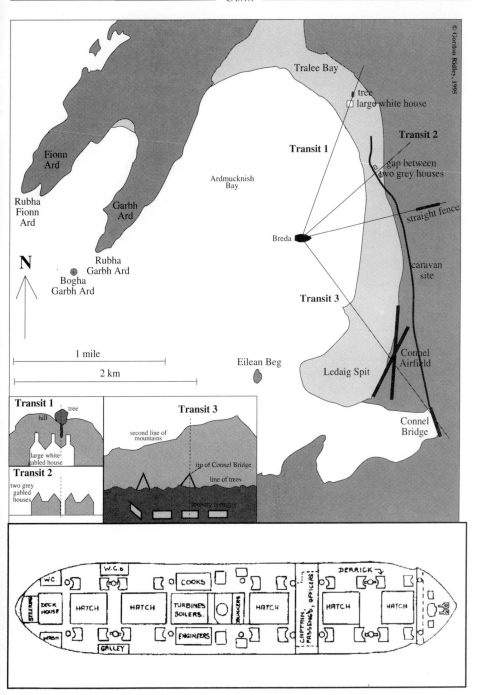

Transits for and sketch plan of the Breda

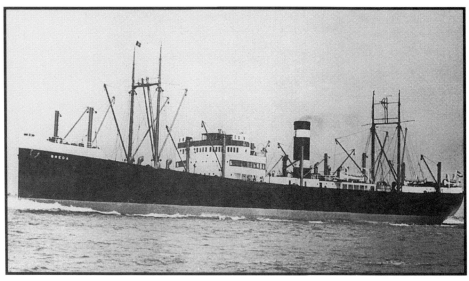

The Breda *(Photograph courtesy of Loet Steeman).*

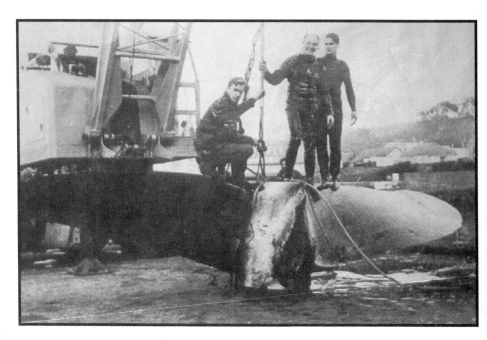

The prop of the Breda on the quay at Oban with Dave Tye (centre), Dave Whitton (kneeling) and Norman O'Neill in 1966. (Photograph:Dave Tye).

drifter *Lupina* was also damaged in this raid.

The *Breda* was the only ship to sink as a result of the bombing raid. Although the bomb was not a direct hit, the *Breda* suffered damage in the form of a fractured cooling water inlet pipe, and taking in water, made her way to the East shore of Ardmucknish Bay. There, Captain Johannis Fooy beached her on a shelf which extends 600 yards out to sea, where the depth is still only 6 metres. Beyond that, the bottom slopes quickly to over 30 metres. She remained on this shelf long enough for some of her cargo to be removed, but soon slid back into deeper water and came to rest with her bows in 24 metres and her stern in 30 metres. Her goalpost foremasts were visible above the surface at low tide until 1961 when the Navy removed them, along with the bridge, funnel, and forepeak to give a swept clearance of 28 ft.

The remains of the bridge and a small part of the forepeak, including the foremasts, now lie in the mud off the port side of the ship, while a large part of the forepeak lies about 40-50 ft. off the starboard bow. The gun mounted on a platform structure at the stern was presumably also removed at that time.

Registered in Rotterdam and belonging to the Royal Netherlands Steamship Co., the *Breda* was built in Schiedam, Holland in 1921. Apart from being laid up in Amsterdam in 1923 and 1924, the normal route for the ship was between Europe and South America. At 6941 tons gross, she was 418' 6" long, 58' wide, and had a moulded depth of 37'. From the keel to the top of the foremast measured 117' 6". She had 3 decks, a cruiser stern and a flat bottom. The bridge lay between the second and third of the *Breda*'s five holds, and contained the radio and navigation rooms, officers' accommodation and cabins for 16 passengers. Aft of hold 3 lay the engine room whose four boilers were originally coal fired, but were converted to oil in 1938. These produced steam for two turbines with double reduction gearing to a single screw. Her service speed was 11.8 knots, and fuel consumption ran at 36 tons of oil per day. The stern housed accommodation for the 37 crew. On the main deck is the steering gear, with the emergency steering position on the deck above. This had originally been open to the elements, but a platform was erected above this position to carry the gun which was fitted during the war. This structure was home to a forest of sea anemones and was easily the most picturesque part of the wreck until it was demolished with explosives by the Royal Navy in 1990, in an attempt to prevent divers reaching the magazine of shells for the stern gun. It was considered that the shells themselves may have been too unstable to risk removing them.

In 1966 the wreck was rediscovered by Edinburgh BSAC divers, and despite the loss of her bridge, derricks and funnel, still looked undamaged and ready to sail again, if she could be raised to the surface. Blasting by Oban Divers removed the bronze propeller in 1968, and further blasting has since removed most of the remaining superstructure, improving access to the lower decks and engine room. Most of the copper degaussing cable, for protection against magnetic mines, was also recovered by Oban Divers, and the insulation burned off on Eilean Mor.

At the time of her sinking, the *Breda* was carrying a very mixed cargo, consisting of 3000 tons of cement, (now set solid), 175 tons of tobacco and cigarettes, 3 *Hawker*

This page:
Above: Oil lamp recovered from the Engineer's store of the Breda.
Below: Parts of the engine of a Tiger Moth aircraft recovered from Hold 3 of the Breda.

Opposite:
Above: The compass from a Tiger Moth aircraft recovered from Hold 3 of the Breda.
Below: The maker's plate off a Dunlop trolley air compressor (for inflating aircraft tyres) recoved from Hold 4 of the Breda.

(All photographs: Bob Baird).

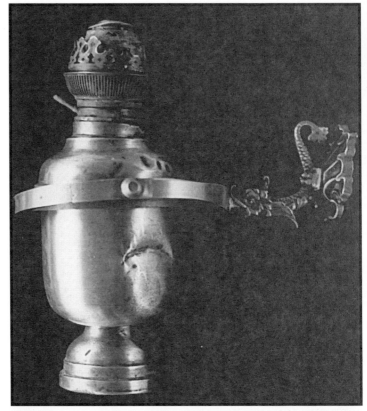

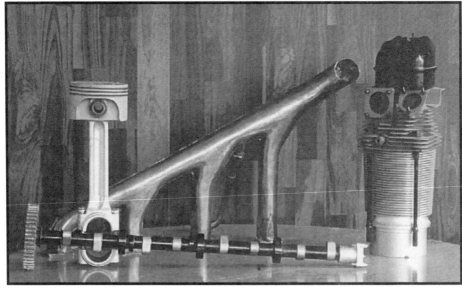

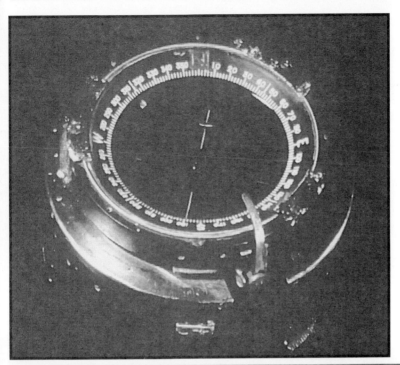

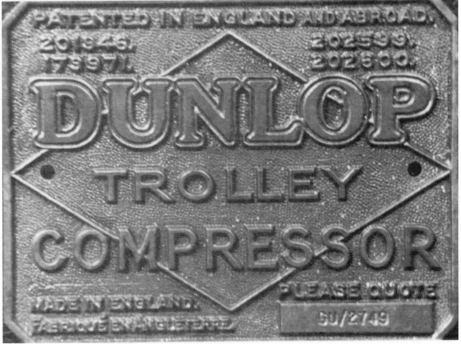

biplanes and 30 *de Havilland Moths.* Aircraft engines, propellers, windscreens, instruments and various other parts have been recovered. The aircraft, which are now hard to recognise, are stored in holds one two and three. Sandals with leather uppers and rubber soles, medical supplies, including kaoline in square-shaped, waisted bottles, (like square *Coca Cola* bottles), batteries, wide strips of leather, tyres, telephone pole insulators, lengths of solder, black boot polish and innumerable other items have been recovered from hold No. 1. On the deck alongside hold No. 2 lies an upside down 4 x 4 vehicle with the tyres still fully-inflated. Another similar vehicle has fallen from the deck to the bottom of hold 2, which also contains aircraft and beer bottles. Hold 3 contains aircraft, tin lids, tyres, barrels containing stoneware bottles of Stephens blue ink, (how many divers can claim to have dived in ink?), dental supplies, including what appear to be drinks coasters, but which are actually material for taking dental impressions, and the pink material for making the gums of false teeth. Regretfully, I have so far failed to find the material for making gold fillings! Hold 4 contains truck spares, gas masks, spectacle lenses, fire hoses, the spare propeller, (cast iron), trolley compressors with brass, double-acting cylinders, (for inflating tyres), brass fire extinguishers, aircraft batteries, and between holds 4 and 5, the 3000 tons of cement. Spare porthole glasses of two different diameters, individually separated by pages of a 1940 Dutch newspaper were also recovered as recently as 1989. The newspaper was still legible, and included the pages giving the BBC radio programmes. Brass oil lamps with gimballed brackets cast in the shape of dolphins were also recovered at the same time. Apart from more of the cement, hold 5 contains bicycles, electrical equipment including switches, fuses and GEC ceiling fans, thousands of sheets of Indian banknotes watermarked *Ten Rupees,* and bales of hay for the 10 horses, reputedly belonging to the Aga Khan, which were also part of the cargo.

When the *Breda* was beached, the horses were either released to swim ashore, or the horse boxes drifted off with the horses still inside. One of these boxes came ashore near Ledaig Spit, with a horse still inside and a very distraught dog standing on top of the box. They were rescued by Mrs. Mary MacNiven, wife of the caretaker at Dunstaffnage Castle. Not all of the horses survived, but at least one was kept in the old smiddy adjacent to the cemetery at the southern edge of the village of Benderloch. The last survivor of the horses died in the Oban area in 1961. Some time after the sinking, the body of a monkey was found in the grounds of Letterwalton House, a few miles north of Benderloch. Around its neck was a collar bearing the inscription "SS Breda".

A few days before the May Holiday weekend in 1995, the first deaths occurred on the *Breda.* Two experienced Welsh divers took a novice down with them. The novice surfaced alone, having lost his two companions underwater. These two never resurfaced.

Not having dived the *Breda* before, the novice was unable to say exactly where they were or what had happened to them, but by describing what he had seen around him when he lost his companions, it was possible to deduce that they had been in hold four.

During the following two weeks, about 70 divers, including Alan Campbell of Nervous Wreck Divers, Oban, the Strathclyde Police Underwater Unit and the Royal Navy, were involved in searching the *Breda* for the lost divers. An ROV with a video camera was also used to penetrate parts of the wreck which were either inaccessible, or considered too dangerous to enter, but no trace of the missing divers could be found. The shores of Ardmucknish Bay and the surrounding area were also searched without result, and the search was eventually abandoned.

Some two weeks later, I heard a most bizarre story about a clairvoyant woman who apparently telephoned from Australia to say that over the years she had had a number of visions and had contacted various police forces throughout the world to give them information to help them find bodies which they had been unable to locate.

She purportedly offered the information that two divers had been lost on a wreck near Oban, and that one of them was very badly crushed beneath machinery, or a plate from either the side of the ship, or from a bulkhead which had fallen on them, and the other had either a broken spine or neck.

When I first heard this story, I was highly dubious about its authenticity, and repeated it to a police contact who checked it out and reported back that this amazing story was indeed true. Oban Police have a report of the Australian woman's call, passed on to them by Strathclyde Police Headquarters, and a further search of the wreck was carried out following her telephone call, but with no more success that hitherto.

It was certainly my belief that something had fallen on the lost divers, as that appeared to offer the most plausible explanation for their simultaneous disappearance, and I was surprised that none of the searchers had apparently noticed any difference in the position of anything on the wreck.

Some of the divers involved in the searching had probably never dived the *Breda* before, and others were insufficiently familiar with the wreck to be aware of anything having recently fallen or changed position.

Having dived the *Breda* myself over 500 times in the past 16 years, I am at least as familiar with the wreck as anyone else, and considerably more so that most.

Whatever fell must be of some significant size to completely cover the two divers, or block their exit from one of the compartments they may have entered, and I should have thought this would be obvious to someone with my experience and knowledge of the wreck.

The starboard after corner of hold four is where the spare propellor is located. I can remember virtually the entire propellor being visible, but over the years there has been collapsing of the wreck in this area, and the propellor is now almost totally buried and inaccessible.

The huge I-beam of the port edge of the hold has an angled crack right through it, compromising its mechanical integrity and strength. The weight of the beam is mainly supported by its other end, fastened to the forward edge of the hold, and another, smaller I-beam which has fallen into a position where it is wedged beneath the large beam.

Immediately forward of this is a very dark, almost totally enclosed area, still part of hold four, extending forward to the aft engine room bulkhead, and running the full width of the ship. It was from within here that the trolley compressors, aircraft batteries and brass fire extinguishers were recovered a number of years ago.

There are several places at which access may be gained to this area, but relatively few visiting divers would be likely to attempt this.

One of the points of access is from the engine room, through a hole near the port side of the ship, where the steel plates of the aft engine room bulkhead have parted due to severe buckling. This is close to a hole in the side of the ship where the hull plates have been blown outwards by an explosion within the engine room. The severe buckling of the bulkhead plates may have been caused by the same explosion.

My first opportunity to dive the *Breda* after the loss of the two divers was on 1st August 1995, and I was struck by the extent of the deterioration in the state of the wreck since my last dive about a year before.

A considerable amount of further buckling and collapsing had obviously occurred during the previous year or so, particularly in the area of hold four, the engine room and the after part of hold three.

Despite evidence of collapsing having occurred over the years, the *Breda* has generally been considered a fairly safe wreck, but it would be advisable to bear in mind that, apart from occasional blasting by salvors (mainly Harry Hemsley, who owns the wreck), the structure has been weakened by corrosion resulting from 55 years of immersion.

PLOVER

Wreck No : 167	**Date Sunk :** 11 11 1893
Latitude : 56 35 30 N PA	**Longitude :** 05 24 00 W PA
Decca Lat : 5635.50 N	**Decca Long :** 0524.00 W
Location : Shuna Island, Loch Linnhe	**Area :** Oban
Type : Steamship	**Tonnage :** 62 gross.
Length : ft. **Beam :** ft.	**Draught :** ft.
How Sunk : Ran aground	**Depth :** metres

The iron steamship *Plover*, of 62 tons net, with a cargo of slates from Easdale to Dundee, was lost by stranding on Shuna Island in Loch Linnhe on 11th November 1893. An officer from the Glasgow Salvage Association was sent to the scene, and reported that the vessel had slipped off the rocks into 7 fathoms (13 metres).

MARTHA

Wreck No : 168	**Date Sunk :** 26 12 1877
Latitude : 56 35 45 N	**Longitude :** 05 23 20 W
Decca Lat : 5635.75 N	**Decca Long :** 0523.33 W
Location : Shuna Island, Loch Linnhe	**Area :** Oban
Type : Smack	**Tonnage :** 31 gross.
Length : ft. **Beam :** ft.	**Draught :** ft.
How Sunk : Ran aground	**Depth :** metres

The 31 tons net smack *Martha*, with a cargo of slates from Easdale to Bowling was lost by running on to Shuna Island, Loch Linnhe on 26th December 1877.

A neatly stacked pile of slates lies in about 13 metres about 50 metres off the North west point of Shuna Island, and stands about 3 metres high on a shingle bottom. The pile of slates is about 40 ft long by about 20 ft wide. The scallop diver who found them reported that there was no sign of remains of the vessel, hence these slates are probably the cargo of the wooden-hulled *Martha*, rather than from the iron-hulled *Plover*, which must also be in the vicinity.

STIRLING CASTLE

Wreck No : 169	**Date Sunk :** 14 01 1828
Latitude : 56 43 20 N PA	**Longitude :** 05 14 30 W PA
Decca Lat : 5643.33 N	**Decca Long :** 0514.50 W
Location : Near Ardgour, Loch Linnhe	**Area :** Oban
Type : Paddle steamer	**Tonnage :** gross
Length : 68.0 ft. **Beam :** ft.	**Draught :** ft.
How Sunk : Ran aground	**Depth :** metres

Henry Bell's wooden paddle steamer *Stirling Castle* built in 1814 was wrecked at Inverscadail near Ardgour, Argyll, in the vicinity of the Corran lighthouse on 14th January 1828.

CHAPTER 6

THE WRECKS OF MULL

INTRODUCTION

Tobermory (*Tobhar Moire*, Mary's Well), at the northern end of the Sound of Mull was developed as a fishing village in 1788. It is very picturesque, with its row of brightly painted stone houses, and fine sheltered harbour. Mull has a mild climate, with high rainfall in the mountains.

The magnificent terraced Italian Garden at Torosay Castle includes a statue walk between 19 figures by the 18th century master Antonio Bonazza. They were originally from a derelict villa near Padua. The cost of transporting them by puffer and horse-drawn cart from Glasgow docks exceeded the cost of their purchase and shipment from Italy to Glasgow! There is also a water garden, a rock garden and a Japanese garden.

During the summer months, a miniature railway carries passengers between Craignure and Torosay castle, through masses of rhododendrons. Torosay Castle itself dates from 1858, and belongs to Mr. David and the Hon. Mrs. Guthrie James. The grounds included the ruin of the 14th century Duart Castle in its prominent position at the southern entrance to the Sound of Mull. Duart Castle had originally been the stronghold of the Clan Maclean, who were staunch Jacobites.

The castle was taken by the Duke of Argyll in 1674, and was garrisoned by government troops during the Jacobite uprisings. In 1691 the castle was burned down, and it was not until 1910 that the ruin was sold back to Sir Fitzroy Maclean, and the restoration of the castle commenced in 1911.

Frank Lockwood's Island is named after the brother-in-law of the 21st MacLean of Lochbuie. He was Solicitor General in Lord Rosebery's administration in 1894-5.

The poem overleaf, located on a visit to Torosay Castle in Mull, is very apt. The poem originally appeared in the *Oban Times* (author unknown).

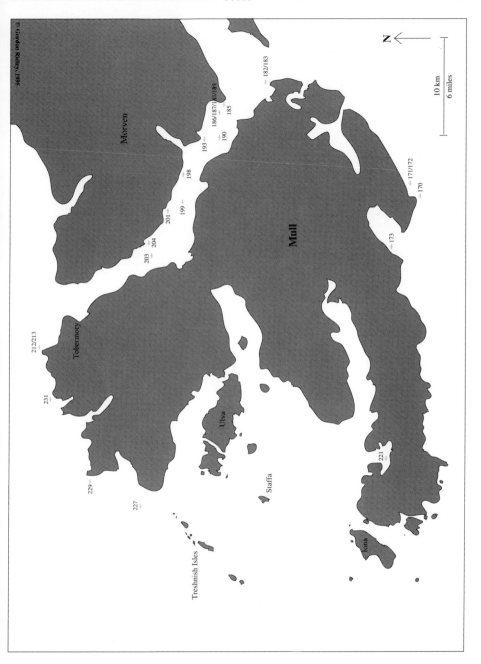

*Chart showing the location of wrecks
lying off the coast of Mull*

MULL WEATHER
by a summer visitor

It rained and rained and rained and rained
The average was well maintained
And when our fields were simply bogs
It started raining cats and dogs
After a drought of half an hour
There came a most refreshing shower
And then the queerest thing of all
A gentle rain began to fall.

Next day 'twas pretty fairly dry
Save for a deluge from the sky
This wetted people to the skin
But after that the rain set in
We wondered what's the next we'd get
As sure as fate we got more wet
But soon we'll have a change again
And we shall have a drop of rain.

THE WRECKS

MAINE

Wreck No : 170   **Date Sunk :** 17 06 1914
Latitude : 56 18 38 N   **Longitude :** 05 50 20 W
Decca Lat : 5618.63 N   **Decca Long :** 0550.33 W
Location : Frank Lockwood's Island   **Area :** Mull
Type : Steamship   **Tonnage :** 2395 gross.
Length : 302.7 ft.   **Beam :** 44.0 ft.   **Draught :** 17.5 ft.
How Sunk : Ran aground   **Depth :**   metres

The 1505 tons net steel steamship *Maine* was built in 1892 by Harlan & Hollingsworth of Wilmington, Delaware, and during the First World War became HMS *Maine*, a hospital ship which ran aground in dense fog at 2.00 am on 17th June 1914.

She had been heading for Oban to collect patients from the mine-laying fleet exercising in Loch Linnhe when she ran aground on the small island of Eilean Straide Eun, which lies close to Mull, about two miles East of the entrance to Loch Buie in South east Mull. This island is now known as Frank Lockwood's Island. So dense was the fog that it was difficult for vessels to leave Oban, but the *Princess Louise*, an excursion steamer, proceeded to the scene to render assistance, as did the MacBrayne steamer *Cavalier*, which had been intercepted at Blackmill Bay, Luing. On arrival at the scene, they found torpedo boats from Northern Ireland and mine-laying vessels from Ballachulish already in attendance.

It was discovered that the former American steamer, was badly damaged forward, and lay in a bad position for salving as she could sink into deep water off the ledge on which she had grounded, and salvage was abandoned as uneconomic in view of her age and low value.

BARCOME

Wreck No : 171   **Date Sunk :** 13 01 1958
Latitude : 56 18 51 N   **Longitude :** 05 52 06 W
Decca Lat : 5618.85 N   **Decca Long :** 0552.10 W
Location : W side of Loch Buie, SE Mull   **Area :** Mull
Type : Boom defence vessel   **Tonnage :** 750 gross.
Length : 173.8 ft.   **Beam :** 32.3 ft.   **Draught :** 9.5 ft.
How Sunk : Ran aground   **Depth :**   metres

The 750 ton boom defence vessel HMS *Barcome* was found shortly after 6.00 pm on 14th January by an Oban-bound fishing vessel, ending a 21 hour search by Naval vessels, aircraft, and the Islay lifeboat, *Charlotte Elizabeth*. *Barcome* had been badly holed

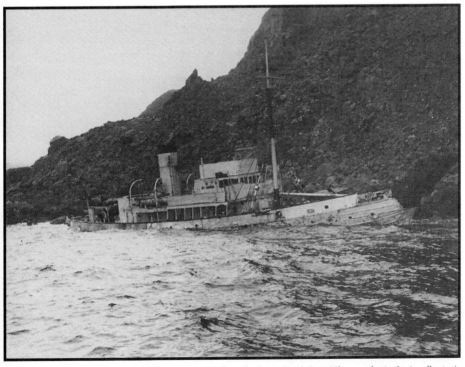

The Barcome *aground on the shore of Loch Buie (Photograph: Author's collection)*

and flooded. The search had been hampered by fog and a series of conflicting reports as to the area in which she had been grounded. Shortly after 9.00 pm on the 13th, *Barcome* had signalled that she was aground near Oronsay Island. The Islay lifeboat was launched at once and searched the Oronsay area all through the night, eventually being sent further north to search the area around the Torran Rocks off South west Mull, over 15 miles from Oronsay. The *Charlotte Elizabeth* and the submarine rescue vessel *Kingfisher* took off the *Barcome*'s crew. At the subsequent court martial of the *Barcome*'s commander, Lt. Cdr. Derek Charles Godfrey, the court recorded that there was a local magnetic anomaly in the Loch Buie area, and extra care should have been taken because of it.

The wreck, which lies broadside at the foot of a 300 ft cliff, was sold to the Northern Shipbreaking Co. in 1959 and is reported to be broken up. Dave Tye has the bell.

GLEN ROSA

Wreck No : 172	**Date Sunk :** 15 01 1958
Latitude : 56 19 31 N	**Longitude :** 05 47 29 W
Decca Lat : 5619.51 N	**Decca Long :** 0547.48 W
Location : NE of Frank Lockwood's Isle	**Area :** Mull
Type : Steam puffer	**Tonnage :** 97 gross.
Length : ft. **Beam :** ft.	**Draught :** ft.
How Sunk : Ran aground	**Depth :** 5 metres

Due to the local magnetic anomaly, which causes compass errors, the puffer *Glen Rosa* went ashore in thick fog 1.5 - 2.0 miles North east of Frank Lockwood's Isle, South east Mull, while en route from Troon to Bunessan with a cargo of coal. The crew left in a boat, and blundered into the grounded HMS *Barcome*, which took them aboard.

MELDON

Wreck No : 173	**Date Sunk :** 03 03 1917
Latitude : 56 19 32 N	**Longitude :** 05 55 33 W
Decca Lat : 5619.53 N	**Decca Long :** 0555.55 W
Location : Loch Buie, NE of Rubha Dubh	**Area :** Mull
Type : Steamship	**Tonnage :** 2514 gross.
Length : 310.0 ft. **Beam :** 43.1 ft.	**Draught :** 20.5 ft.
How Sunk : Mined	**Depth :** 15 metres

The *Meldon*, built in 1902 by R. Stephenson of Newcastle, was a steel screw collier, on hire to the Admiralty at the time of loss, carrying a cargo of anthracite from Cardiff. She hit a mine laid by the U-78.

There is confusion between the *Melbor* and the *Meldon*! The *Melbor* was also reported

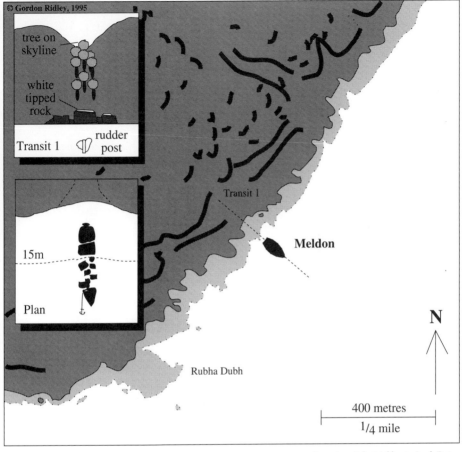

Location of the Meldon in Loch Buie

as a collier which sank in 1938 at the above position in Loch Buie. Another report gives the date of sinking as pre-1951. The similarity between the names seems to be a phonetic or typographical error, as the name Melbor is not recorded by Lloyds, and the discrepancy in the positions results from the original report of the position of hitting the mine, which was described as !/2 mile North of the Garvellachs and !/2 mile West of Isle of the Sea and recorded as 561506N 054500W. The Garvellachs, in the Firth of Lorne, are known as the *Isles of the Sea*.

According to the Hydrographic Department, the wreck charted with a clearance of at least 47 metres in a depth of about 58 metres at 561512N 054500W is the *Meldon*, but the *Meldon* must have made for the shore after hitting the mine, as she sank at the South western edge of the mouth of Loch Buie.

The bow and stern are still intact, but the centre section is broken up. She lies with her stern towards the shore and her rudder post shows above the surface at low water.

SANDA

Wreck No : 174
Latitude : 56 22 00 N PA
Decca Lat : 5622.00 N
Location : At Loch Spelve
Type : Steamship
Length : 197.8 ft.   **Beam :** 25.1 ft.
How Sunk : Ran aground

Date Sunk : 06 12 1887
Longitude : 05 42 00 W PA
Decca Long : 0542.00 W
Area : Mull
Tonnage : 522 gross.
Draught : 14.5 ft.
Depth :   metres

The steamship *Sanda*, built in 1865, went ashore in a gale at Black Head near the entrance to Loch Spelve during a voyage from Gothenburg to Glasgow with a cargo which included 70 tons of pig iron. The vessel broke in two and became a total wreck, but the crew landed safely on Mull. Black Head is not named on the chart or Ordnance Survey map, but is thought to be South of the entrance to Loch Spelve, on the rocky shores of the area of Mull known as Croggan.

Note: *Duart*, (Dubh Ard), is Gaelic for *Black Point*, or *Head*. There is also a Dubh Sgeir, (Black Rock), about 2 miles W by S of the entrance to Loch Spelve.

UNKNOWN - HAFTON?

Wreck No : 175
Latitude : 56 24 36 N
Decca Lat : 5624.60 N
Location : Firth of Lorne
Type :
Length :   ft.   **Beam :**   ft.
How Sunk :

Date Sunk :
Longitude : 05 37 30 W
Decca Long : 0537.50 W
Area : Mull
Tonnage :   gross
Draught : ft.
Depth : 100 metres

On chart No. 2387, which covers the northern part of the Firth of Lorne, a wreck with at least 100 metres over it is shown at 562436N, 053730W.

LCA 1225

Wreck No : 176
Latitude : 56 24 44 N
Decca Lat : 5624.73 N
Location : Off Loch Don, Firth of Lorne
Type : Landing craft
Length : 41.5 ft.   **Beam :** 10.0 ft.
How Sunk : Capsized and foundered

Date Sunk : 18 08 1953
Longitude : 05 37 42 W
Decca Long : 0537.70 W
Area : Mull
Tonnage : 13 gross.
Draught : 2.5 ft.
Depth : 27 metres

ACCORD

Wreck No : 177	**Date Sunk :** 14 04 1928
Latitude : 56 25 18 N PA	**Longitude :** 05 39 00 W PA
Decca Lat : 5625.30 N	**Decca Long :** 0539.00 W
Location : Entrance to Lochdon, E Mull	**Area :** Mull
Type : Drifter	**Tonnage :** gross
Length : ft. **Beam :** ft.	**Draught :** ft.
How Sunk : Ran aground	**Depth :** metres

The steam drifter *Accord* went ashore on a reef at the entrance to Lochdon on 14th April 1928 while en route to Ireland. She was badly holed, and the crew of eight were taken off by the Fraserburgh drifter *Petrilia*.

There are several reefs at the entrance to Lochdon. The PA given is the reef known as Maol Donn, but the *Accord* may have struck one of the other reefs in the area.

MARDI DAN

Wreck No : 178	**Date Sunk :** 10 09 1981
Latitude : 56 29 38 N	**Longitude :** 05 36 48 W
Decca Lat : 5629.63 N	**Decca Long :** 0536.80 W
Location : 1¼ miles NW of Rubha Croin	**Area :** Mull
Type : Fishing vessel	**Tonnage :** 13 gross.
Length : 39.0 ft. **Beam :** ft.	**Draught :** ft.
How Sunk : Fire	**Depth :** 147 metres

The fishing vessel *Mardi Dan* caught fire and sank near the disused ammunition dumping ground in Loch Linnhe on 10th September 1981. She is charted as a wreck with at least 147 metres over it in about 175 metres, 1.25 miles North west of Rubha Croin, the southernmost point of Bernera Island, Loch Linnhe.

ROBERT HEWETT

Wreck No : 179	**Date Sunk :** 24 12 1951
Latitude : N	**Longitude :** W
Decca Lat : N	**Decca Long :** W
Location : Sound of Mull	**Area :** Mull
Type : Trawler	**Tonnage :** 379 gross
Length : 150.5 ft. **Beam :** 25.5 ft.	**Draught :** 13.1 ft.
How Sunk : Ran aground / refloated	**Depth :** metres

The trawler *Robert Hewett* (ex-*Beachflower*) which was built by Cochranes of Selby in 1930 ran aground somewhere in the Sound of Mull on 24 Dec 1951, but was successfully relocated at high tide the following day. I include this information to remove any speculation that this may be one of the *Unknown* wrecks in the area, and to avoid anyone wasting time looking for the wreck.

GOLDEN GLEAM

Wreck No : 180	**Date Sunk :** 1954
Latitude : N	**Longitude :** W
Decca Lat : N	**Decca Long :** W
Location : Sound of Mull	**Area :** Mull
Type : Drifter	**Tonnage :** gross
Length : ft. **Beam :** ft.	**Draught :** ft.
How Sunk :	**Depth :** metres

WHARFINGER

Wreck No : 181	**Date Sunk :** 21 01 1911
Latitude : N	**Longitude :** W
Decca Lat : N	**Decca Long :** W
Location : Off Lochaline, Sound of Mull	**Area :** Mull
Type : Steamship	**Tonnage :** 145 gross.
Length : 90.4 ft. **Beam :** 19.7 ft.	**Draught :** 8.5 ft.
How Sunk : Foundered	**Depth :** metres

The steel steamship *Wharfinger*, a puffer of 57 tons net, was built in 1892 by Anderson & Laverick, Newcastle, engine by Hedley & Boyd of North Shields.

She foundered in the Sound of Mull off Lochaline on 21st January 1911 while en route from Glasgow to Carbost, Skye, after her stern gland burst. Her crew were all saved.

NEW BLESSING

Wreck No : 182	**Date Sunk :** 12 12 1883
Latitude : 56 27 30 N PA	**Longitude :** 05 39 12 W PA
Decca Lat : 5627.50 N	**Decca Long :** 0539.20 W
Location : Duart Point	**Area :** Mull
Type : Brig	**Tonnage :** 158 gross.
Length : ft. **Beam :** ft.	**Draught :** ft.
How Sunk : Ran aground	**Depth :** metres

The 158 tons net brig *New Blessing*, with a cargo of slates from Bangor, Wales, to Aberdeen, was lost on Duart Point on 12th December 1883 in a Force 10 NNW storm.

SWAN (OR SPEEDWELL?)

Wreck No : 183
Latitude : 56 29 45 N
Decca Lat : 5629.75 N
Location : Duart Point
Type :
Length :   ft.   **Beam :**   ft
How Sunk : Ran aground

Date Sunk :
Longitude : 05 39 19 W
Decca Long : 0539.32 W
Area : Mull
Tonnage :   gross
Draught : ft.
Depth :   metres

This is a protected wreck site at Duart Point. Wreckage of a wooden vessel, which is thought to be either the *Swan* or the *Speedwell*, lies between five and ten yards off the point in about 15 metres of water. Both of these vessels were torn from their moorings and dashed ashore on the same day.

GIRL SANDRA

Wreck No : 184
Latitude : 56 29 45 N
Decca Lat : 5629.75 N
Location : At S of Eilean Rubha an Ridire
Type : Tug
Length : 33.0 ft.   **Beam :**   ft
How Sunk : Ran aground

Date Sunk : 25 10 1981
Longitude : 05 42 42 W
Decca Long : 0542.70 W
Area : Mull
Tonnage :   gross
Draught : ft.
Depth : 4 metres

The *Girl Sandra* lies adjacent to the South tip of Eilean Rubha an Ridire with a 45° list to port. The portholes and propeller have gone. She has variously been describes as a tug, or a wooden-hulled fishing boat, used for diving.

On hitting the rocks at mid-day, she immediately sank. The two on board swam to the island and fired flares which were spotted by bird watchers at Craignure. They telephoned the coastguard, and a boat in the Sound of Mull, the *St. Ora*, was despatched to pick them up.

THESIS

Wreck No : 185
Latitude : 56 30 02 N
Decca Lat : 5630.03 N
Location : Nr Barony Point, Sound of Mull
Type : Steamship
Length : 167.0 ft.   **Beam :** 25.0 ft.
How Sunk : Ran aground in fog

Date Sunk : 16 10 1889
Longitude : 05 41 26 W
Decca Long : 0541.60 W
Area : Mull
Tonnage : 500 gross.
Draught : 12.0 ft.
Depth : 30 metres

The *Thesis* was an iron steamship built in Belfast in 1887.

She was wrecked in fog while carrying a cargo of iron ore from Belfast to Middles

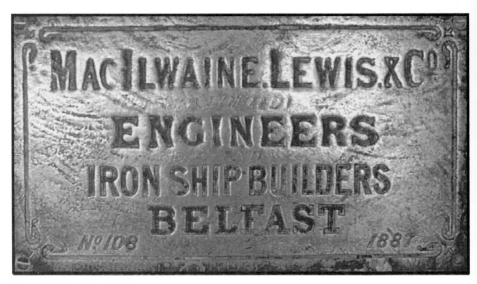

The maker's plate from the Thesis.
(Photograph: Bob Baird)

brough. Captain Wallace and his 11 crew made it safely to Craignure at the opposite side of the Sound of Mull.

The wreck is substantially intact, lying on a slope with the bows pointing towards the shore in 15 metres, and the stern in 30 metres. She lies 350 metres North west of the South tip of Morvern, about 50 metres from the shore, just South of a small bay. The bow is particularly scenic with some of the plates missing, and the frames covered in dead men's fingers. This is definitely a slack water dive only!

The mast of the Ballista *showed for some years after the sinking (Photograph: Bob Baird)*

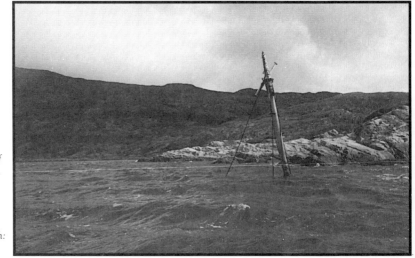

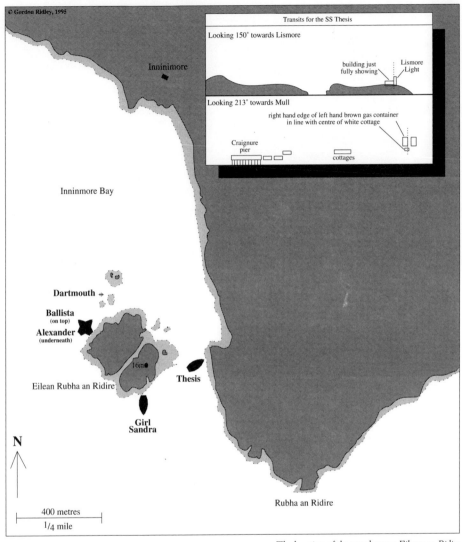

© Gordon Ridley, 1995

Inninimore

Transits for the SS Thesis

Looking 150° towards Lismore

building just
fully showing

Lismore
Light

Looking 213° towards Mull

right hand edge of left hand brown gas container
in line with centre of white cottage

Craignure
pier

cottages

Inninmore Bay

Dartmouth

Ballista
(on top)

Alexander
(underneath)

16m

Thesis

Eilean Rubha an Ridire

**Girl
Sandra**

N

400 metres

1/4 mile

Rubha an Ridire

The location of the wrecks near Eilean an Ridire

BALLISTA

Wreck No : 186
Latitude : 56 30 10 N
Decca Lat : 5630.17 N
Location : SW side of Rubha an Ridire
Type : Puffer
Length : ft.   **Beam :**   ft.
How Sunk : Ran aground

Date Sunk : 06 02 1973
Longitude : 05 41 59 W
Decca Long : 0541.98 W
Area : Mull
Tonnage :   gross
Draught : ft.
Depth : 5 metres

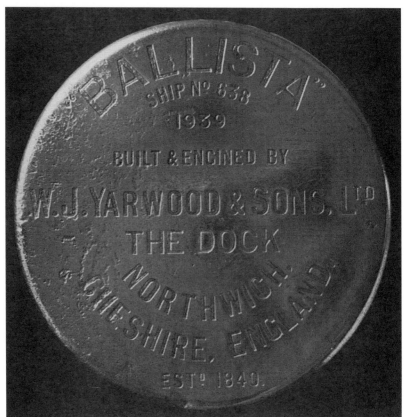

The maker's plate from the Ballista (Photograph : Bob Baird).

The *Ballista* was attempting to recover coal from a wreck just off the South west of Rubha an Ridire. Between 11.00 pm and midnight on 5th February, 1973, her stern mooring snapped in the high wind. Attempts to use the engine to keep the vessel off the rocks failed, and the three crew quickly abandoned her in their dinghy, and let the wind take them to the shore of the rocky islet of Rubha an Ridire, where they landed without any supplies. Several vessels passed during the night, but the men were unable to attract attention with a torch. At dawn they discovered some flares which had been washed ashore from the *Ballista*. When fired, these were seen by the MacBrayne ferry *Bute*. Oban radio was notified, and the Inverness fishing boat *Eminent* headed to the scene, fired a line ashore, and hauled the men and their dinghy to safety.

The *Ballista* now lies almost directly on top of another puffer from which she had been attempting to recover a cargo of coal. Until 1988, her mast was visible above the surface at all states of the tide. Parts of the superstructure at the stern are still visible at low water. The 18" diameter brass manufacturers plate was recovered in 1980, giving the builders name as W. J. Yarwood & Sons of Northwich, Cheshire. The *Ballista* was their Ship No. 638, built in 1939.

RIVER TAY

Wreck No : 187
Latitude : 56 30 10 N
Decca Lat : 5630.17 N
Location : Rubha an Ridire, Sound of Mull
Type : Trawler
Length : 115.4 ft.   **Beam :** 22.1 ft.
How Sunk : Ran aground

Date Sunk : 30 11 1943
Longitude : 05 42 00 W
Decca Long : 0542.00 W
Area : Mull
Tonnage : 203 gross.
Draught : 12.1 ft.
Depth :   metres

The *River Tay*, (ex-*Henry Butcher*), was a trawler built by Hall Russell in 1918. She went aground in 1943 in almost exactly the same place as the *Dartmouth*, but got off the rocks by dumping the coal for her boiler. I suspect the *Alexander* subsequently attempted to recover the coal and suffered the same fate. The *Ballista* made an attempt to recover the coal in 1973, and history repeated itself once more!

The *Alexander* will probably be the vessel upon which the *Ballista* sits today.

ALEXANDER

Wreck No : 188
Latitude : 56 30 10 N
Decca Lat : 5630.17 N
Location : Rubha an Ridire, Sound of Mull
Type : Puffer
Length :   ft.   **Beam :**   ft.
How Sunk : Ran aground? Raised?

Date Sunk : 1970
Longitude : 05 42 00 W
Decca Long : 0542.00 W
Area : Mull
Tonnage :   gross
Draught :   ft.
Depth : 10 metres

I suspect the *Alexander* was attempting to recover the coal which was dumped by the *River Tay* while trying to free herself from the rocks above the *Dartmouth*. The *Alexander* went aground and sank in the same place, and may therefore, be the vessel lying beneath the *Ballista*.

A search through the files of the *Oban Times* may provide further information to confirm this theory. (Try the 1970 file). Another suggestion is that one of the wrecks beneath the *Ballista* may be a vessel named *Ardfern*, possibly sunk in 1950.

DARTMOUTH

Wreck No : 189
Latitude : 56 30 12 N
Decca Lat : 5630.20 N
Location : SW side of Rubha an Ridire
Type : 32 gun frigate

Date Sunk : 09 10 1690
Longitude : 05 41 59 W
Decca Long : 0541.98 W
Area : Mull
Tonnage : 260 gross.

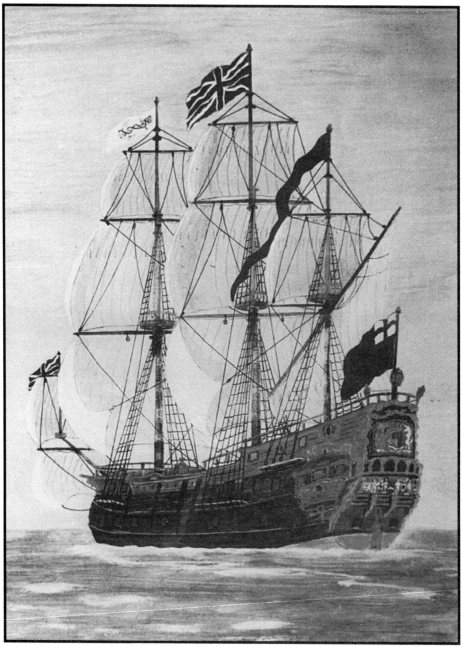

HMS Dartmouth
(*From a painting in the Author's collection*)

Length : 86.0 ft.   **Beam :** 25.0 ft.   **Draught :** 12.0 ft.
How Sunk : Ran aground   **Depth :** 10 metres

The English 32-gun 5th Rate frigate *Dartmouth* was driven ashore in a storm with the loss of Captain Pottinger and 132 men. There were apparently about six survivors. In 1690 she was part of the English force attempting to suppress the Jacobites, whose stronghold of Duart Castle overlooks this wreck site.

Worm-eaten timbers, (now very light), iron cannon and mortar shells have been found. Other artefacts recovered from this historic wreck are in the Royal Scottish Museum of Antiquities in Edinburgh. The remains lie in 10 - 30 ft of water.

BUITENZORG

Wreck No : 190   **Date Sunk :** 14 01 1941
Latitude : 56 30 15 N   **Longitude :** 05 44 28 W
Decca Lat : 5630.25 N   **Decca Long :** 0544.47 W
Location : Sound of Mull   **Area :** Mull
Type : Steamship   **Tonnage :** 7073 gross.
Length : 446.5 ft.   **Beam :** 54.3 ft.   **Draught :** 34.2 ft.
How Sunk : Ran aground   **Depth :** 77 metres

The Dutch vessel *Buitenzorg* sank at 16.12 hrs on 14th January 1941, minutes after striking rocks off Grey Isle. She was en route from Calcutta to Dundee via Oban, where she joined a convoy heading north-about around Scotland for the North Sea. Part of the cargo consisted of bales of latex.

An attempt to recover them with grabs and underwater video cameras was made around 1987. Many of the bales were washed ashore on the Mull and Morvern coasts, and one of the latex bales lay ashore at North Ledaig caravan site, Ardmucknish Bay in 1989.

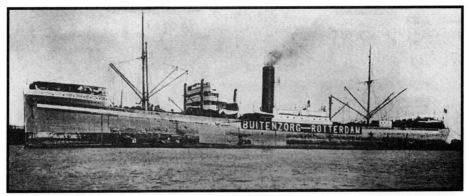

The Buitenzorg *(Photograph courtesy of the World Ship Society)*

The *Buitenzorg* was built in Flushing in 1918, and registered in Rotterdam. She had a cruiser stern and three decks.

An eyewitness to the sinking told me that she sank by the stern, and suggested that tin may have been part of the cargo. Salvage efforts lasting several weeks suggest that there must have been something of value to recover.

The wreck is probably fairly broken up by explosives used during the salvage attempts. Her position has been described as 155° 9.2 cables from Ardtornish light and also given as 563018N 054424W.

SHACKLETON AIRCRAFT

Wreck No : 191	**Date Sunk :** 11 12 1953
Latitude : 56 30 25 N	**Longitude :** 05 44 05 W
Decca Lat : 5630.42 N	**Decca Long :** 0545.08 W
Location : Sound of Mull	**Area :** Mull
Type : Aircraft	**Tonnage :** gross
Length : ft. **Beam :** ft.	**Draught :** ft.
How Sunk : Exploded in flight over the Sound of Mull	**Depth :** 60 metres

A Coastal Command Shackleton aircraft on a training flight from Ballykelly, Northern Ireland, was lost in Scallastle Bay on Friday 11th December 1953. At 5.30 pm, Duncan Campbell, a farmer at Craignure, heard an aircraft engine stalling, followed by a terrific explosion. He and his wife rushed to the window and saw lights like flares on the water. George Clyne, the Craignure ferryman searched between Craignure and Lochaline in his 15 ft launch, assisted by the MacBrayne vessel *Lochnell*, which left Oban within 20 minutes, and the *Lochbuie*, from Tobermory. Nothing was found on the waters of the Sound that night, but next day, Mr. Clyne found a partly submerged body off Garmony Point, Mull, and a second body was found on the Morvern shore, about 3 miles North of Lochaline, by the RAF Mountain Rescue team from Kinloss, who were operating on that side of the Sound. The anti-submarine frigate HMS *Volage* made wide sweeps of the Sound, while some of her crew also searched the hills around Craignure.

Wreckage from the aircraft was found at several points on both sides of the Sound, and a rubber dinghy was found close to the spot where the first body had been discovered. Two helicopters later joined the search, but the bodies of the other eight members of the crew were never found. A conical buoy used to mark the position of some of the wreckage, but it is no longer there, and as this area has been worked by scallop dredgers, there is probably little, if any, of the aircraft left intact, particularly as it would seem the aircraft blew up in flight.

An in-line aircraft engine complete with propeller with unbent blades has been found in Scallastle Bay, along with scattered aluminium wreckage from the aircraft. George Foster, the Lochaline-based scallop diver, found this engine in about 25 metres, to the South of the position given.

JANE SHEARER

Wreck No : 192
Latitude : 56 30 30 N PA
Decca Lat : 5630.50 N
Location : Off Garmony Pt, Scallastle Bay
Type : Brigantine
Length : ft.   **Beam :** ft.
How Sunk : Foundered

Date Sunk : 28 12 1879
Longitude : 05 44 00 W PA
Decca Long : 0544.00 W
Area : Mull
Tonnage :   gross
Draught : ft.
Depth : 18 metres

During a ferocious storm on Sunday night, 28th December 1879, a brigantine was seen riding at anchor in Scallastle Bay, but next morning all that could be seen were the tips of her masts. On 7th February, the owners of the *Jane Shearer* visited the scene and found a sail with the name *George Frew, Sailmaker* floating near the surface. This evidence enabled the vessel to be identified as the *Jane Shearer* which was six weeks overdue from Liverpool to Arisaig with a cargo of coal. Her crew of four were lost. George Foster has recovered the compass.

EVELYN ROSE

Wreck No : 193
Latitude : 56 31 08 N
Decca Lat : 5631.13 N
Location : 15 yds N of Ardtornish Point
Type : Trawler
Length : 138.5 ft.   **Beam :** 23.7 ft.
How Sunk : Ran aground

Date Sunk : 31 12 1954
Longitude : 05 45 24 W
Decca Long : 0545.40 W
Area : Mull
Tonnage : 327 gross.
Draught : 12.8 ft.
Depth : 60 metres

The trawler *Evelyn Rose* (ex-*William Jackson*), built by Cochrane's of Selby in 1918, and owned by the Cevic Steam Fishing Co. of Fleetwood, was en route from Fleetwood to Faröe, when at about 1.00 am on New Years Eve 1954, she struck the shore North of Ardtornish Point, having taken a route to the wrong side of the light. All on board were asleep, except the skipper and two deckhands who were on watch. Before a lifeboat could be launched, she slipped astern off the steeply sloping rocks and went right down into 20 fathoms of water. Two survivors from the crew of 14 were more or less washed off the deck and managed to reach the shore at Ardtornish Point. Two bodies were subsequently washed ashore, but the remaining 10 were never found.

This version of the events came mainly from the *Oban Times*, and appears to suggest that the wreck must lie in Ardtornish Bay, probably between the lighthouse and the *pier*, (which is, in reality, stone steps down the rocks on the shore), but no trace of the wreck was found during a fairly thorough search of that area by echo sounder down to 90 metres. I have heard a rumour that she lies in 50 metres off Rubha an t-Sasunnaich at the South east of Ardtornish Bay, some half a mile E by S of Ardtornish Light.

The transcript of the court of enquiry revealed that she was proceeding North west up the Sound in darkness, and was being navigated by radar. Ardtornish Point, which is low-lying, was obscured on the radar screen by the hills and high cliffs a few hundred yards inshore of the point. This led to an overestimation of the distance to the light, and she struck the rocks just 15 yards North west of the lighthouse. The court of enquiry concluded that she is in, but probably only just in, the red sector of Ardtornish Light.

It is claimed that she has been seen on an echo sounder, lying almost vertically, (like the *Rondo*), with her bows in at least 60 metres, and the rest of the vessel extending down to even deeper depths. The slope underwater at this side of the lighthouse is much steeper than at the Ardtornish Bay side of the light, with unusual geological rock formations in the form of huge cubes of rock half the size of a house.

The *Evelyn Rose* made several crossings between Dunkirk and Ramsgate during the evacuation of Dunkirk in 1940. During her last crossing she was so badly damaged that she had to be beached at Ramsgate. After being repaired she was used by the Admiralty as a mine-sweeper until released in 1946.

JANET

Wreck No : 194	**Date Sunk :** 29 10 1977
Latitude : 56 31 12 N	**Longitude :** 05 37 06 W
Decca Lat : 5631.20 N	**Decca Long :** 0537.10 W
Location : Camas Gorm, Loch Linnhe	**Area :** Mull
Type : MFV	**Tonnage :** gross
Length : 40.0 ft. **Beam :** ft.	**Draught :** ft.
How Sunk : Ran aground	**Depth :** metres

This position is adjacent to the shore 2.5 miles ENE of Rubha an Ridire.

CESSNA 150 AIRCRAFT

Wreck No : 195	**Date Sunk :** 24 12 1975
Latitude : 56 31 22 N	**Longitude :** 05 51 12 W
Decca Lat : 5631.37 N	**Decca Long :** 0551.20 W
Location : NE of entrance to Fishnish Bay	**Area :** Mull
Type : Aircraft	**Tonnage :** gross
Length : ft. **Beam :** ft.	**Draught :** ft.
How Sunk : Crashed into the sea	**Depth :** 25 metres

A *Cessna 150* aircraft from Glenforsa airstrip on Mull went missing late on 24/12/1975. A search was carried out, but no trace of the aircraft could be found on land, and it was presumed to have crashed into the sea.

Four months later, on 21st April, 1976, the undamaged body of the pilot, Peter Gibbs, was found 400 ft up a hillside near Pennygown Quarry, about one mile East of the airstrip. His clothing bore no trace of sea water, and he had apparently died of exposure, rather than having fallen from the aircraft. Did the rain and snow during that winter wash away all traces of salt? On October 5th 1976, a tyre and partially inflated inner tube, positively identified as from that aircraft, were found on the shore of the Sound of Mull at Kentallen, Mull.

In 1987, about 12 years after its disappearance, George Foster, a scallop diver, came across the wreckage of the aircraft 300 yards off the shore, near the rocks at the North east of the entrance to Fishnish Bay in the Sound of Mull. How did the pilot get from the aircraft in the Sound to a hillside on Mull? Presumably he landed the *Cessna* on the water, was able to get out of the aircraft before it sank, swam ashore in a confused state, not knowing exactly where he was in the dark, (no mean feat in itself!), and set off to find civilisation, only to die of exposure on a remote hillside.

If the above scenario is even partially correct, he would have had to cross the main Tobermory to Craignure road in order to get to where his body was found. Why did he leave the road and climb a mountain? Did he not realise he had crossed the narrow road in the darkness? The *Great Mull Air Mystery* was the subject of several television programmes, all produced before the aircraft was found, hence the suppositions and conjectures made at that time were based on incomplete evidence.

JOHANNA

Wreck No : 196	**Date Sunk :** 29 04 1968
Latitude : 56 31 52 N	**Longitude :** 05 46 57 W
Decca Lat : 5631.87 N	**Decca Long :** 0546.95 W
Location : 200 yds SSE of Lochaline Pier	**Area :** Mull
Type : Trawler	**Tonnage :** gross
Length : 32.0 ft. **Beam :** ft.	**Draught :** ft.
How Sunk :	**Depth :** 100 metres

Johanna was a wooden fishing vessel.

LOGAN

Wreck No : 197	**Date Sunk :** 15 12 1961
Latitude : 56 31 55 N	**Longitude :** 05 46 58 W
Decca Lat : 5631.92 N	**Decca Long :** 0546.97 W
Location : 100 yds SSE of Lochaline Pier	**Area :** Mull
Type : Puffer	**Tonnage :** 98 gross.
Length : ft. **Beam :** ft.	**Draught :** ft.
How Sunk : Foundered	**Depth :** 100 metres

While proceeding up the Sound of Mull, en route from Troon to Skye with a cargo of

105 tons of coal, the puffer *Logan* sprang a leak near the stern. In a force 7 to 8 gale off Craignure, she became unmanageable, with her engine room awash. Five distress rockets were fired, but not seen. The crew's sixth, (and last!), rocket was spotted by the Oban-bound fishing boat *Artemis* which took the *Logan* in tow to Lochaline pier, where she was made fast. Fort William Fire Brigade was summoned, and pumped water out of the vessel for some hours until it was realised that the task was hopeless, as the *Logan* continued to settle in the water, and was obviously going to sink. Despite the 100 metres depth of water at the pier, the *Logan* was moved about 100 yards away, where she sank in deep water.

JOHN PRESTON

Wreck No : 198	**Date Sunk :** 02 12 1882
Latitude : 56 32 00 N	**Longitude :** 05 48 16 W
Decca Lat : 5632.00 N	**Decca Long :** 0548.27 W
Location : Rubha Dearg, Morvern shore	**Area :** Mull
Type : Schooner	**Tonnage :** 116 gross.
Length : ft. **Beam :** ft.	**Draught :** ft.
How Sunk : Ran aground	**Depth :** 21 metres

The remains of a wooden vessel with a tightly-packed cargo of slates lies in 21 metres, about 100 yds off the shore at Rubha Dearg, which is ⅔ mile west of Lochaline pier at National Grid Reference NM 661445.

Two white-painted squares on the rocks on the shore are an aid to finding the wreck which is about 100 yds directly out from that mark. The bottom drops off steeply just beyond the wreck, which is known as *The Slate Wreck*. Very little remains of the vessel itself.

On 2nd December 1882 the 116 tons net schooner *John Preston* of Caernarvon, with a cargo of slates from Port Dinorwic to Fraserburgh anchored in Scallastle Bay, to shelter from a south-westerly storm, Force 10. The force of the storm tore her from her mooring and blew her on to the rocks at the Morvern side of the Sound of Mull near Lochaline. Her crew were all saved. The tops of her masts showed above water for a time after she sank.

RONDO

Wreck No : 199	**Date Sunk :** 25 01 1935
Latitude : 56 32 17 N	**Longitude :** 05 54 40 W
Decca Lat : 5632.28 N	**Decca Long :** 0554.67 W
Location : Eileanan Glasa, Sound of Mull	**Area :** Mull
Type : Steamship	**Tonnage :** 2363 gross.
Length : 250.8 ft. **Beam :** 42.0 ft.	**Draught :** 24.0 ft.
How Sunk : Ran aground	**Depth :** 5 metres

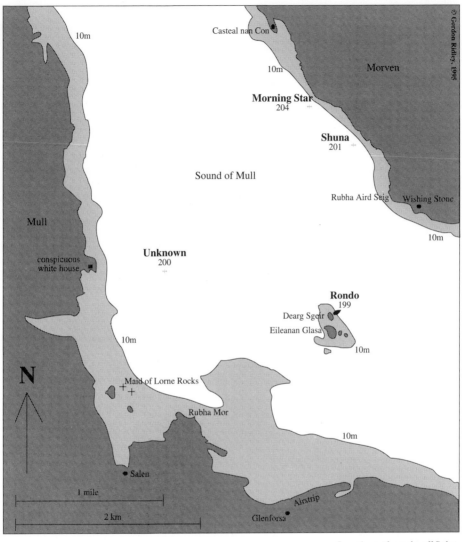

Locations of wrecks off Salen

The Norwegian steamship *Rondo* was sheltering in Aros Bay in the Sound of Mull, en route from Glasgow to Oslo when her anchor dragged, and she was driven on to Eileanan Glasa (Green Isle), in the middle of the Sound. She rode right up on to the low-lying rocky island, demolished the lighthouse, and remained perched on the rock in its place. The fishery cruiser *Minna* and two Fleetwood trawlers failed to pull her off, and after a fortnight her crew were taken off and she was abandoned. For several weeks thereafter, salvage work progressed until, with her centre of gravity affected by the

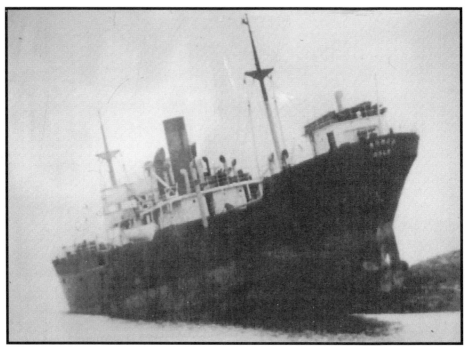

The Rondo *aground on Eileanan Glasa. (Photograph: Author's collection)*

salvage work, and the further effect of the waves, she began to rock back and forth. The salvage crew then moved on to the rock, working aboard by day and camping on the rock at night. Eventually, she slipped off the rock and down the steep slope at the other side until her bows came to rest on the bottom at 55 metres, with her stern still only 5 metres below the surface!

It is possible to swim right under the wreck through a gap between the rock and the keel at about 20 metres. An anchor lies on the rock, adjacent to the port side, at the gap. Her propeller lies amongst the kelp in shallow water at the edge of the rock about 25 yards to the North west of the stern, and is visible at low water. With excellent visibility and a profusion of marine life, this is a most spectacular wreck to dive on.

UNKNOWN - PRE-1947

Wreck No : 200
Latitude : 56 32 22 N
Decca Lat : 5632.37 N
Location : 2 miles N of Salen Pier
Type :
Length :   ft.   **Beam :**   ft.

Date Sunk : Pre - 1947
Longitude : 05 56 50 W
Decca Long : 0556.83 W
Area : Mull
Tonnage :   gross
Draught : ft.

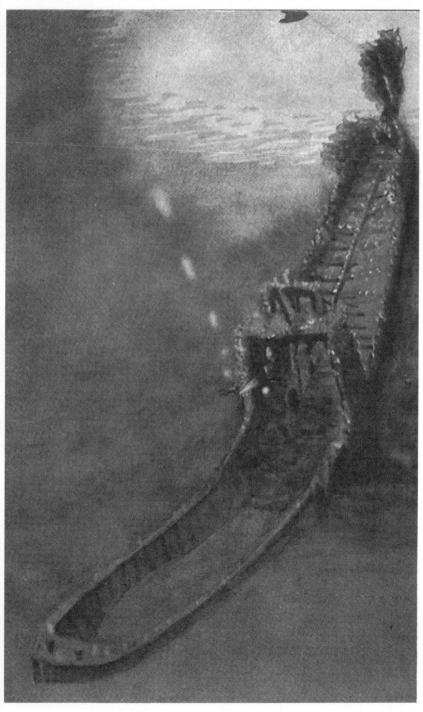

An
artist's
impression
of the
Rondo
(Painting
courtesy
of Robert
Sproul
Cran)

How Sunk :   **Depth :** 32 metres

A wreck was first reported in this position in 1947. During her fifty years of service from 1908-1958, the MacBrayne steamer *Lochinvar* ran into a fishing boat anchored off Craignure in fog, and cut through the anchored vessel with her bow. Although it is hardly appropriate to describe this position as *off Craignure*, this is the nearest *Unknown* wreck I am aware of, and might possibly be that fishing boat.

The *Lochinvar* apparently suffered little more than scratched paint, which suggests the fishing boat had a wooden hull. There was no loss of life. In 1943, the *Lochinvar* also ran into the *Golden Gift* in Oban Bay and sank her, again with no loss of life.

SHUNA

Wreck No : 201   **Date Sunk :** 09 05 1913
Latitude : 56 33 24 N   **Longitude :** 05 54 48 W
Decca Lat : 5633.40 N   **Decca Long :** 0554.80 W
Location : 1½ miles SE of Casteal nan Con   **Area :** Mull
Type : Steamship   **Tonnage :** 1426 gross.
Length : 240.9 ft.   **Beam :** 35.2 ft.   **Draught :** 16.5 ft.
How Sunk : Ran aground   **Depth :** 23 metres

Shuna was a British steamship built for Glen & Co. in 1909 by A. Vuick, Holland, storm, and with water coming in, tried to make for Tobermory. When it was realised that the rate of water ingress was greater than her pumps could cope with, she was instead, run towards the nearest shore to be beached. When the fore part of the vessel was beached, the seas were breaking over the bridge. Her anchors were dropped, and she was also made fast with a hawser to the shore at a headland named Rhu Riddrie. (Iron eyes set in the rocks are still visible on the shore). The crew of 18 got off in three boats about two hours before the hawser broke, the hatches blew off, and the *Shuna* sank with a loud report. The shipwrecked crew were taken aboard the MacBrayne steamer *Chieftain*, at 5.00 am, and landed at Tobermory.

The wreck was found intact by a scallop diver in late 1990, sitting upright on a level sandy bottom at 32 metres, about 150 yds off the Morvern shore, in a bay about 1.5 miles South east of Casteal nan Con (Castle of the Dogs), and a little over half a mile North west of the Wishing Stone. Depth to the deck is 23 metres. The engine plate, recovered in July 1991, gives the name of the engine builder as G. T. Grey, Holburn Works, South Shields, Engine No. 426. Her holds are full of coal, and the outside of the wreck is covered in a beautiful profusion of marine growths, although inside the wreck is a thick layer of silt. She can be dived at any state of the tide, and unusually for the Sound of Mull tidal streams are not a problem.

By July 1991, salvage operations by divers had demolished the wheelhouse. The spare compass, still in its wooden box, was recovered that month. The main compass, bridge telegraph, and all of the portholes are now gone. The spare propeller lies horizontally on the deck near the stern, with a spare anchor immediately adjacent on the starboard side. Her port bow anchor chain runs down to the sand.

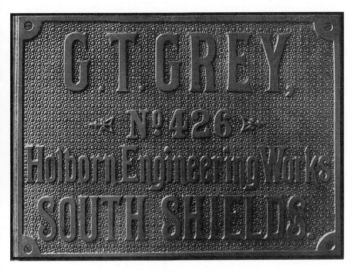

Left: The maker's plate from the engine, recovered from the wreck of the Shuna. *(Photograph: Bob Baird).*

Below: The location of and transits for the Shuna

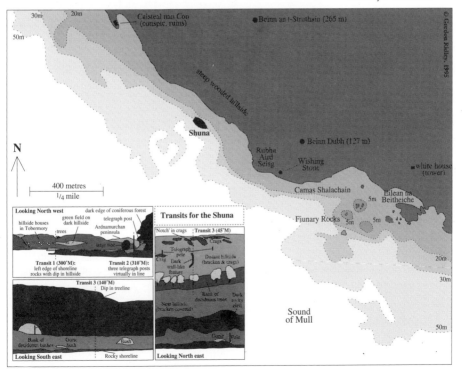

WHITE HEAD

Wreck No : 202
Latitude : 56 34 18 N PA
Decca Lat : 5634.30 N
Location : Ardnacross Point
Type : Steamship
Length : 247.5 ft.   **Beam :** 29.7 ft.
How Sunk : Ran aground

Date Sunk : 1902
Longitude : 05 58 53 W PA
Decca Long : 0558.88 W
Area : Mull
Tonnage : 1145 gross.
Draught : 16.5 ft.
Depth :   metres

The 1145 tons gross iron steamship *White Head* was stranded on Ardnacroish (Ardnacross) Point in the Sound of Mull in 1902. The vessel had a cargo of coal. This point is shown on the Ordnance Survey map as Rubh'a Ghlaisich, and lies between Salen and Tobermory, directly across the Sound of Mull from Rhemore.

HISPANIA

Wreck No : 203
Latitude : 56 34 51 N
Decca Lat : 5634.85 N
Location : Sound of Mull
Type : Steamship
Length : 266.8 ft.   **Beam :** 37.3 ft.
How Sunk : Ran aground

Date Sunk : 18 12 1954
Longitude : 05 59 13 W
Decca Long : 0559.22 W
Area : Mull
Tonnage : 1337 gross.
Draught : 15.5 ft.
Depth : 23 metres

The Swedish steamship *Hispania*, built in 1912, struck Sgeir More reef head on in heavy weather, during a voyage from Liverpool to Varberg, near Gothenburg. By running astern, she came off the reef with a 25° list to port, and the crew of 21 took to the boats before she sank, except for Captain Dahn who could not be persuaded to leave, and went down with the ship. The position has also been recorded as 563447N, 055913W. Her cargo of steel was recovered during the 1950s.

The least depth to her bows, which are pointing towards the South east is 15 metres. This substantially intact wreck, sitting upright on the bottom, with a slight list to starboard, and covered in marine life, is considered by many to be one of the finest wrecks to dive in Scottish waters. The wreck is usually buoyed, but can be found by taking a line from Glenmorven Cottage through the red can buoy off Rubh an Sean Chaisteal. Follow this line for approximately 30 yds towards the shore, and you should be over the wreck.

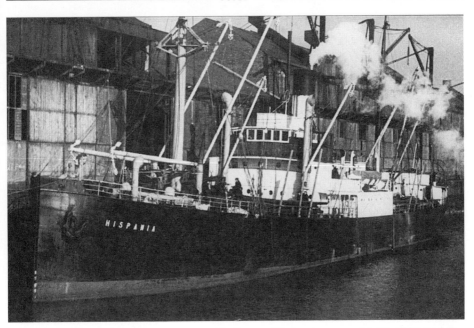

The Hispania (Photograph courtesy of the World Ship Society)

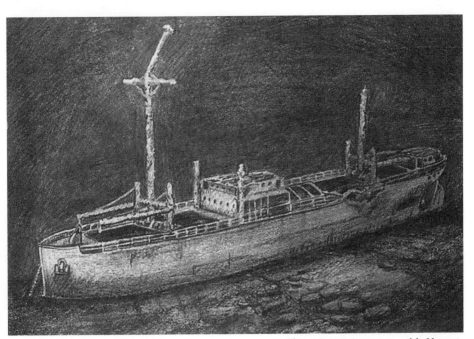

Above: An artist's impression of the Hispania
(Painting courtesy of Robert Sproul Cran)

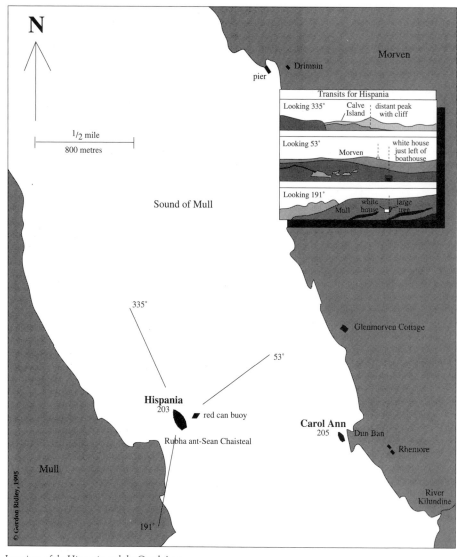

Locations of the Hispania *and the* Carol Ann

MORNING STAR

Wreck No : 204
Latitude : 56 34 57 N
Decca Lat : 5634.95 N
Location : Kilundine Point, Sound of Mull
Type : Fishing Boat

Date Sunk : 16 04 1973
Longitude : 05 57 34 W
Decca Long : 0557.57 W
Area : Mull
Tonnage :   gross

Length : ft.　　**Beam :** ft.　　**Draught :** ft.
How Sunk : Ran aground　　　　　　**Depth :** 7 metres

The wooden-hulled Fraserburgh fishing boat *Morning Star* suffered engine failure, and was being towed to Oban for repair by the *Golden Quest*, another Fraserburgh fishing boat. In the early hours of Monday April 16, 1973, both vessels went aground on the rocks at Kilundine Point in the Sound of Mull. The *Golden Quest* managed to free herself and took on board the six crewmen from the *Morning Star*, which could not be freed, and became a total loss.

The wreck charted at 563457N, 055734W in 0.2 metres, very close inshore on the South west corner of Dun Ban ledge has been assumed to be the *Morning Star*, but the very broken up, kelp-covered wreckage there consists mainly of steel hull plating which is not consistent with the wooden construction of the *Morning Star*. The bows of this wreck are reported to lie in 7 metres, pointing North east.

Part of a wooden hull which looks very like that of a fishing boat, along with some steel parts, are visible on the shore about ¼ mile to the South east at 563444N, 055712W, and I strongly suggest this to be from the *Morning Star*, and would expect to find the rest of the wreck lying under water close by that location. Kilundine Point is not named on the chart, nor on the Ordnance Survey map, but would seem to be more appropriately applicable to the promontory at Casteal nan Con, or the point mid way between Dun Ban and Casteal nan Con. It is hardly the most obvious choice of words to describe Dun Ban or An Corr Eilean.

There are persistent rumours of another wreck near here with a cargo of sewing machines and bicycles. I have been aware of these rumours since 1979, and have personally spoken to an aged local who claimed in 1991 to have seen her sink during the war, but was unable to obtain a precise location.

CAROL ANN

Wreck No : 205　　　　　　**Date Sunk :** 18 11 1971
Latitude : 56 35 02 N　　　　**Longitude :** 05 57 38 W
Decca Lat : 5635.03 N　　　　**Decca Long :** 0557.63 W
Location : Off Rehmore, NW of Lochaline　　**Area :** Mull
Type : Fishing Boat　　　　　**Tonnage :** gross
Length : 56.0 ft.　　**Beam :** ft.　　**Draught :** ft.
How Sunk : Ran aground　　　　**Depth :** metres

The three man crew of the Belfast fishing boat *Carol Ann* swam ashore when their boat struck Rhemore Point, two miles from Drimnin late on Wednesday night, 17th November 1971, while en route from Campbeltown to Tobermory. Two of the crew were strong swimmers, and assisted their non-swimming friend, who supported himself on a suitcase, which was the only article they were able to save. Richard Shaw, the farm manager at Drimnin Estate was returning from Lochaline when he saw a torch being waved in a field below the road. On stopping to investigate, he was surprised to find a pyjama-clad figure who told him about the wreck.

Mr. Shaw took the three men to his home where they had a bath and were given beds for the night. Next morning he kitted them out with clothes of his own and took them by car to Lochaline. They hoped to return with diving gear to investigate the possibility of refloating their boat, which is in shallow water - the mast showed above the surface - about 6 miles North west of Lochaline, between An Corr Eilean and the shore in about 4 metres.

She is visible above the surface at low water, has an iron or steel hull, and her bows point East towards the shore.

STRATHBEG

Wreck No : 206	**Date Sunk :** 03 05 1984
Latitude : 56 36 44 N	**Longitude :** 06 02 00 W
Decca Lat : 5636.73 N	**Decca Long :** 0602.00 W
Location : Calve Sound	**Area :** Mull
Type : MFV	**Tonnage :** gross
Length : 70.0 ft. **Beam :** ft.	**Draught :** ft.
How Sunk : Foundered at moorings	**Depth :** metres

The fishing vessel *Strathbeg* sank at her moorings during a gale on 3rd May 1984. The tops of her masts were visible above the surface at low water.

LOHADA

Wreck No : 207	**Date Sunk :**
Latitude : 56 37 02 N	**Longitude :** 06 02 35 W
Decca Lat : 5637.03 N	**Decca Long :** 0602.58 W
Location : Calve Island	**Area :** Mull
Type :	**Tonnage :** gross
Length : ft. **Beam :** ft.	**Draught :** ft.
How Sunk : Ran aground?	**Depth :** 7 metres

This has been reported to be the wreck of a small iron or steel vessel with a clipper bow. There is some doubt about the name - possibly due to somebody being unable to decipher someone else's handwriting? The position given is very close to the *Pelican*, and the description of the wreck is also similar to that vessel.

Are there really two wrecks here, or are the *Lohada* and *Pelican* one and the same wreck? *Lohada* is the name commonly used in the Tobermory area for this wreck. It may possibly be a phonetic corruption of *Lowlander*, which is another name that has been suggested, or even of *Bondja* which sank outside Tobermory harbour in 1946, about a mile away from this position. On the other hand, a wreck was reported close by at 563654N, 060230W in 1884.

PELICAN

Wreck No : 208

Latitude : 56 37 14 N

Decca Lat : 5637.23 N

Location : SW end Calve Island, Tobermory

Type : Steamship

Length : 205.6 ft.   **Beam :** 28.3 ft.

How Sunk : Ran aground

Date Sunk : 05 12 1895

Longitude : 06 02 50 W

Decca Long : 0602.83 W

Area : Mull

Tonnage : 638 gross.

Draught : 15.8 ft.

Depth : 15 metres

This wreck was first located in 1957 at the head of the inlet between Calve Island and Mull. Permission was sought to disperse the wreck with explosives on 1st June 1961, and the stern section does seem to have blasted apart.

There appears to be a certain amount of confusion over the name of this wreck. She is sometimes, (incorrectly), referred to as the *Anna Bhan*, which seems to me to be a phonetic corruption of the name *Pelican*.

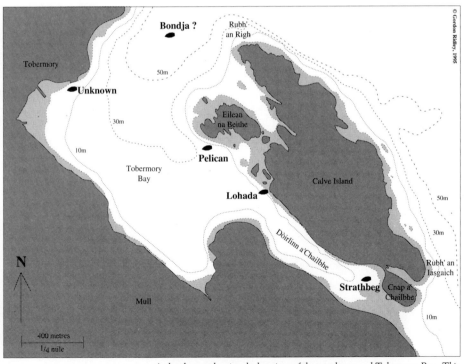

A sketch map showing the locations of the wrecks around Tobermory Bay. This will shed light on the confusion over the Lohada, Pelican *and* Anna Bhan.

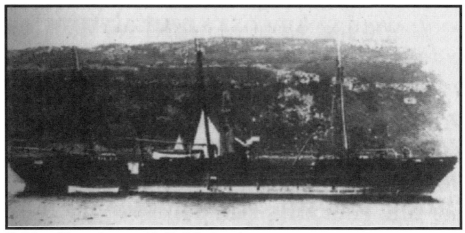

The Pelican *(Photograph courtesy of the World Ship Society).*

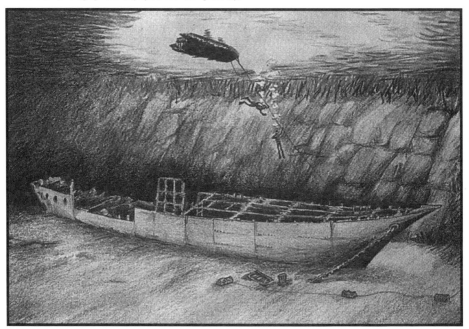

An artist's impression of the Pelican, *though this was originally thought to be the* Lowlander
(Painting courtesy of Robert Sproul Cran)

She was built in Cork in 1850, with an iron hull fastened to a wooden frame, and had a clipper bow. In 1888 she was bought by MacBrayne for a service to Iceland, but by 1895 was laid up, first at Portree, then in Tobermory Bay as a coal hulk. During a NNW Force 10 storm on 5th December 1895, she broke from her moorings and was driven on to rocks at the South west of Calve Island at high water. The steamers *Handa* and *Fingal* of the West Highland Fleet visited the scene of the wreck, but for their own safety, had to leave this hazardous location. As the tide receded, the *Pelican* gradually listed to starboard, slipped from the rocks and became totally submerged. The only thing on board was a quantity of bunker coal. The position has been recorded by the Hydrographic Dept. as 563656N, 060228W.

UNKNOWN - PRE-1932

Wreck No : 209	Date Sunk : Pre - 1932
Latitude : 56 37 21 N	Longitude : 06 03 53 W
Decca Lat : 5637.35 N	Decca Long : 0603.88 W
Location : Alongside Tobermory Pier	Area : Mull
Type : Lighter	Tonnage : gross
Length : ft. Beam : ft.	Draught : ft.
How Sunk :	Depth : metres

A small wooden vessel apparently sank alongside Tobermory pier, and must have been there in 1932. The pier in those days was the one in the centre of the harbour, not the one at the north of the bay, presently used by MacBrayne vessels. At low water, the area around the old pier dries out, and there is no longer any sign of a wreck. The wreck which was there might possibly have been the *Inchmurren*.

BONDJA

Wreck No : 210	Date Sunk : 18 08 1946
Latitude : 56 37 48 N PA	Longitude : 06 03 12 W PA
Decca Lat : 5637.80 N	Decca Long : 0603.20 W
Location : Outside Tobermory harbour	Area : Mull
Type : Yacht	Tonnage : 15 gross.
Length : ft. Beam : ft.	Draught : ft.
How Sunk : Collision with *John Gatling*	Depth : 71 metres

The 15 ton yacht *Bondja* was approaching Tobermory harbour at about 4.00 am on Sunday 18th August 1946 after a cruise around the West Coast and Western Islands, when it was in collision with the Fleetwood trawler *John Gatling*, which had left Tobermory a few minutes earlier, bound for the West Coast fishing grounds.

The *Bondja* sank almost immediately, the skipper of the yacht and the navigator managing to climb aboard the *John Gatling* before their boat sank. The four others on board the yacht were asleep below. Three of them were thrown into the sea, and succeeded in getting into the yacht's dinghy which had floated free as the *Bondja* sank. The *John Gatling* hove to immediately the impact was felt, and lowered a boat, but despite an intensive search, the one remaining member of the yacht's crew could not be found. The *John Gatling* took the survivors to Oban.

CRANE

Wreck No : 211
Date Sunk : 25 02 1908
Latitude : 56 38 48 N PA
Longitude : 06 01 18 W PA
Decca Lat : 5638.80 N
Decca Long : 0601.30 W
Location : Big Stirk, Sound of Mull
Area : Mull
Type : Steamship
Tonnage : 209 gross.
Length : 118.2 ft.   **Beam :** 21.5 ft.
Draught : 11.2 ft.
How Sunk : Ran aground /refloated
Depth :   metres

The Grimsby steam trawler *Crane* was built in 1902 by Cooper of Hull, engine by C. D. Holmes of Hull. She ran aground on the Stirks, off Tobermory on 25th February 1908. The crew were saved, and the vessel was refloated.

MAID OF HARRIS

Wreck No : 212
Date Sunk : 10 09 1974
Latitude : 56 39 22 N
Longitude : 06 07 37 W
Decca Lat : 5639.37 N
Decca Long : 0607.62 W
Location : Just E of Ardmore Point, Mull
Area : Mull
Type : Trawler
Tonnage :   gross
Length :   ft.   **Beam :**   ft.
Draught : ft.
How Sunk : Ran aground
Depth :   metres

The *Maid of Harris* went aground just East of Ardmore Point and stuck fast on the rocks. Her radio call for help was answered by the prawn fishing vessel *Ros Guill* which attempted to pull her off, but became stuck on the rocks herself. The *Maid of Harris* was so close in that the crew could get ashore.

ROS GUILL

Wreck No : 213
Date Sunk : 10 09 1974
Latitude : 56 39 42 N
Longitude : 06 07 12 W
Decca Lat : 5639.70 N
Decca Long : 0607.20 W
Location : 0.4 miles 35° Ardmore Point
Area : Mull
Type : Trawler
Tonnage : 21 gross.
Length :   ft.   **Beam :**   ft.
Draught : ft.
How Sunk : Ran aground
Depth :   metres

The prawn fishing vessel *Ros Guill* (OB63) went aground just East of Ardmore Point, the most northerly point of Mull, while attempting to haul the *Maid of Harris* off the rocks where she had gone aground. The two vessels were stranded on the rocks, touching by the bows. Other boats arrived on the scene and in their efforts to pull the *Ros Guill* clear, her stern opened up, and she sank into 53 fathoms (96 metres), according to the *Oban Times*.

RIANT

Wreck No : 214
Latitude : 56 40 30 N PA
Decca Lat : 5640.50 N
Location : Loch Sunart
Type : Trawler
Length : ft.   **Beam :** ft.
How Sunk : Foundered

Date Sunk : 25 01 1940
Longitude : 05 50 30 W PA
Decca Long : 0550.50 W
Area : Mull
Tonnage : 95 gross.
Draught : ft.
Depth : metres

HMS *Riant* was a motor trawler built in 1919. She was hired by the Admiralty for use as a mine-sweeper in November 1939, and foundered in a storm on 25th January 1940. All on board were lost

The position given, 564030N 055030W PA, is close ashore ¼ mile North west of Eilean nan Gillean on the North shore of Loch Sunart.

She has also been reported to have sunk on 27th January 1940 at 554000N 055000W PA, which is close ashore about a mile North of Tayinloan. Note that these positions are almost identical, apart from one being recorded as 55° North and the other as 56° North. This suggests a typographical error in one of them - but which one?

Both of the above positions are close ashore, which would tend to suggest that she was lost through running aground rather than foundering.

ELI

Wreck No : 215
Latitude : 56 09 30 N PA
Decca Lat : 5609.50 N
Location : 144° 12 miles Skerryvore Light
Type : Motor vessel
Length : 380.8 ft.   **Beam :** 54.2 ft.
How Sunk : Bombed

Date Sunk : 10 09 1940
Longitude : 06 54 00 W PA
Decca Long : 0654.00 W
Area : Mull
Tonnage : 4332 gross.
Draught : 24.5 ft.
Depth : metres

The Norwegian steamship *Eli*, built in 1931, was bombed and sunk by German aircraft on 10th September 1940, 144° 12 miles from Skerryvore. She was not located during a search in 1967.

ROSEBUD II

Wreck No : 216
Latitude : 56 14 00 N PA
Decca Lat : 5614.00 N
Location : On Torran Rocks, SW Mull
Type : Trawler
Length : ft.   **Beam :** ft.

Date Sunk : 14 12 1970
Longitude : 06 25 00 W PA
Decca Long : 0625.00 W
Area : Mull
Tonnage : gross
Draught : ft.

How Sunk : Ran aground   **Depth :**   metres

All vessels in the area of the Ross of Mull were alerted at 8.30 pm on Monday 14th December 1970 when a Birmingham radio ham picked up a Mayday from the Burghead fishing boat *Rosebud II* which had grounded on the Torran Rocks in a strong South west wind. Fishing boats already in the vicinity, and others which cast off from the railway pier in Oban, headed for the scene to search in the darkness for the crew of seven, including two brothers, who had taken to the life rafts.

A *Shackleton* aircraft circled the area, and in the early light of dawn on Tuesday, a deflated life raft was spotted near Erraid, which is at the South west extremity of Mull, some two miles North of the Torran Rocks. When recovered, it was found not to be from the stricken vessel. Some twelve hours after the alert, the fishing boat *Reliant* came across wreckage from the *Rosebud II*, drifting half a mile WSW of Eilean a Chalmain, and later the body of one of the crew was found in the same area.

The Burghead fishing boat *Accord* found a second body floating off the Dutchman's Cap in the Treshnish Isles, a few miles to the North. All seven of the crew were lost.

NYLAND

Wreck No : 217   **Date Sunk :** 05 12 1940
Latitude : 56 14 18 N   **Longitude :** 06 27 39 W
Decca Lat : 5614.30 N   **Decca Long :** 0627.65 W
Location : W Rock of Iona, Torran Rocks   **Area :** Mull
Type : Steamship   **Tonnage :** 1375 gross.
Length : 250.9 ft.   **Beam :** 41.3 ft.   **Draught :** 14.8 ft.
How Sunk : Ran aground   **Depth :**   metres

The Norwegian steamship *Nyland*, built in 1940, was en route from the Tyne to Mackenzie, and was last seen by another Norwegian steamship, the *Marga*, near Skerryvore on the evening of 5th December 1940. She was reported to have run on to the West Rock of Iona the following day. A piece of wreckage bearing her name was washed up two weeks later. West Reef is the western outlier of the Torran Rocks, South west of Mull.

CATHCART PARK

Wreck No : 218   **Date Sunk :** 15 04 1912
Latitude : 56 15 00 N PA   **Longitude :** 06 30 00 W PA
Decca Lat : 5615.00 N   **Decca Long :** 0630.00 W
Location : Torran Rocks   **Area :** Mull
Type : Steamship   **Tonnage :** 840 gross.
Length : 208.2 ft.   **Beam :** 29.7 ft.   **Draught :** 13.6 ft.

How Sunk : Ran aground   **Depth :**   metres

The 453 tons net steel steamship *Cathcart Park* was built in 1897 by Carmichael, Maclean & Co. of Greenock. While en route from Runcorn to Wick with a cargo of salt, she ran on to the Sheep Rock, in the centre of the Torran Rocks, on 15th April 1912. The 11 crew escaped in two of the ship's boats and were picked up and landed at Oban by the MacBrayne vessel *Dirk*. It was impossible to approach the wreck because of breaking seas on the surrounding rocks, and the vessel quickly broke up. The wreck was apparently visible from Iona for a short time after she ran aground.

LABRADOR

Wreck No : 219   **Date Sunk :** 01 03 1899
Latitude : 56 17 30 N   **Longitude :** 07 10 10 W
Decca Lat : 5617.50 N   **Decca Long :** 0710.17 W
Location : Mackenzie's Rocks, Skerryvore   **Area :** Mull
Type : Steamship   **Tonnage :** 2998 gross.
Length : 399.3 ft.   **Beam :** 46.2 ft.   **Draught :** 29.7 ft.
How Sunk : Ran aground   **Depth :** 16 metres

The Liverpool-registered steel steamship *Labrador*, 2998 tons net, was lost when she ran on to Mackenzie's Rock, 3 miles South west of Skerryvore on 1st March 1899. She had been on her way from St. Johns, New Brunswick to Liverpool with a general cargo and 64 passengers. Mackenzie's Rock dries 2.2 metres at low water, and is the most south-westerly of a series of rocks which extend for 12 miles towards the South west from the southern point of Tiree. For a considerable part of this area, depths are less than 20 metres, with a further large adjacent area where depths range from 20 to 30 metres.

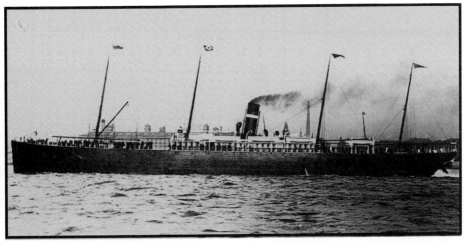

The Labrador *(Photograph courtesy of the World Ship Society)*

That was the good news. The bad news is that this is a very exposed place, and because of the relatively shallow depths around these rocks, there are overfalls in the tidal stream, and the whole area breaks heavily in north west gales.

Because of the distance from land, it would be prudent to visit this extremely remote site with more than one boat.

MAID OF LORNE

Wreck No : 220
Latitude : 56 17 48 N
Decca Lat : 5617.80 N
Location : N point of Eilean Ura, Iona
Type : Steamship
Length :   ft.   **Beam :**   ft.
How Sunk : Ran aground/refloated

Date Sunk : 17 04 1896
Longitude : 06 25 40 W
Decca Long : 0625.67 W
Area : Mull
Tonnage : 42 gross.
Draught :   ft.
Depth :   metres

Maid of Lorne was a small steel steamship of 42 tons net, lost by stranding on 17th April 1896 at the North point of Eilean Ura, off Iona. The spelling of the name *Ura* may be incorrect, perhaps resulting from an incorrect interpretation of a verbal description given by someone with an accent not totally familiar to the listener. Could it be Sgeir an Oir, or Eilean na h-Uamha? The former suggestion is a rock lying just South of Iona at 561748N, 062540W. The latter is a small islet off the South of Ulva at 562745N, 061300W. At 563133N, 055702W in Salen Bay in the Sound of Mull, a group of rocks named Maid of Lorne Rocks are almost awash at low water. Why are they so named? A report in the *Oban Times* says the crew were safe on Iona, and that their vessel was refloated on 28th August 1896.

OSTENDE

Wreck No : 221
Latitude : 56 19 18 N
Decca Lat : 5619.30 N
Location : Bunessan, SW Mull
Type : Steamship
Length : 375.1 ft.   **Beam :** 50.5 ft.
How Sunk : Explosion

Date Sunk : 17 01 1943
Longitude : 06 15 50 W
Decca Long : 0615.83 W
Area : Mull
Tonnage : 4438 gross.
Draught : 27.4 ft.
Depth : 4 metres

The Belgian steamship *Ostende* (ex-*Ehrenfels*), built by Swan Hunter & Wigham Richardson in 1903 was en route from New York to Liverpool with 5374 tons of general cargo including 1830 tons of steel when she either hit a mine or was torpedoed at 5613N 0700W and set on fire. She was then taken to the sheltered, shallow Bunessan Bay where a further massive explosion blew the ship asunder. Large parts of the ship are

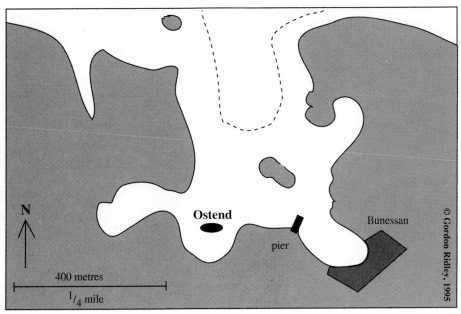

Location of the Ostend

still visible on the surrounding hillside to the North west of Bunessan, and wreckage is scattered over a wide area on the bottom of the bay.

After the explosion, the inhabitants of Bunessan all got something from the wreck - spanners and pliers with names on them, bags of flour, still in perfectly good condition, the water having penetrated only half an inch, and innumerable other items.

Apparently the Royal Navy spent 6 or 7 months during 1984 on the site of the wreck, clearing it of all the ammunition and guns, etc., because Irish divers had taken some recovered items of that nature back to Ireland. Crates of pistols coated in grease and still in good working order had previously been recovered, and some divers had even left rifles lying on the beach, to the concern of the local police constable. It seems unlikely that much can be left after such a concentrated effort by the Navy, unless some items still lie buried in sand at the bottom of the bay.

In 1987 the seabed was reported examined by Bendoran Boatyard and found to be free of wreckage and obstructions, but in 1991 the Navy was still seeking confirmation that the site is clear.

UNKNOWN

Wreck No : 222
Latitude : 56 21 48 N
Decca Lat : 5621.80 N
Location : N side of Loch Scridain
Type :

Date Sunk : Pre - 1972
Longitude : 06 05 06 W
Decca Long : 0605.10 W
Area : Mull
Tonnage :   gross

Length :   ft.   Beam :   ft.   Draught :   ft.
How Sunk :   Depth :   metres

An obstruction thought to be a wreck, close to the North shore of Loch Scridain, between Sgeir Mhor and Scobull Point was located in 1972, and buoyed by the Royal Navy in October of that year. No further details are known.

PROTESILAUS

Wreck No : 223   **Date Sunk :** 13 09 1940
Latitude : 56 22 13 N   **Longitude :** 07 15 29 W
Decca Lat : 5622.22 N   **Decca Long :** 0715.48 W
Location : 295° 4.9 miles Skerryvore Lt.   **Area :** Mull
Type : Steamship   **Tonnage :** 9577 gross.
Length : 484.9 ft.   **Beam :** 60.4 ft.   **Draught :** 39.5 ft.
How Sunk : Gunfire   **Depth :** 60 metres

On 13th November 1939, U-28 (Kuhnke) laid mines in the approach to Swansea. Just over two months later, on 21st January 1940, the steamship *Protesilaus* struck one of these mines at 5131N, 0404W. Severely damaged, and in a sinking condition, she was beached and later cut in two to aid refloating. The bow section was refloated on 26th July and towed to Briton Ferry for scrapping. The stern section was later towed toward Scapa Flow, where it had been intended to use it as a blockship

En route, the stern section started to leak, and was sunk by gunfire from HMS *King Sol* on 13th September 1940. The wreck of the stern section is charted at 42 metres in 562213N, 071529W. It was located by sonar in 60 metres on 13th January 1986, 295° 4.9 miles Skerryvore Light.

This is perhaps not the most useful information in an area with a magnetic anomaly, where magnetic compass readings are unreliable. Gyro compasses, however, would not be affected, and their readings are in degrees true. In fact, 295° (true), 4.9 miles Skerryvore Light plots in 562130N, 071500W. The wreck was not found during a search on 14th August 1989.

RAVENSHEUGH

Wreck No : 224   **Date Sunk :** 29 10 1911
Latitude : 56 25 00 N PA   **Longitude :** 07 05 00 W PA
Decca Lat : 5625.00 N   **Decca Long :** 0705.00 W
Location : Off Skerryvore   **Area :** Mull
Type : Steamship   **Tonnage :** 1781 gross.
Length : 263.0 ft.   **Beam :** 35.2 ft.   **Draught :** 22.4 ft.
How Sunk : Ran aground   **Depth :**   metres

The British steamship *Ravensheugh* was built in 1881 by Palmers Co., and owned by Robertson, Mackie & Co. of Glasgow. On 29th October 1911, while en route from the Clyde to Riga, Latvia, with a cargo of coal and herrings, she struck a submerged object during the night, supposedly a derelict, about 4 miles off Skerryvore. (Note that there are many dangerous rocks close to the surface in this area, and a local magnetic anomaly which affects compass readings!)

The forepeak immediately filled with water, and the captain decided to make for Tobermory, but after the vessel had proceeded about 8 miles, the holds also filled. At the same time the weather worsened, and at about 4.00 am it was decided to take to the boats. Nine of the crew got away in the starboard lifeboat, and after many hours of buffeting, landed on Gigha, from where they were picked up by the Duke of Bedford's steam yacht *Sapphire*. The port lifeboat could not be lowered because of the list in the ship, and the remainder of the crew, including Captain Daniels, were drowned. The Hydrographic Dept. has recorded position 561924N, 070700W.

CRETAN

Wreck No : 225	**Date Sunk :** 07 01 1939
Latitude : 56 29 17 N	**Longitude :** 06 07 08 W
Decca Lat : 5629.28 N	**Decca Long :** 0607.13 W
Location : Rubh an Dobhrain, Loch na Keal	**Area :** Mull
Type : Steam lighter	**Tonnage :** 39 gross.
Length : ft. **Beam :** ft.	**Draught :** ft.
How Sunk : Ran aground	**Depth :** metres

The steam lighter *Cretan* was driven ashore at the rocky headland of Rubh an Dobhrain in Loch na Keal in the West of Mull in the early hours of Saturday 7th January, 1939. The boat, owned by Hay & Sons of Glasgow, was on her way to Inchkenneth to collect the furniture and effects of the late Lady Boulton who had died in Oban the previous October. She was the widow of Sir Harold Boulton, composer of the Skye Boat Song. When the *Cretan* had reached Loch na Keal a blizzard was blowing, and as a precaution, the boat was anchored. The weather worsened, however, and she dragged her anchor and was driven on the rocks. With difficulty, Captain MacIlwaine and his crew got ashore in their boat and obtained shelter at a farmhouse. The *Cretan* was so badly damaged that she became a total wreck.

UNKNOWN - JASON?

Wreck No : 226	**Date Sunk :**
Latitude : 56 33 00 N	**Longitude :** 06 28 00 W
Decca Lat : 5633.00 N	**Decca Long :** 0628.00 W
Location : 4 ½ miles W of Treshnish Point	**Area :** Mull

Type :

Length : ft.   **Beam :** ft.

How Sunk :

Tonnage : gross

Draught : ft.

Depth : 48 metres

A wreck is charted here with at least 18 metres clearance in about 60 metres. It is obviously only an approximate position, and was originally intended to represent the loss of HMS *Jason* in this area in 1917 (see *Jason* entry)

TEUNIKA

Wreck No : 227

Latitude : 56 35 42 N PA

Decca Lat : 5635.70 N

Location : 223° 2.5 miles Caliach Point

Type : Motor vessel

Length : 112.0 ft.   **Beam :** 22.0 ft.

How Sunk : Foundered

Date Sunk : 16 05 1969

Longitude : 06 23 36 W PA

Decca Long : 0623.60 W

Area : Mull

Tonnage : 199 gross.

Draught : 8.0 ft.

Depth : 30 metres

Teunika, (ex-*Marken*, ex-*Willem*, ex-*Velocitas*, ex-*Wilhelmina*), was a Dutch motor vessel built in 1936. While carrying a cargo of gravel from Corpach to Tiree she sprang a leak and suffered engine failure.

She was taken in tow, but foundered 11 miles West of Tobermory or 2.5 miles from Caliach Point, where there is a wreck charted at 563542N, 062336W PA, just over the 30 metre isobath with an estimated clearance of at least 18 metres. This position is also about 4 miles North west of Lunga, in the Treshnish Isles (between Mull and Coll).

A further wreck position has been added to the chart 1.5 miles to the North east at 563654N 06224W PA, with an estimated clearance of at least 65 metres in about 70 metres. It is not clear to me whether this is an additional wreck or a more accurate position for the same wreck.

I have no further information to offer.

JASON

Wreck No : 228

Latitude : 56 35 45 N PA

Decca Lat : 5635.75 N

Location : N of Fladda

Type : Mine-sweeper

Length : 230.0 ft.   **Beam :** 27.0 ft.

How Sunk : Mined

Date Sunk : 07 04 1917

Longitude : 06 28 15 W PA

Decca Long : 0628.25 W

Area : Mull

Tonnage : 810 gross.

Draught : 12.5 ft.

Depth : 42 metres

HMS *Jason* was a gunboat/mine-sweeper built in 1893, and was armed with two 4.7" guns, four 3-pounders and three 18" torpedo tubes. She struck a mine North of Fladda at 11.10 am on 7th April 1917, and sank in less than five minutes with the loss of 25 of

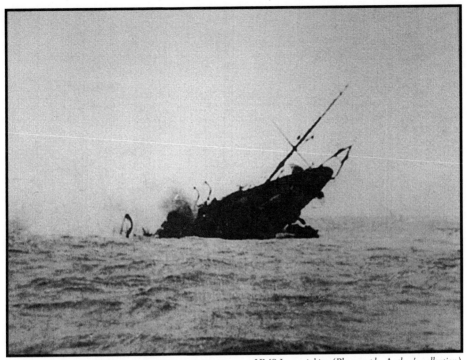

HMS Jason sinking (Photograph: Author's collection)

her crew of 98. The mine she struck had been laid on 11th February by *U-78*.

The position given in 1917 by HMS *Circe*, one of her sister ships of the *Alarm* Class, which was in company with HMS *Jason*, was 563545N, 062815W. A wreck with an estimated clearance of at least 60 metres in about 73 metres is charted as PA in that position, 5 miles West of Caliach Point.

AURANIA

Wreck No : 229	**Date Sunk :** 06 02 1918
Latitude : 56 36 00 N	**Longitude :** 06 19 36 W
Decca Lat : 5636.00 N	**Decca Long :** 0619.60 W
Location : Caliach Point, NW Mull	**Area :** Mull
Type : Steamship	**Tonnage :** 13984 gross.
Length : 520.5 ft. **Beam :** 65.3 ft.	**Draught :** 42.6 ft.
How Sunk : Torpedoed by *UB-67*	**Depth :** 25 metres

The twin screw Cunard Liner *Aurania*, built in 1924 by Swan Hunter, was torpedoed by the *UB-67*, 15 miles N !/2 W of Inishtrahull, County Donegal, off the North of Ireland and abandoned while on a voyage in ballast from Liverpool to New York. Eight lives were lost. She did not sink immediately, but drifted ashore in County Donegal but was

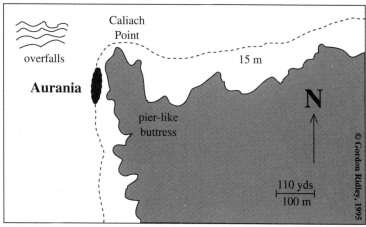

The location of the Aurania.

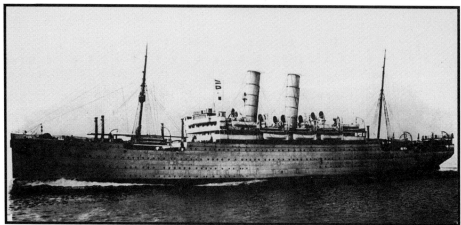

The Aurania *(Photograph courtesy of Maritime Photo Library)*

refloated and taken in tow. Off Mull, the tow broke, and *Aurania* drifted in a gale before running aground at Caliach Point, Mull.

The remains are now very broken up in 20-25 metres, and scattered over an area 550 ft x 80 ft, lying in a North/South direction, 40 metres out from the cliff face, running North from a conspicuous flat-topped rock outcrop to the South of Caliach Point.

UNKNOWN

Wreck No : 230
Latitude : 56 36 54 N PA
Decca Lat : 5636.90 N
Location : 1.5 miles NW of Caliach Point

Date Sunk :
Longitude : 06 21 48 W PA
Decca Long : 0621.80 W
Area : Mull

				Tonnage :	gross
Type :					
Length :	ft.	**Beam :**	ft.	**Draught**	ft.
How Sunk :				**Depth :** 65 metres	

Charted as Wk PA with at least 65 metres over it in 80 metres, 1.5 miles North west of Caliach Point, Mull.

ROBERT LIMBRICK

Wreck No : 231		**Date Sunk :** 05 02 1957	
Latitude : 56 38 02 N		**Longitude :** 06 13 40 W	
Decca Lat : 5638.03 N		**Decca Long :** 0613.66 W	
Location : Quinish Point, NW Mull		**Area :** Mull	
Type : Trawler		**Tonnage :** 273 gross.	
Length : 137.7 ft.	**Beam :** 23.7 ft.	**Draught :** 11.5 ft.	
How Sunk : Ran aground		**Depth :**	metres

The trawler *Robert Limbrick*, (ex-*Sir Galahad*, ex-*Star of Freedom*), built 1942 by Hall Russell of Aberdeen, struck a rock and foundered off Quinish Point, North west Mull, during the worst storm in Scottish seas in living memory. Although the vessel was only 25 yards from the shore, coastguards were unable to reach her because of the heavy swell. All 14 of the crew, who came from Milford Haven, were lost. The ship's lifeboat was washed up on the shore, almost undamaged, with its protective covering intact, not having been used. Quinish Point is at 563802N, 061340W.

INCHMURREN

Wreck No : 232		**Date Sunk :** 06 04 1895	
Latitude : 56 38 10 N PA		**Longitude :** 06 12 15 W PA	
Decca Lat : 5638.17 N		**Decca Long :** 0612.25 W	
Location : Laorin Bay, N Mull		**Area :** Mull	
Type : Steam Lighter		**Tonnage :** gross	
Length : ft.	**Beam :** ft.	**Draught :** ft.	
How Sunk : Ran aground		**Depth :**	metres

The steam lighter *Inchmurren* of Glasgow became stranded on the rocks *at Lourin, North of Mull*, while attempting to discharge a general cargo on 6th April 1895. The wind was blowing strongly from the North at the time. About ½ mile to the East of Quinish Point there is a rocky headland named Rubh an Laorin, and a further ½ mile East is Laorin Bay, a small inlet with a sandy beach at its head, from which a track leads inland to Glengorm Castle. Both the headland and the bay are exposed to North winds. The *Inchmurren* was later refloated and towed to Tobermory. She might possibly have been the unknown lighter sunk alongside Tobermory pier at 563721N, 060353W.

CHAPTER 7

THE WRECKS OF TIREE AND COLL

INTRODUCTION

Tiree is about 10 miles long by 6 miles wide, and lies 15 miles West of Treshnish Point, Mull. Apart from two hills at its South end, Tiree is a flat, fertile island.

The climate is mild, with a low average rainfall. In springtime it has the highest number of hours of sunshine in Scotland, but because it is low-lying and flat, there is no shelter from the wind. Living on Tiree has been likened to living on the deck of an aircraft carrier! The prominent weather station on Tiree is the first one to be mentioned every day in the shipping forecasts broadcast by the BBC.

Skerryvore lighthouse, on a group of drying rocks ten miles SSW of Tiree, is surrounded by strong tides with overfalls, and there is also a local magnetic anomaly. Tidal streams of up to 3 knots run in the two mile wide Gunna Sound, between Coll and Tiree. With an opposing tide there can be heavy overfalls at the windward end of the Sound.

Coll is about 13 ½ miles long by 4 miles wide, and lies 7 ½ miles west of Caliach Point, Mull.

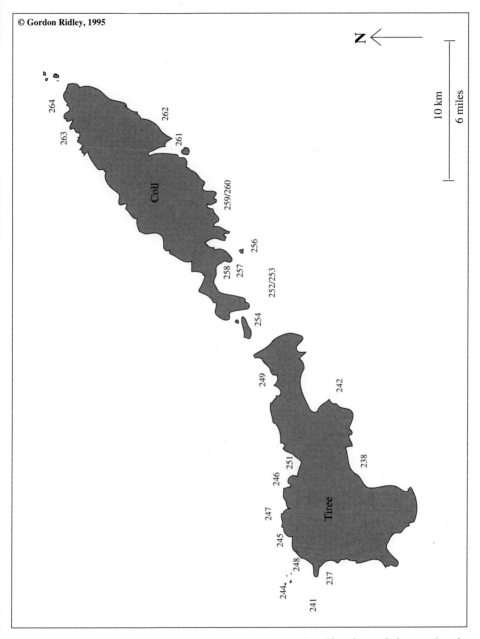

© Gordon Ridley, 1995

Chart showing the location of wrecks
lying off the coast of Tiree and Coll

THE WRECKS

KENMORE

Wreck No : 233	**Date Sunk** : 26 08 1917
Latitude : 56 06 06 N	**Longitude** : 07 30 18 W
Decca Lat : 5606.10 N	**Decca Long** : 0730.30 W
Location : Off Skerryvore	**Area** : Tiree
Type : Steamship	**Tonnage** : 3919 gross
Length : 356.4 ft. **Beam** : 49.5 ft.	**Draught** : 23.1 ft.
How Sunk : Torpedoed	**Depth** : 99 metres

This wreck, charted in 99 metres, 18.5 miles South west of Skerryvore is possibly broken in two, but the dimensions of the wreck closely match the British steamship *Kenmore* which was torpedoed by a U-Boat off Skerryvore on 26th August 1917.

KINGSTON BERYL

Wreck No : 234	**Date Sunk** : 25 12 1943
Latitude : 56 12 00 N PA	**Longitude** : 07 30 00 W PA
Decca Lat : 5612.00 N	**Decca Long** : 0730.00 W
Location : 12 miles WSW of Skerryvore	**Area** : Tiree
Type : Trawler	**Tonnage** : 356 gross.
Length : 151.5 ft. **Beam** : 24.0 ft.	**Draught** : 12.9 ft.
How Sunk : Mined	**Depth** : metres

The trawler *Kingston Beryl*, built in 1928 by Cook, Welton & Gemmel of Beverley, engine by C. D. Holmes, was requisitioned in September 1939. While on convoy escort duty on Christmas Day 1943, she ran on to some floating mines which had broken free from a British minefield. British mines were supposed to go *safe* automatically when they broke loose from their mooring wires, but the automatic safety mechanism failed to operate, and she was sunk with all hands about 12 miles WSW of Skerryvore.

ARANDA

Wreck No : 235	**Date Sunk** : 05 08 1916
Latitude : 56 19 24 N PA	**Longitude** : 07 06 45 W PA
Decca Lat : 5619.40 N	**Decca Long** : 0706.75 W
Location : Off W coast of Scotland	**Area** : Tiree
Type : Steamship	**Tonnage** : 1838 gross.
Length : 270.0 ft. **Beam** : 36.6 ft.	**Draught** : 16.5 ft.
How Sunk : Mined	**Depth** : metres

The Norwegian steamship *Aranda*, built in 1890 by Richardson, Duck & Co., struck a mine and sank on 5th August, off the West coast of Scotland. The Norwegian Maritime

Directorate gives *Atlantic Ocean, Skerryvore light*. Skerryvore light is at 561924N, 070645W. *Lloyds War Losses* gives 12 miles W by N of Skerryvore. According to the Hydrographic Dept., the *Aranda* is at 550900N, 070300W, which is in Lough Foyle, Northern Ireland. Was she still under her own power or was she taken in tow after striking the mine, only to founder after 70+ miles? (9th September 1916?) Her mast apparently showed above water for a time after sinking opposite Saltpans.

PECTEN

Wreck No : 236	**Date Sunk :** 25 08 1940
Latitude : 56 22 00 N PA	**Longitude :** 07 55 00 W PA
Decca Lat : 5622.00 N	**Decca Long :** 0755.00 W
Location : 15 miles W of Skerryvore	**Area :** Tiree
Type : Tanker	**Tonnage :** 7468 gross.
Length : 435.6 ft. **Beam :** 59.4 ft.	**Draught :** 33.0 ft.
How Sunk : Torpedoed by *U-57*	**Depth :** metres

The motor tanker *Pecten*, built in 1927 by Palmers Co., and owned by the Anglo Saxon Petroleum Co., was torpedoed and sunk by the *U-57* (KL Erich Topp), at 7.48 pm on 25th August 1940. The position of attack has been variously described as 15 miles West of Skerryvore, 40 miles West of Skerryvore, and a third report gives the position as 562200N, 075500W PA, where a wreck is charted in about 170 metres, and this is 26 miles West of Skerryvore. Captain Dale and 48 of the 57 crew were lost. The eight survivors included the radio operator, an apprentice and six Chinese.

STURDY

Wreck No : 237	**Date Sunk :** 30 10 1940
Latitude : 56 29 00 N PA	**Longitude :** 06 59 00 W
Decca Lat : 5629.00 N	**Decca Long :** 0659.00 W
Location : Sandaig, W Tiree	**Area :** Tiree
Type : Destroyer	**Tonnage :** 905 gross.
Length : 276.0 ft. **Beam :** 26.7 ft.	**Draught :** 10.9 ft.
How Sunk : Ran aground in fog	**Depth :** metres

HMS *Sturdy*, built in 1918, ran aground on the West of Tiree in heavy weather. She is now reported to be completely broken up. Another report suggests she ran aground on the East coast of Tiree. Two lives were lost.

UNKNOWN

Wreck No : 238	**Date Sunk :** Pre - 1986
Latitude : 56 29 12 N	**Longitude :** 06 52 24 W
Decca Lat : 5629.20 N	**Decca Long :** 0652.40 W

Location : W end of Crossapol beach   **Area :** Tiree
Type : Trawler   **Tonnage :**   gross
Length :   ft.   **Beam :**   ft.   **Draught :** ft.
How Sunk : Ran aground   **Depth :**   metres

At the West end of Crossapol beach, the wreck of what is known locally as a Russian trawler just shows above water. The wreck is mostly buried in sand.

LADY ISLE

Wreck No : 239   **Date Sunk :** 10 08 1956
Latitude : 56 29 58 N   **Longitude :** 06 48 02 W
Decca Lat : 5629.97 N   **Decca Long :** 0648.03 W
Location : 115° 0.12 miles Scarinish Lt.   **Area :** Tiree
Type : Puffer   **Tonnage :** 96 gross.
Length :   ft.   **Beam :**   ft.   **Draught :**   ft.
How Sunk : Ran aground /refloated   **Depth :**   metres

Lady Isle was a Clyde puffer. Some reports suggest she broke up where she ran aground, but another suggests she was subsequently refloated and finally broken up at North Queensferry in 1986.

U-484

Wreck No : 240   **Date Sunk :** 09 09 1944
Latitude : 56 30 00 N PA   **Longitude :** 07 40 00 W PA
Decca Lat : 5630.00 N   **Decca Long :** 0740.00 W
Location : Off Inner Hebrides   **Area :** Tiree
Type : Submarine   **Tonnage :** 769 gross.
Length : 221.4 ft.   **Beam :** 20.5 ft.   **Draught :** 15.4 ft.
How Sunk : Depth-charged   **Depth :** 170 metres

U-484 (KL Schafer), was depth-charged by the RCN frigate *Dunver* and the RN corvette *Hespeler* and RCAF aircraft of *423 Squadron,* "off the Inner Hebrides" at 5630N, 0740W on 9th September 1944. There were no survivors. A wreck is charted in this position in about 160 metres, 21 miles North west of Skerryvore, and 17 miles South of Barra Head. The Type VIIC Atlantic U-Boat displaced 769 tons surfaced, 871 tons submerged.

CAIRNSMUIR

Wreck No : 241   **Date Sunk :** 06 07 1885
Latitude : 56 29 57 N   **Longitude :** 07 01 36 W
Decca Lat : 5629.95 N   **Decca Long :** 701.60 W

Location : 2½ miles off Craiguish Point   **Area :** Tiree
Type : Steamship   **Tonnage :** 1123 gross.
Length : 290.3 ft.   **Beam :** 33.7 ft.   **Draught :** 23.9 ft.
How Sunk : Ran aground   **Depth :** 8 metres

The 1123 ton iron steamship *Cairnsmuir* stranded 2.5 miles off Craiguish (Craiginish) Point, Tiree on 6th July 1885 while en route from Hamburg to Glasgow. Her cargo appears to have been mainly cases of spirits and beer, which the Customs and Excise, along with the Captain and two officers from the vessel attempted to retrieve as it was washed ashore. Mostly empty bottles and wooden cases were discovered. The Customs men found their task very difficult due to non-co-operation from the locals, who were carrying out their own recovery operation. (What a surprise!)

At low water, the kelp on Bo Mor reef is visible as a dark area in the water. The broken remains of the wreck are scattered among the gullies in the reef.

MARY STUART

Wreck No : 242   **Date Sunk :** Pre - 1969
Latitude : 56 30 07 N   **Longitude :** 06 48 14 W
Decca Lat : 5630.12 N   **Decca Long :** 0648.23 W
Location : Near Scarinish Light, Tiree   **Area :** Tiree
Type : Sailing vessel   **Tonnage :**   gross
Length : 70.0 ft.   **Beam :**   ft.   **Draught :**   ft.
How Sunk : Ran aground   **Depth :**   metres

The *Mary Stuart* is lying on the beach near Scarinish harbour. One report suggests she was laid up there circa 1938. By June 1985, the wreck had largely disintegrated, but wooden ribs still stood several feet above the sand.

SAXON

Wreck No : 243   **Date Sunk :** 21 08 1930
Latitude : 56 31 20 N PA   **Longitude :** 07 01 00 W PA
Decca Lat : 5631.33 N   **Decca Long :** 0701.00 W
Location : Hough Skerries, West of Tiree   **Area :** Tiree
Type : Trawler   **Tonnage :** 239 gross.
Length : 120.3 ft.   **Beam :** 21.6 ft.   **Draught :** 11.6 ft.
How Sunk : Ran aground   **Depth :**   metres

Built in 1907 by Smiths Dock, Middlesbrough, the Fleetwood steam trawler *Saxon* was wrecked on Hough Skerries, Tiree on 21st August 1930.

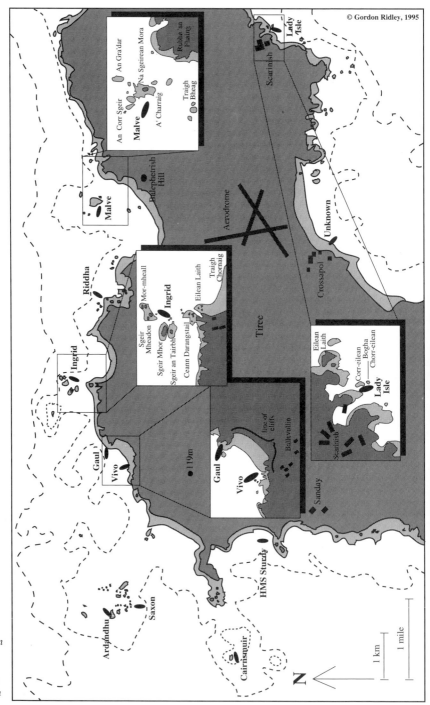

© Gordon Ridley, 1995

Location of wrecks off West & North Tiree

ARDANDHU

Wreck No : 244	**Date Sunk :** 17 09 1891
Latitude : 56 31 20 N PA	**Longitude :** 07 01 00 W PA
Decca Lat : 5631.33 N	**Decca Long :** 0701.00 W
Location : Hough Skerries, W of Tiree	**Area :** Tiree
Type : Steamship	**Tonnage :** 1148 gross.
Length : 235.9 ft. **Beam :** 31.1 ft.	**Draught :** 17.0 ft.
How Sunk : Ran aground	**Depth :** metres

The 732 tons net iron steamship *Ardandhu* ran on to Hough Skerries on 17th September 1891 in dense fog while en route from Riga to Fleetwood with a cargo of sleepers. She was holed in the forehold and engine room, and had 15 ft of water over her afterdeck. The wreck quickly disappeared in a southerly gale.

The vessel was built in 1879 by H. Murray & Co. of Port Glasgow, engine by W. King & Co. of Glasgow.

GAUL

Wreck No : 245	**Date Sunk :** 29 03 1926
Latitude : 56 31 30 N PA	**Longitude :** 06 57 30 W PA
Decca Lat : 5631.50 N	**Decca Long :** 0657.50 W
Location : Traigh Bailamhuillin, NW Tiree	**Area :** Tiree
Type : Trawler	**Tonnage :** gross
Length : ft. **Beam :** ft.	**Draught :** ft.
How Sunk : Ran aground	**Depth :** metres

This PA is just off the sandy beach of Traigh Bail a Mhuillin in North west Tiree. The Fleetwood trawler *Gaul* ran aground here in a gale on 29th March 1926. Seven of the crew of nine were lost when their small boat was overturned by huge breaking waves as they attempted to make for the shore. Despite being dashed against rocks, the two others succeeded in swimming ashore through the heavy surf. Depths here vary from 2.2 metres to 12.3 metres.

RIDDHA

Wreck No : 246	**Date Sunk :** 01 12 1902
Latitude : 56 32 00 N	**Longitude :** 06 53 00 W
Decca Lat : 5632.00 N	**Decca Long :** 0653.00 W
Location : Near Cornaigbeg Point, Tiree	**Area :** Tiree
Type : Steamship	**Tonnage :** 701 gross.
Length : ft. **Beam :** ft.	**Draught :** ft.
How Sunk : Ran aground	**Depth :** metres

The German steamship *Riddha* stranded on a sunken rock near Cornaigbeg Point, Tiree on 1st December 1902. The ship was en route from Sundswall to Preston with a cargo of wood pulp and one passenger. Those aboard abandoned ship and were saved. The *Riddha* was only six months old at the time of loss.

INGRID

Wreck No : 247	**Date Sunk :** 19 01 1942
Latitude : 56 32 04 N	**Longitude :** 06 56 00 W
Decca Lat : 5632.07 N	**Decca Long :** 0656.00 W
Location : Off Tiree	**Area :** Tiree
Type : Steamship	**Tonnage :** 2607 gross.
Length : 251.0 ft. **Beam :** 43.7 ft.	**Draught :** 25.8 ft.
How Sunk : Ran aground	**Depth :** 8 metres

The Norwegian steamship *Ingrid*, built in 1920, was sunk off Tiree en route from the Tyne to Cuba on 19th January 1942.

The wreck is reported to lie close in behind the central island of Mor Mheall in a general depth of 7.5 metres, and is badly broken up with the boiler showing above the surface at low water.

The word *stranded* was used to describe the circumstances of loss. The report in *DODAS* uses the word *wrecked*. Both of these words can normally be interpreted as *ran aground*.

VIVO

Wreck No : 248	**Date Sunk :** 12 12 1890
Latitude : 56 31 21 N	**Longitude :** 06 57 31 W
Decca Lat : 5631.35 N	**Decca Long :** 0657.52 W
Location : Balevulin, Tiree	**Area :** Tiree
Type : Steamship	**Tonnage :** 1139 gross.
Length : 240.9 ft. **Beam :** 34.3 ft.	**Draught :** 13.6 ft.
How Sunk : Ran aground	**Depth :** metres

The 739 ton net Newcastle iron steamship *Vivo* ran aground at Balevulin, Tiree on 12th December 1890 in a South west gale, Force 8. The lat/long is only an approximation in the area of the North of Tiree. The *Vivo* was built in 1883 by T&W Smith of North Shields, engine by Hawks, Crawshay & Sons.

FISHER QUEEN

Wreck No : 249	**Date Sunk :** 13 04 1973
Latitude : 56 32 30 N PA	**Longitude :** 06 46 45 W PA
Decca Lat : 5632.50 N	**Decca Long :** 0646.75 W
Location : Salum Beach, NE Tiree	**Area :** Tiree

Type : Trawler		**Tonnage** :	gross
Length : ft.	**Beam** : ft.	**Draught** : ft.	
How Sunk : Ran aground ?		**Depth** :	metres

Salum is near the North east tip of Tiree.

ADAMTON ?

Wreck No : 250	**Date Sunk** : 08 04 1916
Latitude : 56 32 30 N PA	**Longitude** : 07 26 30 W PA
Decca Lat : 5632.50 N	**Decca Long** : 0726.50 W
Location : 17 miles NW of Skerryvore	**Area** : Tiree
Type : Steamship	**Tonnage** : 2304 gross.
Length : 295.2 ft. **Beam** : 46.0 ft.	**Draught** : 19.2 ft.
How Sunk : By submarine - gunfire	**Depth** : 140 metres

The British steel steamship *Adamton* was built in 1904 by Northumberland S. B. Co., engine by Richardsons & Westgarth, Sunderland. En route in ballast from Scapa Flow to Barry, she was captured by the U-22 and sunk by gunfire on 8th April 1916. One member of the crew was killed.

The position given by the Hydrographic Department was 5633N, 0719W, about 15 miles North of Skerryvore. *Lloyds War Losses* gives the position of attack as 18 miles S by E ½E of Barra Head, and the wreck charted in 165 metres at 563230N, 072630W, about 17 miles North west of Skerryvore, very closely matches that description. *British Vessels Lost at Sea 1914-18* describes the position of attack as 15 miles South of Skerryvore. (Skerryvore is at 5618N, 0706W).Another report gives her position as 15 miles South of Skerryvore, and 10 miles South west of Tiree.

It has also been suggested that the wreck in this position may be a steamship named *Gloucester*, sunk in March 1903, but there is another wreck charted in the area at 563548N, 071112W at 126 metres, which may be the *Gloucester*.

MALVE

Wreck No : 251	**Date Sunk** : 14 02 1931
Latitude : 56 31 57 N	**Longitude** : 06 52 15 W
Decca Lat : 5631.95 N	**Decca Long** : 0652.25 W
Location : Balephetrish Bay, Tiree	**Area** : Tiree
Type : Steamship	**Tonnage** : 2412 gross.
Length : 251.0 ft. **Beam** : 43.0 ft.	**Draught** : 26.0 ft.
How Sunk : Ran aground	**Depth** : metres

The Finnish steamship *Malve* (ex-*Monique Vieljeux*, ex-*Roubaix*, ex-*Warfish*) was built in 1917 by Port Arthur S. B. Co. She ran aground on the North end of Tiree on 14th February 1931 while carrying a cargo of timber and pulp from Tallin to Manchester. She was refloated that evening, but broke down shortly afterwards, and sank after drifting on to rocks near Balephetrish Bay.

On 12th April 1931, the Belfast salvage vessel *Glen Lyon*, which was working on the wreck of the *Malve*, dragged her anchors and struck rocks in Balephetrish Bay, and sank in 7 fathoms (13 metres), alongside the *Malve*. Later, these two wrecks were joined by the *St. Anthony*, which also attempted salvage and suffered the same fate.

ST. CLAIR

Wreck No : 252	**Date Sunk :** 22 10 1880
Latitude : 56 32 24 N	**Longitude :** 06 40 00 W
Decca Lat : 5632.40 N	**Decca Long :** 0640.00 W
Location : Gunna Sound, Coll/Tiree	**Area :** Coll
Type : Steamship	**Tonnage :** 130 gross.
Length : 84.1 ft. **Beam :** 20.0 ft.	**Draught :** 8.0 ft.
How Sunk : Ran aground	**Depth :** metres

563300N, 064400W was the approximate position given for several years, but that position plots ashore on North east Tiree. It was not until 1986 that the 18th century steamship wreck was finally located at 563224N, 064000W, just to the East of Roan Bogha Rock.

The 67 tons net iron steamship *St. Clair* was built in 1876 by Birrell Stenhouse & Co., Dumbarton, engine by Walker Henderson & Co., Glasgow. She was owned by John McCallum & Co. of Glasgow which was one of the companies eventually absorbed by Caledonian MacBrayne, and plied between Glasgow and the West Highlands via the Crinan Canal.

On 20th June 1877 she was stranded in Loch Bracadale, Skye, but was refloated after a fortnight. She went aground again at Salen in Loch Sunart on 25th September 1878 and filled with water, but was successfully raised. While en route from Glasgow to North Uist with a general cargo on 22nd October 1880, she was finally lost when she ran on to Roan Bogha Rock in Gunna Sound between Coll and Tiree. The vessel sank within 15 minutes, giving the crew barely enough time to escape in the small boats with only the clothes they were wearing.

The wreck lies just East of Roan Bogha, very broken up, with a clipper type bow pointing to the East, and counter stern to the West.

HURLFORD

Wreck No : 253	**Date Sunk :** 29 04 1917
Latitude : 56 32 30 N	**Longitude :** 06 40 05 W
Decca Lat : 5632.50 N	**Decca Long :** 0640.08 W
Location : Gunna Sound, Coll/Tiree	**Area :** Coll

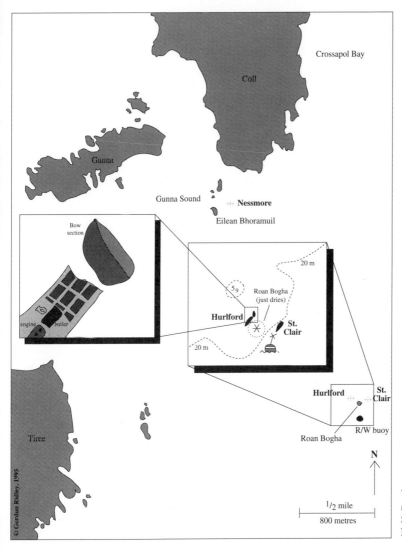

The locations of the Hurlford, *St. Clair &* Nessmore

Type : Steamship
Length : 155.3 ft. **Beam :** 25.6 ft.
How Sunk : Ran aground

Tonnage : 444 gross.
Draught : 11.1 ft.
Depth : 20 metres

Hurlford (ex-*Abington*) was a 178 tons net steel screw steamer built in 1905 by Murdoch & Murray, Port Glasgow, engine by Renfrew Bros., Irvine. She was on hire to the Admiralty as a collier when she was wrecked on Roan Bogha Rock off the North coast of Tiree on 29th April 1917. Her nine crew were all saved. She is reported to lie off the North west of Roan Bogha, which just dries at low water.

NESSMORE

Wreck No : 254
Latitude : 56 33 38 N
Decca Lat : 5633.63 N
Location : Caoles Reef, SE Coll
Type : Steamship
Length : 340.0 ft.   **Beam :** 40.4 ft.
How Sunk : Ran aground

Date Sunk : 21 11 1895
Longitude : 06 41 33 W
Decca Long : 0641.55 W
Area : Coll
Tonnage : 3377 gross.
Draught : 24.2 ft.
Depth :   metres

Nessmore was a British cargo ship built in 1882 by Barrow S. B. Co. Four days out from Montreal bound for Liverpool ,with a general cargo which included 555 cattle, cheese, flour, apples and American organs, she encountered gales which made navigational observations impossible. Off course, she entered the sound between Tiree and Coll - a place where even the local steamers will navigate only in daylight - and ran on to Roan Bogha Rock and broke in two. The crew took to their small boats and landed safely on Coll, but only after one of their boats capsized, those on board having to swim ashore.

Salvage attempts were frustrated by storms during the following weeks, which battered the *Nessmore* to pieces. Wreckage and large quantities of her cargo were washed ashore on the North west coast of Mull, the shores of Gometra and the Treshnish Isles. Gometra was favoured with one of the musical instruments, Quinish with cheese and a vast abundance of apples. The flour which was washed ashore was said to be in a wonderfully preserved state, the salt water having penetrated no more than half an inch. The wreck is now very broken up, partially buried in sand, and lies immediately adjacent to a rock which dries 1.7 metres at low water.

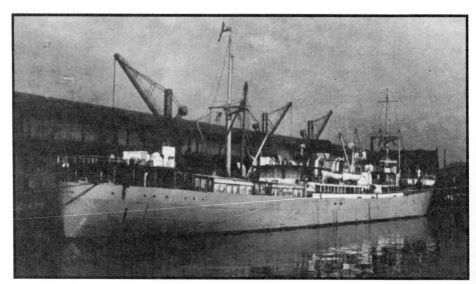

The Tapti *(Photograph courtesy of Glasgow Museums and Art Galleries).*

FARADAY

Wreck No : 255
Latitude : 56 33 38 N
Decca Lat : 5633.63 N
Location : S side of Coll
Type : Trawler
Length : ft. **Beam :** ft.
How Sunk : Ran aground

Date Sunk : 1907
Longitude : 06 41 33 W
Decca Long : 0641.55 W
Area : Coll
Tonnage : gross
Draught : ft.
Depth : metres

The steam trawler *Faraday* was wrecked when she ran aground on the South side of Coll in 1907. The engine and boiler, along with fittings, were recovered in salvage operations during August 1908. The remains lie near the *Nessmore*.

She was reported to have gone aground on Tumbla Island, off Coll.

TAPTI

Wreck No : 256
Latitude : 56 33 40 N
Decca Lat : 5633.67 N
Location : Off Soa Island, SE Coll
Type : Motor vessel
Length : 415.6 ft. **Beam :** 55.2 ft.
How Sunk : Ran aground

Date Sunk : 17 01 1951
Longitude : 06 37 53 W
Decca Long : 0637.88 W
Area : Coll
Tonnage : 6609 gross.
Draught : 33.9 ft.
Depth : 23 metres

The *Tapti* was in ballast, en route from Irwell to the Tyne, when she ran aground on Bac Beg Bank on 17th January, 1951. Four days later, she slipped off and sank in deeper water, very close west of the most southerly point of Eilean Iomalloch, which is just off the South of Soa Island at the South east of Coll. The wreck is breaking up, particularly around the bow which is lying on its port side, pointing towards the surface. The depth varies from 10-15 metres. Some salvage has been carried out, and the propeller and some non-ferrous fittings have been removed.

ARNOLD

Wreck No : 257
Latitude : 56 33 42 N
Decca Lat : 5633.70 N
Location : Wrecked at Soa Island
Type : Steamship
Length : 231.0 ft. **Beam :** 35.0 ft.
How Sunk : Ran aground

Date Sunk : 18 01 1925
Longitude : 06 38 00 W
Decca Long : 0638.00 W
Area : Coll
Tonnage : 1179 gross.
Draught : 14.7 ft.
Depth : metres

A wreck, which was thought possibly to be a large trawler, was reported in 1981 to lie

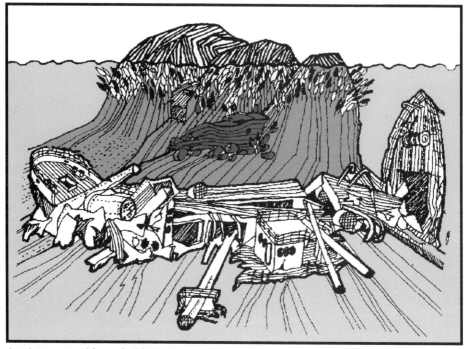

Artist's impression of the wreck of the Tapti.
(Drawing courtesy of Maurice Davidson).

west of Soa, and North west of the wreck of the *Tapti*. I suspect this wreck is actually the Swedish steamship *Arnold* which was built at Sunderland in 1881. The crew were all saved when she was wrecked at Soa, off the South east of Coll on 18th January 1925. The vessel had sailed from Belfast, and was in ballast at the time of loss.

BICKLEY

Wreck No : 258
Latitude : 56 34 45 N PA
Decca Lat : 5634.75 N
Location : Crossapol Bay, Coll
Type : Steamship
Length :   ft.   **Beam :**   ft.
How Sunk : Ran aground

Date Sunk : 06 10 1884
Longitude : 06 40 00 W PA
Decca Long : 0640.00 W
Area : Coll
Tonnage : 401 gross.
Draught :   ft.
Depth :   metres

The 401 tons net iron steamship *Bickley* ran aground in Crossapol Bay, Coll on 6th October 1884 while en route from Liverpool to Copenhagen with a general cargo. The master of the West Highland steamer *Claymore* reported that a boat containing the *Bickley's* five crew had left for the nearest telegraph station to report the loss of their

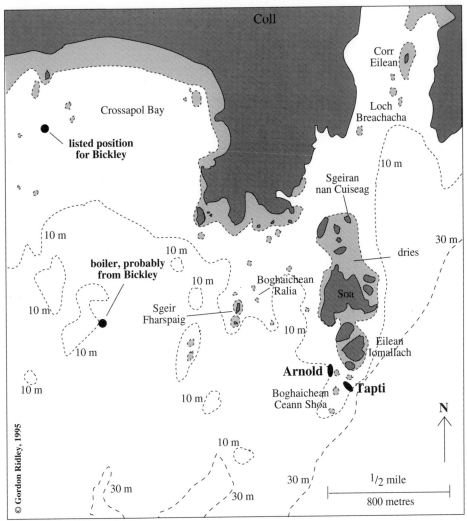

Locations of the Tapti, Arnold *and* Bickley

vessel, but the boat with the five men was never seen again. It was presumed that the boat had been swamped, and the occupants drowned.

At low water, the bow of the *Bickley* was in five fathoms (9 metres), but the stern remained high upon the reef. The forehold was submerged, but lighters took off her cargo and landed it at Tobermory. On 25th October it was reported that hopes were still high that she could be got off the reef. Steamers with recovery apparatus were lying at Arinagour, awaiting favourable weather for an attempt at refloating her.

It is not known whether she was safely recovered, but there have been many instances in which hopes of success in similar ventures have proved to be over-optimistic.

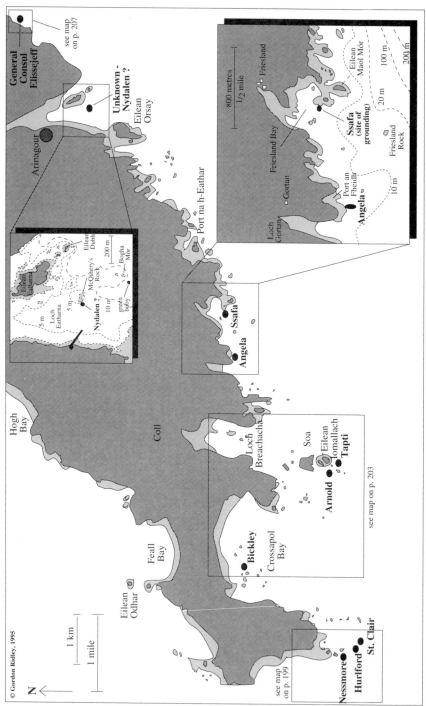

The
location of
wrecks off
South
west Coll.

© Gordon Ridley, 1995

ANGELA

Wreck No : 259

Latitude : 56 35 06 N

Decca Lat : 5635.10 N

Location : NE side of Friesland Head

Type : Motor vessel

Length : 167.3 ft.   **Beam :** 27.1 ft.

How Sunk : Ran aground

Date Sunk : 10 04 1953

Longitude : 06 35 30 W

Decca Long : 0635.50 W

Area : Coll

Tonnage :   gross

Draught : 8.8 ft.

Depth :   metres

Very little remains of this vessel. Plating and other parts of the hull are scattered amongst the rocks on the North east side of the southern fringe of Friesland Head. Some of the wreckage is on the shore above high water mark. The remains of the stern extend 50 yards out to sea, but only as fragments on the seabed. As it was possible to approach the vessel at low water shortly after she went ashore, everything salvageable was removed at that time.

SSAFA

Wreck No : 260

Latitude : 56 35 10 N

Decca Lat : 5635.17 N

Date Sunk : 17 01 1961

Longitude : 06 34 50 W

Decca Long : 0634.83 W

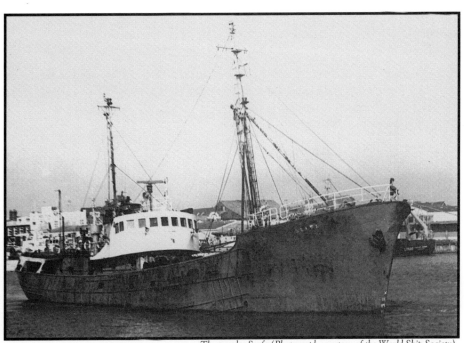

The trawler Ssafa (Photograph courtesy of the World Ship Society)

Location : NE of Friesland Head, Coll   Area : Coll
Type : Trawler   Tonnage : 427 gross.
Length : 138.8 ft.   Beam : 28.5 ft.   Draught :   ft.
How Sunk : Ran aground / refloated   Depth :   metres

On 17th January, 1961, the Fleetwood trawler *Ssafa*, en route to the Shetland fishing grounds, ran aground in a gale on rocks in Friesland Bay, in the South west of Coll. Distress signals from the *Ssafa* were sighted at dawn, and immediately three other ships and the Mallaig lifeboat raced to the bay, but they found the *Ssafa* was too close to the shore for any salvage attempt. For nine hours, skipper Harry Pook, together with three members of his crew stayed on board in the hope of refloating her, but eventually they had to be ordered by the owners to abandon the vessel. Earlier, the other twelve members of the crew were all pulled ashore through the surf by the island's lifesaving team. The trawler, which was owned by the Boston Deepsea Fishing Co. of Fleetwood, was subsequently refloated and repaired to fish again.

UNKNOWN - NYDALEN?

Wreck No : 261   Date Sunk :
Latitude : 56 36 52 N   Longitude : 06 30 33 W
Decca Lat : 5636.87 N   Decca Long : 0630.55 W
Location : Off Arinagour, Loch Eatharna   Area : Coll
Type :   Tonnage :   gross
Length :   ft.   Beam :   ft.   Draught :   ft.
How Sunk :   Depth :   metres

An obstruction, which dries 2.9 metres, lies 0.12 miles East of the flashing red light at the head of the pier at Arinagour, Loch Eatharna, on the East side of Coll. Could this be the 625 ton Norwegian steamship *Nydalen* (ex-*Grevelingen*), built in 1920, and lost about one mile from Arinagour on 31st March 1940?

GENERAL CONSUL ELISSEJEFF

Wreck No : 262   Date Sunk : 20 02 1914
Latitude : 56 37 45 N   Longitude : 06 29 29 W
Decca Lat : 5637.75 N   Decca Long : 0629.48 W
Location : 400 yds NE of Eil. Nam Muc   Area : Coll
Type : Steamship   Tonnage : 1457 gross.
Length : 250.5 ft.   Beam : 35.8 ft.   Draught : 16.1 ft.
How Sunk : Ran aground   Depth : 15 metres

The 890 tons net Danish steel steamship *General Consul Elissejeff* was built in 1902 by J. Crown of Sunderland, engine by MacColl & Pollock of Sunderland. She is very broken

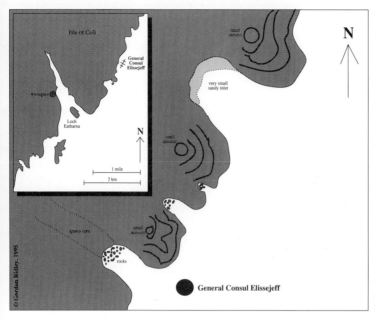

The location of the General Consul Elissejeff

up as a result of salvage and sea action. The propeller and other non-ferrous fittings have been removed. The wreck lies very close to the shore with 25 ft. of water over the bows, which point towards the shore, and 50 ft. of water over the stern, 1 mile North east of Loch Eatharna, and 400 yds North east of Eilean nam Muc. She had a cargo of agricultural machinery.

Apparently it had been originally intended to name her *Ada*, and the brass centre cap of her steering wheel recovered from the site of the wreck has this name engraved on it.

ST. BRANDAN

Wreck No : 263
Latitude : 56 40 46 N
Decca Lat : 5640.77 N
Location : On reefs S of Rubha Mor, N Coll
Type : Steamship
Length : ft. **Beam :** ft.
How Sunk : Ran aground

Date Sunk : 20 10 1928
Longitude : 06 31 12 W
Decca Long : 0631.20 W
Area : Coll
Tonnage : gross
Draught : ft.
Depth : metres

The steam coaster *St. Brandan*, belonging to J & A Gardner of Glasgow was en route from Skye to Glasgow with a cargo of 200 tons of grain and a quantity of whisky valued at £8000, when she struck a rock near the North tip of Coll at about 10.00 pm on 20th October 1928. Pitch darkness and a strong south-easterly wind with rain and hail, made visibility so bad that it was impossible to see Ardnamurchan light. The crew remained

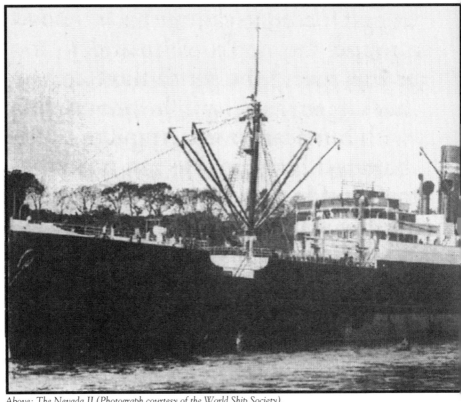

Above: The Nevada II (Photograph courtesy of the World Ship Society).

Below: The location of the Nevada II

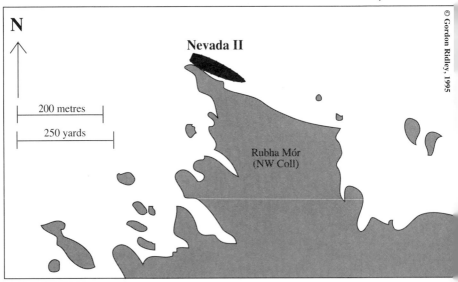

aboard as long as they dared, but at about 5.00 am they took to two lifeboats. For three hours they were buffeted about until the Fleetwood trawler *City of York* came on the scene, took them on board, and later landed them in Tobermory.

The wreck is charted as visible above water close ashore 1 mile South west of Rubha Mor near the northern tip of Coll at 564048N, 063100W PA. The wreck at 564046N, 063112W was for years assumed to be the *Nevada II*, but it is, in fact, the *St. Brandan*.

NEVADA II

Wreck No : 264	**Date Sunk :** 19 07 1942
Latitude : 56 41 24 N	**Longitude :** 06 29 27 W
Decca Lat : 5641.40 N	**Decca Long :** 0629.45 W
Location : NE side of Rubha Mor, N Coll	**Area :** Coll
Type : Steamship	**Tonnage :** 5693 gross.
Length : 420.0 ft. **Beam :** 56.0 ft.	**Draught :** 28.0 ft.
How Sunk : Ran aground	**Depth :** 16 metres

Built in 1918, the *Nevada II* ran aground during a voyage to Bathurst, Gambia, with a general cargo, some of which has been salvaged. The propeller was removed in 1957. Despite sea action and salvage work, the hull is still in one piece. The bows face East and lie in about 10 ft. of water, and the stern in 50 ft. At low water, the deck beams are nearly one metre above the surface. Part of the cargo included West African currency, and recovered coins circulating on the Island of Coll sparked off an investigation by HM Customs many years after the sinking.

The wreck lies parallel to the shore at the North east side of Rubha Mor peninsula, between the shore and a reef visible at low water 250 ft off the shore. For many years the position of the *Nevada II* was recorded as 564046N, 063112W, but the wreck in that position at the south of Rubha Mor is the *St. Brandan*, and the position of the *Nevada II* has been amended by the Hydrographic Department to 564124N, 062927W.

STINA

Wreck No : 265	**Date Sunk :** 02 03 1918
Latitude : 56 48 00 N PA	**Longitude :** 06 30 00 W PA
Decca Lat : 5648.00 N	**Decca Long :** 0630.00 W
Location : 6 miles N by E Cairns of Coll	**Area :** Coll
Type : Steamship	**Tonnage :** 1136 gross.
Length : ft. **Beam :** ft.	**Draught :** ft.
How Sunk : Torpedoed	**Depth :** 36 metres

The wreck of the Swedish steamship *Stina* is charted at 564800N, 063000W PA, which is 6 miles N by E of Cairns of Coll. The Cairns of Coll is the group of rocks at 564242N, 062700W, about two miles North of the northern tip of Coll. The vessel was captured by a German submarine then sunk 8 miles N by E from Cairns of Coll.

CHAPTER 8

THE WRECKS OF MUCK, EIGG, RUM AND MALLAIG

Introduction

Muck, Eigg, Rum and Canna are collectively known as the Small Isles.

Rum is the largest of these islands, and measures about 8 ½ x 8 miles. It has been run as a private estate for several centuries, and is now owned by the Nature Conservancy Council who use it as an open-air laboratory for the study of red deer, wild goats, Highland cattle and ponies. Surprisingly, attempts in the past to farm sheep here have never been successful. The wild ponies are reputedly descended from animals which swam ashore from a wrecked Spanish galleon, presumably at Wreck Bay, but another theory is that they originally came from Eriskay. Only about 40 people live on the island.

Although only about one third the size of Rum, the population of Eigg is almost double that of its neighbour. Half a mile South west of the main village of Galmisdale is MacDonalds cave, where, in the winter of 1577, 395 MacDonalds took refuge from the attacking MacLeods of Skye. When their hiding place was discovered, the MacLeods burned brushwood at the cave entrance, and all of the MacDonalds were suffocated.

Muck (Pig Island), has a population of about 25, and lies two and a half miles South west of Eigg and eight miles North of Ardnamurchan, the most westerly point of the British mainland.

Mallaig is a busy fishing and ferry harbour from which Caledonian MacBrayne serves the Small Isles with a thrice-weekly boat.

Hyskeir (Oigh Sgeir), is a group of low rocky islets 5 miles South west of Canna with a 39 metres high, unmanned, white lighthouse, built in 1902.

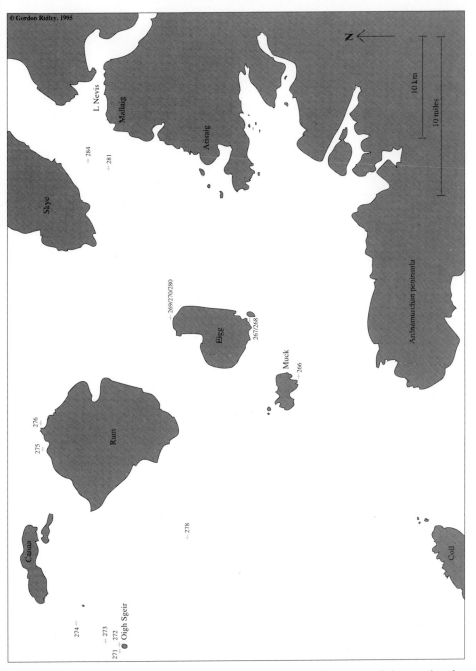

© Gordon Ridley, 1995

N

10 km

10 miles

L. Nevis

Mallaig

Arisaig

Skye

++ 284

++ 281

269/270/280

Eigg

267/268

Muck

++ 266

Ardnamurchan peninsula

276 ++

275 ++

Rum

++ 278

Canna

Coll

274 ++

++ 273

272

271 ++

Oigh Sgeir

Chart showing the location of wrecks lying off the coasts of the Small Isles

THE WRECKS

TARTAR

Wreck No : 266	**Date Sunk :** 13 03 1895
Latitude : 56 49 40 N PA	**Longitude :** 06 13 30 W PA
Decca Lat : 5649.67 N	**Decca Long :** 0613.50 W
Location : In S harbour of Muck	**Area :** Muck
Type : Steamship	**Tonnage :** 173 gross.
Length : 120.4 ft. **Beam :** 19.6 ft.	**Draught :** 9.3 ft.
How Sunk : Ran aground	**Depth :** metres

The iron puffer *Tartar* ran aground on rocks in the South harbour of Muck on 13th March 1895 while carrying a general cargo. The vessel was built by Scotts of Bowling in 1885, engine by Muir & Houston, Glasgow.

HERMANN

Wreck No : 267	**Date Sunk :** 03 12 1904
Latitude : 56 52 39 N PA	**Longitude :** 06 07 36 W PA
Decca Lat : 5652.65 N	**Decca Long :** 0607.60 W
Location : Off Galmisdale pier, Eigg	**Area :** Eigg
Type : Steamship	**Tonnage :** 992 gross.
Length : 217.8 ft. **Beam :** 33.5 ft.	**Draught :** 13.0 ft.
How Sunk : Ran aground	**Depth :** metres

The 621 tons net steel steamship *Hermann* ran aground at Eigg on 3rd December 1904. She was bound from Fleetwood to Fredericia, Denmark with a cargo of rock salt. In 1992, what was described as a large iron ship was found near the wreck of the *South Esk* of Montrose, off Eigg. The wreck lies adjacent to the shore, smashed to pieces, about 150 yards South of the pier, which is on the East side of Eigg. *Hermann* was built in 1890 by Rostocker A. G. at Rostock, and was registered in Preston.

SOUTH ESK

Wreck No : 268	**Date Sunk :** 28 12 1879
Latitude : 56 52 39 N PA	**Longitude :** 06 07 36 W PA
Decca Lat : 5652.65 N	**Decca Long :** 0607.60 W
Location : Off Galmisdale pier, Eigg	**Area :** Eigg
Type : Brigantine	**Tonnage :** 157 gross.

Length : ft.   **Beam :** ft.   **Draught :** ft.
How Sunk : Ran aground   **Depth :** metres

The brigantine *South Esk* of Montrose was lost off Galmisdale pier, Eigg on 28th December 1879.

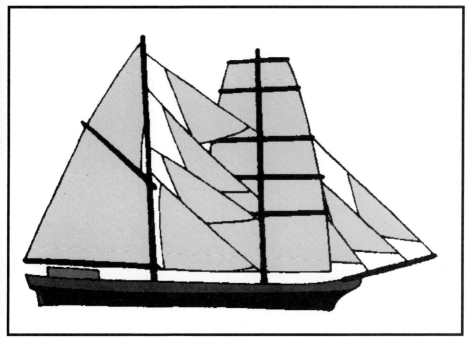

A typical 19th Century brigantine, similar to the South Esk.

JENNIE

Wreck No : 269   **Date Sunk :**
Latitude : 56 56 30 N   **Longitude :** 06 07 37 W
Decca Lat : 5656.50 N   **Decca Long :** 0607.62 W
Location : Near the N tip of Eigg   **Area :** Eigg
Type : Puffer   **Tonnage :** gross
Length : ft.   **Beam :** ft.   **Draught :** ft.
How Sunk : Ran aground   **Depth :** metres

The puffer *Jennie* is reported to be high and dry on the North tip of Eigg.

LYTHE

Wreck No : 270
Latitude : 56 56 30 N
Decca Lat : 5656.50 N
Location : Near N tip of Eigg
Type : Puffer
Length : ft.   **Beam :** ft.
How Sunk : Ran aground

Date Sunk : 1954
Longitude : 06 07 38 W
Decca Long : 0607.63 W
Area : Eigg
Tonnage : gross
Draught : ft.
Depth : metres

The puffer *Lythe* was wrecked in 1954 while endeavouring to recover the cargo of coal from the puffer *Jennie* which stranded here.

ANNA MOORE

Wreck No : 271
Latitude : 56 58 00 N PA
Decca Lat : 5658.00 N
Location : Hyskeir Reef, off Rum
Type : Steamship
Length : 316.0 ft.   **Beam :** 40.5 ft.
How Sunk : Ran aground

Date Sunk : 24 08 1914
Longitude : 06 40 30 W PA
Decca Long : 0640.50 W
Area : Rum
Tonnage : 2825 gross.
Draught : 20.9 ft.
Depth : metres

The 1794 tons net steel steamship *Anna Moore* was built in 1890 by J. L. Thompson of Sunderland. She ran on to Hyskeir Reef, off Rum on 24th August 1914, while on Admiralty service with a cargo of coal from Barry.

GRANFOS

Wreck No : 272
Latitude : 56 58 00 N PA
Decca Lat : 5658.00 N
Location : Hyskeir Rocks
Type : Steamship
Length : 254.0 ft.   **Beam :** 38.0 ft.
How Sunk : Ran aground

Date Sunk : 21 04 1912
Longitude : 06 40 30 W PA
Decca Long : 0640.50 W
Area : Rum
Tonnage : 849 gross.
Draught : 16.4 ft.
Depth : metres

The Norwegian steel steamship *Granfos*, (ex-*Ariel*), was built in 1906 by Wood, Skinner. En route from Drammen to Manchester with a cargo of timber and one passenger, she struck Hyskeir Rocks off Rum and was lost on 21st April 1912.

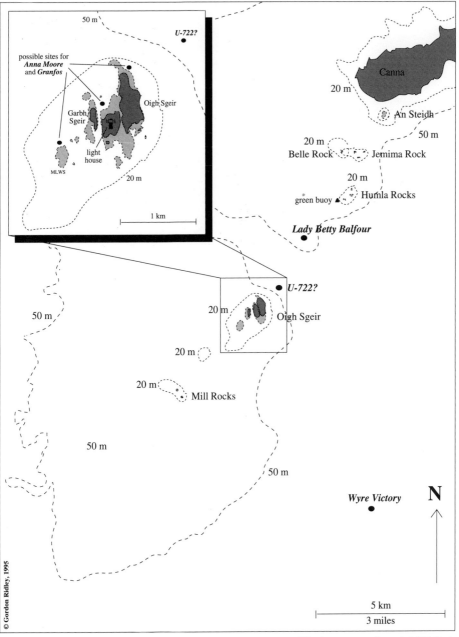

Wrecks on or near the reef of Oigh Sgeir
(also called Hyskeir), South west of the
island of Canna.

© Gordon Ridley, 1995

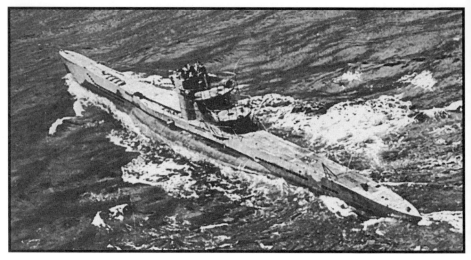

A Type VIIC U-boat, similar to U-722. The vessel is seen manned by a British crew on its way to be scuttled during Operation Deadlight after WW2. Note that the guns have been removed. (Photograph courtesy of Conway Maritime Press).

UNKNOWN - U-722?

Wreck No : 273	**Date Sunk :**
Latitude : 56 58 45 N	**Longitude :** 06 39 48 W
Decca Lat : 5658.75 N	**Decca Long :** 0639.80 W
Location : ½ mile NE of Oigh Sgeir	**Area :** Rum
Type : Submarine	**Tonnage :** gross
Length : ft. **Beam :** ft.	**Draught :** ft.
How Sunk :	**Depth :** 60 metres

According to local fishermen, this is the wreck of a submarine.

Despite an intensive search through U-boat records from both WW1 and WW2, no trace has been found of any U-boat recorded as having been sunk in this position. The nearest U-boat is *U-722* (see wreck number 286 on page 224), which is consistently recorded as sunk at 5709N 0655W, about 10 miles from this position. Perhaps that was the position in which she was first located, and maybe she was pursued for some distance from that position before being destroyed by depth charges. If this is the *U-722*, one would have thought the descriptive position would have been related to Oigh Sgeir, rather than *23 miles South west of Dunvegan*.

It may be significant that the fishermen apparently use the word *submarine* rather tha the word *U-boat*. Perhaps this implies that they consider this to be a British submarine, but I am unable to suggest a possible identity. As the fishermen's information came to me through a third party, I do not know what reason they have to think the wreck here is that of a submarine.

LADY BETTY BALFOUR?

Wreck No : 274
Latitude : 56 59 48 N
Decca Lat : 5659.80 N
Location : 1 ½ miles NE of Oigh Sgeir
Type : Trawler
Length : 120.0 ft.   **Beam :**   ft.
How Sunk :

Date Sunk :
Longitude : 06 38 36 W
Decca Long : 0638.60 W
Area : Rum
Tonnage :   gross
Draught : ft.
Depth : 27 metres

This wreck was identified by fishermen as a trawler about 120 ft long. It may be the *Lady Betty Balfour* which was lost on 8th October 1922.

MIDAS

Wreck No : 275
Latitude : 57 03 30 N PA
Decca Lat : 5703.50 N
Location : Near Kilmory, N Rum
Type : Barque
Length :   ft.   **Beam :**   ft.
How Sunk : Ran aground

Date Sunk : 27 12 1896
Longitude : 06 21 00 W PA
Decca Long : 0621.00 W
Area : Rum
Tonnage : 823 gross.
Draught : ft.
Depth :   metres

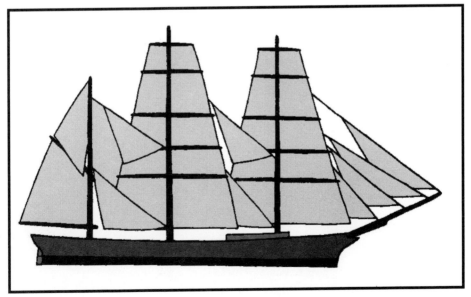

A typical 19th Century barque, similar to the Midas.

The 823 tons net Norwegian barque Midas was wrecked near Kilmory, at the North of Rum on 27th December 1896 while en route from Londonderry to Sapelo, USA. A severe gale, Force 9 was blowing from the North west at the time.

BOUNTEOUS

Wreck No : 276

Latitude : 57 03 00 N PA

Decca Lat : 5703.00 N

Location : N shore of Rum

Type : Drifter

Length :   ft.   **Beam :**   ft.

How Sunk : Ran aground

Date Sunk : 04 12 1917

Longitude : 06 20 00 W PA

Decca Long : 0620.00 W

Area : Rum

Tonnage : 63 gross.

Draught :   ft.

Depth :   metres

The drifter *Bounteous* was wrecked on the North shore of Rum on 4th December 1917.

CYGNET

Wreck No : 277

Latitude : 56 52 00 N PA

Decca Lat : 5652.00 N

Date Sunk : 1882

Longitude : 05 45 00 W PA

Decca Long : 0545.00 W

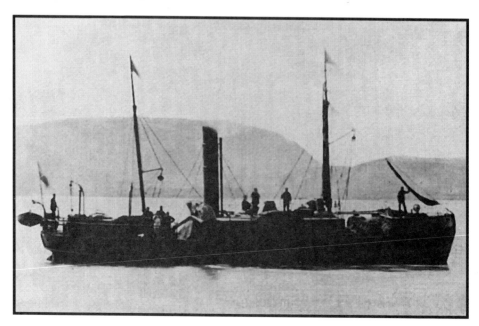

The paddle steamer Cygnet seen in Oban Bay. (Photograph courtesy of McIsaac & Riddle).

Location : Wrecked in Loch Ailort　　　**Area :** Mallaig
Type : Paddle Steamer　　　　　　　　**Tonnage :** 101 gross.
Length : 77.5 ft.　　**Beam :** 14.5 ft.　　**Draught :** 10.0 ft.
How Sunk : Ran aground?　　　　　　**Depth :**　　metres

Iron paddle steamer launched as the *Ben Nevis* in 1848. The cause of her loss has been given as *wrecked in Loch Ailort*. This can normally be interpreted as *ran aground*.

WYRE VICTORY

Wreck No : 278　　　　　　　　　　　**Date Sunk :** 14 01 1976
Latitude : 56 54 06 N　　　　　　　　　**Longitude :** 06 36 00 W
Decca Lat : 5654.10 N　　　　　　　　**Decca Long :** 0636.00 W
Location : 5 miles SE of Oigh Sgeir　　**Area :** Mallaig
Type : Trawler　　　　　　　　　　　　**Tonnage :** 398 gross.
Length : 140.0 ft.　　**Beam :** 28.0 ft.　　**Draught :** 14.0 ft.
How Sunk : Ran aground/Foundered　　**Depth :** 97 metres

The steel trawler *Wyre Victory*, built in 1960 ran aground on Mill Rocks, but drifted off and sank about 4.5 miles South east of Oigh Sgeir lighthouse, after being abandoned in gale force winds. The crew were all saved by the use of four life rafts. The wreck is charted as PA with at least 64 metres over it in about 97 metres.

UNKNOWN - PRE-1982

Wreck No : 279　　　　　　　　　　　**Date Sunk :**
Latitude : 56 54 35 N　　　　　　　　　**Longitude :** 05 51 57 W
Decca Lat : 5654.58 N　　　　　　　　**Decca Long :** 0551.95 W
Location : Close ashore　　　　　　　　**Area :** Mallaig
Type :　　　　　　　　　　　　　　　　**Tonnage :**　　gross
Length :　　ft.　　**Beam :**　　ft.　　**Draught :**　ft.
How Sunk : Ran aground　　　　　　　**Depth :**　　metres

NELLIE

Wreck No : 280　　　　　　　　　　　**Date Sunk :** 1954
Latitude : 56 56 30 N　　　　　　　　　**Longitude :** 06 07 45 W
Decca Lat : 5656.50 N　　　　　　　　**Decca Long :** 0607.75 W
Location : Ashore near NE tip of Eigg　**Area :** Mallaig
Type :　　　　　　　　　　　　　　　　**Tonnage :**　　gross
Length :　　ft.　　**Beam :**　　ft.　　**Draught :**　ft.

How Sunk : Ran aground   **Depth :**   metres

This may be the puffer *Jennie* which ran aground on the North tip of Eigg.

ROTCHE

Wreck No : 281   **Date Sunk :** 08 07 1977
Latitude : 56 57 32 N   **Longitude :** 05 55 00 W
Decca Lat : 5657.53 N   **Decca Long :** 0555.00 W
Location : 4 miles SW by W from Mallaig **Area :** Mallaig
Type : MFV   **Tonnage :** 40 gross.
Length :   ft.   **Beam :**   ft.   **Draught :** ft.
How Sunk : Collision with *Stroma II*   **Depth :** 55 metres

The crews of the motor fishing vessels *Rotche* and *Stroma II* had all been drinking in the Clachan Bar, and left Mallaig almost together after the pub shut. In the darkness, at about 2.30 am, the *Stroma II* struck the *Rotche* with a severe impact from an angle of 45° abaft her starboard beam at a point forward of her wheelhouse.

The *Rotche* was badly holed and went down in five minutes, with both members of her crew. After the collision, *Stroma II* proceeded in an easterly direction, taking in water, back to Mallaig harbour, assisted by the *Arctic Star* and *Ocean Starlight*, who took off the crew of the *Stroma II* about 75 yards off Mallaig harbour, where she sank. She was later raised.

The survey vessel *Challenger* observed debris and a large oil slick in an area South west of Mallaig, whose centre was about 3.5 miles from Mallaig, in the proximity of 246° true, Mallaig light 3 miles.

The cause of the collision was inadequate watchkeeping and alcohol consumption by the crews of both vessels.

FAIR MORN

Wreck No : 282   **Date Sunk :** 02 08 1969
Latitude : 56 58 30 N   **Longitude :** 05 53 30 W
Decca Lat : 5658.50 N   **Decca Long :** 0553.50 W
Location : 3 miles SW of Mallaig   **Area :** Mallaig
Type : Trawler   **Tonnage :**   gross
Length :   ft.   **Beam :**   ft.   **Draught :** ft.
How Sunk : Ran aground   **Depth :** 23 metres

The trawler *Fair Morn* sank while being taken off Anshay Point, about 1.75 miles West of Morar Bay. Decca Red E22.45, Purple A62.65, North Scottish Chain.

CRAIGENROAN

Wreck No : 283
Latitude : 57 00 00 N PA
Decca Lat : 5700.00 N
Location : Mallaig
Type : Drifter
Length : ft.   **Beam :** ft.
How Sunk : Fire

Date Sunk : 27 04 1977
Longitude : 05 49 40 W PA
Decca Long : 0549.67 W
Area : Mallaig
Tonnage :   gross
Draught : ft.
Depth : 22 metres

Craigenroan was a steam drifter, (BCK 93), which was so badly damaged by fire that she was towed here and sunk.

ARNEWOOD

Wreck No : 284
Latitude : 57 00 42 N PA
Decca Lat : 5700.70 N
Location : 4 miles ESE of Sleat Point
Type : Steamship
Length : 287.0 ft.   **Beam :** 41.0 ft.
How Sunk : Mined

Date Sunk : 13 12 1917
Longitude : 05 54 30 W PA
Decca Long : 0554.50 W
Area : Mallaig
Tonnage : 2259 gross.
Draught : 23.0 ft.
Depth : 120 metres

The collier *Arnewood* was mined 4 miles ESE of Sleat Point, Skye. *Lloyds War Losses* gives the position of striking the mine as 12 miles ESE of Sleat Point.

HIXIE 49

Wreck No : 285
Latitude : 57 01 00 N PA
Decca Lat : 5701.00 N
Location : 400-500 yds N of Mallaig Vaig Bay
Type : Drifter
Length : ft.   **Beam :** ft.
How Sunk :

Date Sunk : 1926
Longitude : 05 49 40 W PA
Decca Long : 0549.66 W
Area : Mallaig
Tonnage :   gross
Draught : ft.
Depth : 40 metres

The drifter *Hixie 49* sank 400-500 yards North of Mallaig Vaig Bay in 1926.

CHAPTER 9

THE WRECKS OF SKYE AND LOCH ALSH

INTRODUCTION

Kyle of Lochalsh is the main gateway to Skye. It is too small to be classed as a town, and only in its surrounding scenery can it be said to match Oban. The highly-photogenic Eilean Donan Castle is probably the most instantly recognised castle in the Western Highlands. It is sometimes referred to as *Castle Shortbread* as a result of the number of tin boxes of that product which have been adorned with its image. The castle sits on a rocky islet, and was the stronghold of the Clan Mackenzie of Kintail. With the assistance of a garrison of Spanish troops, it was held by the Jacobites until 10th May 1719, when 3 men o' war, *Worcester*, *Flamborough* and *Enterprise* attacked and blew up the castle, forcing the Spaniards to surrender. The ruined castle was restored by Colonel and Mrs. MacRae-Gilstrap between 1912 and 1932, the causeway connecting it to the mainland being constructed during that period. Closer to Kyle of Lochalsh, Donald Murchison's Monument is a memorial to the factor of William Dubh Mackenzie, 5th Earl of Seaforth, who supported his High Chief with rents, while he was in exile in France after the failure of the 1719 Jacobite uprising.

Skye is the largest island of the Inner Hebrides, with an area of 690 square miles. It is 49 miles long, and varies from 7 to 25 miles wide, but because of its irregular shape, no part of the island is more than 5 miles from the sea, and its coastline is over 900 miles long! Few would disagree with the statement that Skye contains some of the most magnificent scenery in Britain. Such a statement, however, carries with it the unfortunate implication that the scenery throughout the rest of the area is in some way inferior. Nothing could be further from the truth. Virtually the whole of the Western Highlands is an area of superb scenic beauty and grandeur.

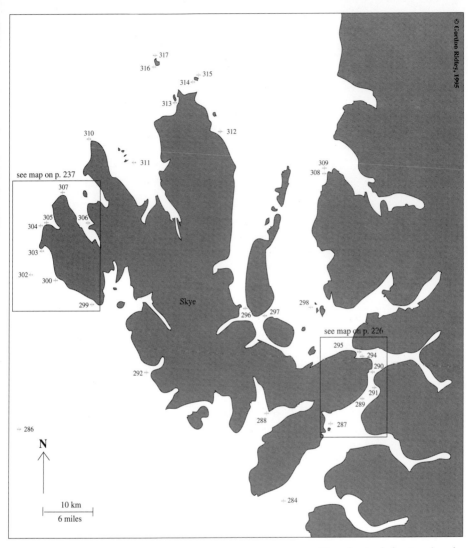

Chart showing the location of wrecks
lying off the coasts of Skye

THE WRECKS

U-722

Wreck No : 286	**Date Sunk :** 27 03 1945
Latitude : 57 09 00 N PA	**Longitude :** 06 55 00 W PA
Decca Lat : 5709.00 N	**Decca Long :** 0655.00 W
Location : 6 miles NW of Canna	**Area :** Skye
Type : Submarine	**Tonnage :** 769 gross.
Length : 221.4 ft. **Beam :** 20.5 ft.	**Draught :** ft.
How Sunk : Depth-charged	**Depth :** 120 metres

Type VIIC Atlantic U-Boat, 769 tons surfaced, 871 tons submerged. Max. diving depth 309 ft. *U-722* (KL Reimers) was depth-charged by RN Frigates *Byron*, *Fitzroy* and *Redmill* on 27th March 1945. The position given is 6 miles North west of Canna in 120 metres. All 44 members of the crew were lost. Five bodies floated to the surface.

According to Skye and Lochalsh District Council, these five bodies, (4 identified and 1 unidentified), were buried at Portree on 11th April 1945. I was unable to find their graves in the cemetery at Portree in June 1992, and wonder if they may, in fact, have been interred at Broadford. Skye and Lochalsh District Council also advised that 12 or 13 bodies from HMS *Curacoa* were buried at Broadford, but I found the graves of five or six of them in Portree cemetery.

The cruiser HMS *Curacoa* was run down by the *Queen Mary* at 5551N, 0838W, 40 miles NNW of Bloody Foreland at the North west of Ireland, while escorting the *Queen Mary* inward-bound from the United States with American troops. Zig-zag manoeuvres to reduce the possibility of torpedo attack by U-Boats were the order of the day, but the accompanying destroyers and the *Curacoa* were unable to conform to the liner's zig-zag pattern because of the heavy seas, and only the liner was zig-zagging. At 14.42 hrs on Friday 2nd October 1942, the *Queen Mary* hit *Curacoa* on the port side, 114 ft from her stern. The impact swung the cruiser 90 degrees to port, and the liner ran right over her, cutting her in two. The fore part went over on its beam ends, then righted itself and sank in 5 minutes, with the loss of 329 lives. A total of 101 survivors, including her commander, Captain John Boutwood, were picked up by the destroyers *Bramham* and *Cowdray*.

Queen Mary's stem was buckled back, but she was still able to do 13 knots, and made for the Clyde. She was patched temporarily in Boston, and 5 years later, in 1947, she was given a new stem at Southampton

The loss of the *Curacoa* was kept secret until May 1945. The Admiralty sued Cunard for £1,200,000 in compensation for the loss of *Curacoa* and her crew, but lost their case. Cunard and the *Queen Mary* were cleared of any blame for the incident.

EMBRACE

Wreck No : 287
Latitude : 57 09 30 N
Decca Lat : 5709.50 N
Location : N of Ornsay, E of Duisdalemore
Type : Drifter
Length : 86.2 ft.   **Beam :** 18.5 ft.
How Sunk : Ran aground

Date Sunk : 02 08 1940
Longitude : 05 47 12 W
Decca Long : 0547.20 W
Area : Skye
Tonnage : 94 gross.
Draught : 9.1 ft.
Depth : 18 metres

Embrace was a steel steam trawler, built in 1907 by Mackie & Thomson, Glasgow, engine by C. Houston & Co., Glasgow, registered in Inverness.

TRITON

Wreck No : 288
Latitude : 57 10 00 N PA
Decca Lat : 5710.00 N
Location : Suisnish Point
Type : Steamship
Length :   ft.   **Beam :**   ft.
How Sunk : Ran aground

Date Sunk : 18 12 1933
Longitude : 05 59 30 W PA
Decca Long : 0559.50 W
Area : Skye
Tonnage :   gross
Draught :   ft.
Depth :   metres

The steamship *Triton* is reported to have gone ashore on Suisnish Point, Skye on 18th December 1933. There are 15 vessels named *Triton* in the 1930/1 edition of *Lloyds Register*! Which one of them was lost on 18th December 1933?

CRYSTALINE

Wreck No : 289
Latitude : 57 12 57 N
Decca Lat : 5712.95 N
Location : 1 cable S Sheepfold Dun Ruaige
Type : Barque
Length :   ft.   **Beam :**   ft.
How Sunk : Ran aground

Date Sunk : 05 05 1894
Longitude : 05 40 05 W
Decca Long : 0540.08 W
Area : Skye
Tonnage :   gross.
Draught :   ft.
Depth :   metres

The iron barque *Crystaline* stranded South of the Kylerhea Narrows on 5th May 1894. This wreck was located in an aerial photograph in 1969. Only a small area of wreckage remains.

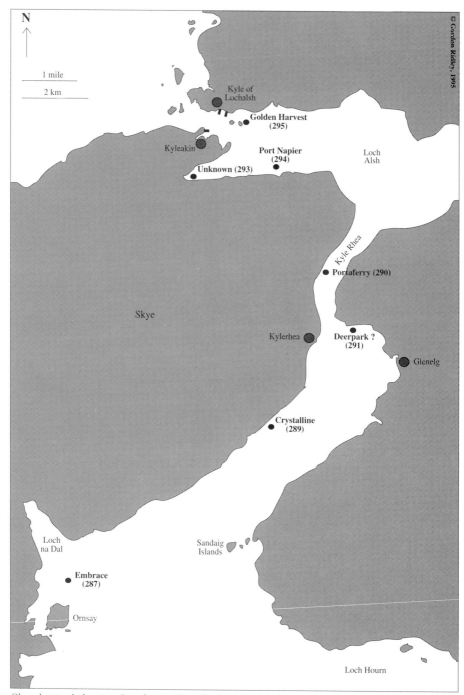

Chart showing the location of wrecks near Kyle of Lochalsh and Kyleakin

PORTAFERRY

Wreck No : 290
Latitude : 57 15 00 N
Decca Lat : 5715.00 N
Location : N of Kylerhea Light
Type :
Length : ft. **Beam :** ft.
How Sunk : Ran aground

Date Sunk : 21 04 1905
Longitude : 05 39 00 W
Decca Long : 0539.00 W
Area : Skye
Tonnage : 74 gross
Draught : ft.
Depth : metres

The 74 ton Irish vessel *Portaferry* (ex-*Ben Nevis*), with a cargo of coal and manure, stranded at Glenelg on 21st April 1905. Notice to Mariners No.521 of 1905 advises that the wreck has been dispersed.

Extremely strong tidal streams flow through the narrows. Any period of slack water will only be of very short duration.

DEERPARK?

Wreck No : 291
Latitude : 57 13 30 N PA
Decca Lat : 5713.50 N
Location : 1.4 m E of Cuil a Inheaunam
Type : Steamship
Length : 215.2 ft. **Beam :** 31.5 ft.
How Sunk :

Date Sunk : 16 11 1912
Longitude : 05 38 30 W PA
Decca Long : 0538.50 W
Area : Skye
Tonnage : 928 gross.
Draught : 14.2 ft.
Depth : 5 metres

The location of this wreck about 1.4 miles East of Cuil a Inheaunam, Bernera Bay, in the Sound of Sleat fits the description of the position of loss of the *Deerpark* on 16th November 1912.

The 549 tons net steel steamship *Deerpark* was built in 1901 by Scott & Co., Greenock. En route from Glasgow to Randers, Denmark, she ran aground one mile South of Kyle Rhea Lighthouse and became a total loss.

ALTAVELA

Wreck No : 292
Latitude : 57 14 30 N PA
Decca Lat : 5714.50 N
Location : Cracknish Point, L. Eynort
Type : Barque
Length : 230.5 ft. **Beam :** 36.3 ft.

Date Sunk : 26 11 1913
Longitude : 06 23 00 W PA
Decca Long : 0623.00 W
Area : Skye
Tonnage : 1220 gross.
Draught : 22.4 ft.

How Sunk : Ran aground   **Depth :**   metres

The Norwegian iron barque *Altavela*, (ex-*Colombo*), of 1157 tons net, was built in 1868 by R. Duncan of Port Glasgow. On 26th November 1913 she ran aground on Cracknish Point, Loch Eynort, Skye, while en route from Ardrossan to Montevideo with a cargo of coal. The current spelling is *Kraiknish*, where, according to the Ordnance Survey map, there are two buildings - probably belonging to the Forestry Commission, in a very remote, mountainous area at the south-western edge of Glen Brittle forest. The rocky headland a mile to the West, at the South side of the mouth of Loch Eynort does not seem to have a name of its own, but Cracknish, (or Kraiknish) Point suits very well.

UNKNOWN

Wreck No : 293	**Date Sunk :**
Latitude : 57 15 45 N	**Longitude :** 05 43 24 W
Decca Lat : 5715.75 N	**Decca Long :** 0543.40 W
Location : Loch na Beiste	**Area :** Skye
Type : Lighter	**Tonnage :** gross
Length : ft. **Beam :** ft.	**Draught :** ft.
How Sunk :	**Depth :** 20 metres

This may be the wreck of a barge, about 100 yds off drying rocks on the South shore of Loch na Beiste, 90° magnetic to the beacon at Corran na Mudlaich, on the South shore of the entrance to Loch na Beiste, and 190° magnetic to the top of Cnoc na Loch, the small hill on the North shore of the loch. According to the Hydrographic Dept. it is the wreck of an ammunition lighter, which dates from some time during the Second World War. The minimum depth is 17 metres.

WARNING: This barge may contain live munitions in an unstable condition.

PORT NAPIER

Wreck No : 294	**Date Sunk :** 27 11 1940
Latitude : 57 15 59 N	**Longitude :** 05 41 12 W
Decca Lat : 5715.98 N	**Decca Long :** 0541.20 W
Location : Loch Alsh	**Area :** Skye
Type : Minelayer	**Tonnage :** 9600 gross.
Length : 360.0 ft. **Beam :** ft.	**Draught :** ft.
How Sunk : Fire and explosion	**Depth :** 18 metres

While under construction for the Port Line in 1940, the *Port Napier* was requisitioned by the Admiralty and completed as a minelayer. Loaded with 550 mines and 6000

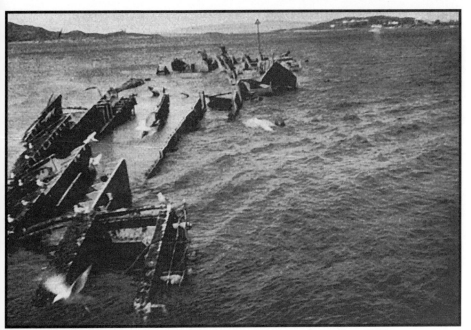

The wreck of the Port Napier *at low tide, taken after the removal of the port side plates late in WW2.*
(Photograph: Author's collection).

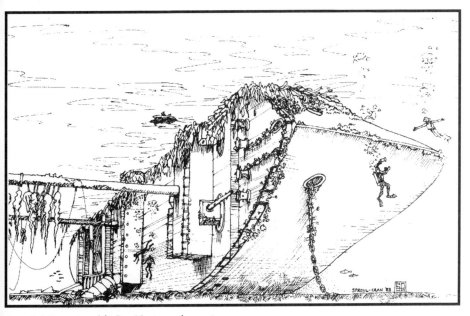

An artist's impression of the Port Napier *as she now is*
(Drawing courtesy of Dr. Robert Sproul-Cran)

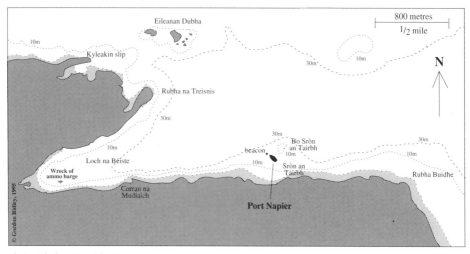

Above: The location of the Port Napier.

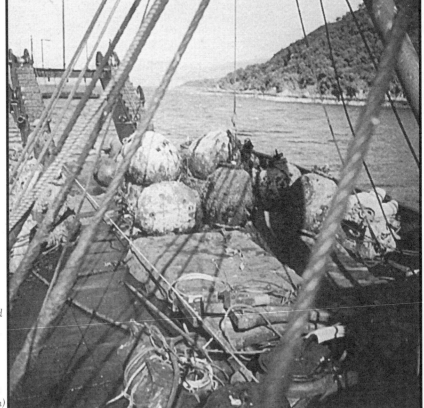

Mines recovered from the wreck of the Port Napier (Photo: Author's collection)

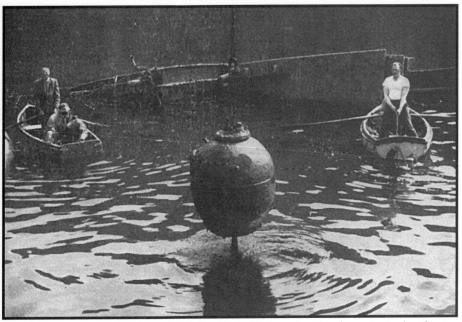

Recovering a mine from the wreck of the Port Napier. *The 'amatol soup' can be seen pouring from the mine.*
(Photograph: Author's collection)

Mine recovery from HMS Port Napier

HMS *Port Napier* was one of a squadron of large minelayers based in Loch Alsh for laying minefields to the North of Shetland. This - the so-called Northern Belt - was intended to prevent U-boats and large surface raiders (such as *Bismarck, Tirpitz*) passing between Shetland and Iceland. The minelayers each carried some 600 anti-submarine moored mines. A quarter-ton sinker moored the mine about 25 feet below the surface, so that light-draught ships could pass safely over it but deep-draught ships and submarines would hit and detonate the mine.

Preparing for minelaying was a complicated process; for detonation the electrical firing gear had to be connected, a primer inserted into the main mine charge and, lastly, a detonator inserted. Then a watertight cover was fastened over the primer/detonator access aperture in the base of the mine. In heavy weather these operations would all be carried out before leaving port.

When the fire broke out, the *Port Napier* was carrying 540 prepared mines. The mining party stayed aboard and probably removed all the detonators. As the fire began to subside, a party boarded the ship and discharged some mines but were forced to leave by the smoke and heat, immediately before the large explosion(s) occurred.

Divers examined the wreck later and 250 feet of the fore part and 250 feet of the after part of the wreck's hull plating reasonably intact, but about 100 feet of the centre portion

on the port side and decks above the engine room was completely blown out. Salvage was impossible. Later in the war shipbreakers removed as much of the port side armour and plating as could be reached at low water. While attempting to salvage the twin 10-ton phosphor-bronze props, a small demolition charge exploded a mine, sinking the diving tender and damaging the salvage ship. Salvage was abandoned.

In May 1952 the Navy ordered Capt. W.R. Fell aboard BDV *Barglow* to remove all mines and ammunition and to sink them in very deep water. The four salvage divers found 73 mines (19 undamaged and 54 variously disintegrating) on the seabed to the seaward of the wreck. These were recovered in two weeks and sunk 800 feet deep between Raasay and Eilean More. By the end of June 90 mines had been recovered from inside the wreck. Finally, by the end of September, the team had found, rendered safe and dumped 527 detonators, 310 primers, 635 rounds of 4" ammunition and 440 mines. Salvage ended on 5th October, 1952.

As probably three mines were lost in explosions, this leaves some 97 mines unaccounted for and probably in the wreck, along with detonators, primers and a large amount of 4" ammunition.

The Navy will not sell the wreck because of this remaining ordnance. Divers are warned accordingly.

The above has been extracted from a 1960 manuscript by Capt. W.R. Fell entitled *The Sea Surrenders*.

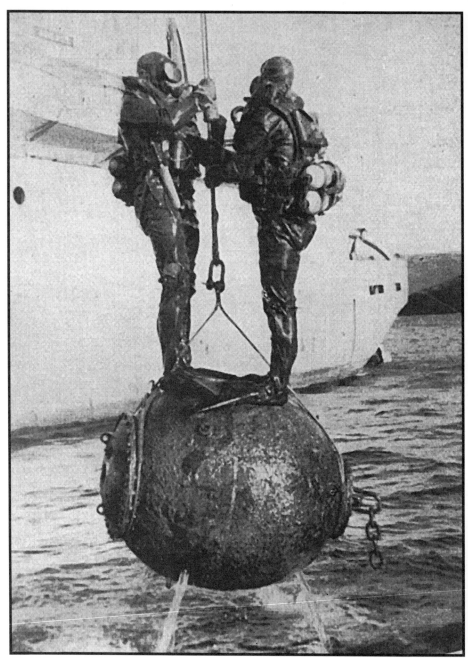

Navy salvage divers being winched aboard BDV Barglow
after recovering a mine from the wreck of the Port Napier.
(Photograph: Author's collection)

rounds of ammunition, she caught fire while tied up at Kyleakin. Efforts to extinguish the fire were not immediately successful, and in view of the nature of the cargo, there was no doubt a particularly acute shortage of time for the fire-fighting efforts to be rewarded with success!

It was realised that if the cargo exploded, Kyleakin would disappear. She was therefore towed away into Loch Alsh, towards Sron an Tairbh, and abandoned, still on fire. Shortly afterwards, a terrific explosion threw large sections of the ship more than quarter of a mile towards Skye, some of the pieces landing half way up a hillside, where they are still visible today.

Most of the mines were later salvaged, part of the port side of the hull being removed in order to achieve this. The total number of mines recovered or destroyed did not quite match the number known to have been aboard. Some 12 or 13 mines are still not accounted for (but see note on previous page).

The wreck lies on her starboard side, with her bow towards Kyleakin. Her two 4" guns are still in place on the now vertical foredeck. At low water, her port side protrudes above the surface. The clarity of the water and shallow depth have resulted in a fantastic variety of marine life, making this one of the most impressive and memorable wrecks to dive.

GOLDEN HARVEST

Wreck No : 295	**Date Sunk :** 02 1977
Latitude : 57 16 38 N	**Longitude :** 05 42 11 W
Decca Lat : 5716.63 N	**Decca Long :** 0542.18 W
Location : Eileanan Dubha, Loch Alsh	**Area :** Skye
Type : Trawler	**Tonnage :** gross
Length : 80.0 ft. **Beam :** ft.	**Draught :** ft.
How Sunk : Ran aground	**Depth :** 5 metres

Golden Harvest was a fishing vessel lost in February 1977. The wreck is charted at 571638N, 054211W PA, close in to the South east of the most easterly of the group of rocks named Eileanan Dubha off Kyle of Lochalsh. This rock, which has a beacon on it, does not appear to have a separate name of its own, and in fact the wreck lies close in to the North side of this rock, a few yards West of its most northerly point, at 571640N, 054213W. At low tide, a cable running in to the water is visible at the North of the rocky islet. It leads to the wreck, which is very broken up.

SPINDRIFT

Wreck No : 296	**Date Sunk :**
Latitude : 57 19 53 N	**Longitude :** 06 03 50 W
Decca Lat : 5719.88 N	**Decca Long :** 0603.83 W
Location : Ferry Pier, S Raasay	**Area :** Skye

Type :		**Tonnage :**	gross
Length : 30.0 ft.	**Beam :** ft.	**Draught :** ft.	
How Sunk : Jammed under pier		**Depth :** 5 metres	

The *Spindrift* jammed under the pier on a rising tide and broke her back. NG 554341.

IRISHMAN

Wreck No : 297		**Date Sunk :** 20 09 1862	
Latitude : 57 20 00 N PA		**Longitude :** 06 00 00 W PA	
Decca Lat : 5720.00 N		**Decca Long :** 0600.00 W	
Location : Skernataid Rock, Scalpay		**Area :** Skye	
Type : Steamship		**Tonnage :** gross	
Length : ft.	**Beam :** ft.	**Draught :** ft.	
How Sunk : Ran aground		**Depth :** metres	

The steamship *Irishman* stranded on Skernataid Rock, between Scalpay and Raasay, on 20th September 1862.

Could this be Sgeir Thraid at 575230N 055624W? This rock has a light on it, and lies about ¾ mile North east of Rubh an Lochain on Scalpay.

SCOMBER

Wreck No : 298		**Date Sunk :** 10 10 1923	
Latitude : 57 21 00 N PA		**Longitude :** 05 51 00 W PA	
Decca Lat : 5721.00 N		**Decca Long :** 0551.00 W	
Location : W of Caolas Beag, Crowlin Is.		**Area :** Skye	
Type : Trawler		**Tonnage :** 321 gross.	
Length : 132.0 ft.	**Beam :** 24.0 ft.	**Draught :** 14.0 ft.	
How Sunk : Ran aground /refloated		**Depth :** 17 metres	

The Fleetwood steam trawler *Scomber* ran aground at speed on rocks immediately below the lighthouse at the North end of Crowlin Island at 4.30 am, one hour before high water on 10th October 1923. The vessel was badly damaged and six of the crew got off in their small boat and were picked up at 7.00 am by a passing car ferry, the *Pioneer*, which was en route from Kyle of Lochalsh to Harris. The master and four crewmen were left to stand by the vessel. Her engine room and cabin were flooded, and the vessel was listing heavily to port. The *Scomber* was in a bad position with a rock through her hull, and salvage did not seem possible. The men standing by left by 3.00 pm. Despite her seemingly hopeless situation, the vessel was subsequently refloated, repaired and returned to service.

IRLANA

Wreck No : 299
Latitude : 57 21 19 N
Decca Lat : 5721.32 N
Location : NW of Idrigill Point, Skye
Type : Steamship
Length :   ft.   **Beam :**   ft.
How Sunk : Ran aground

Date Sunk : 05 09 1943
Longitude : 06 39 20 W
Decca Long : 0639.33 W
Area : Skye
Tonnage : 6852 gross.
Draught :   ft.
Depth : 10 metres

The steamship *Irlana* was built by Wm. Gray of West Hartlepool in 1941 for the British India Steam Navigation Co. En route from Buenos Aires to London with a cargo of wool, she went aground on the Isle of Skye on 5th September 1943. She lies just to the East of a group of underwater pinnacles at Geodha Mor, North west of Idrigill Point, and has been partially dispersed with explosives.

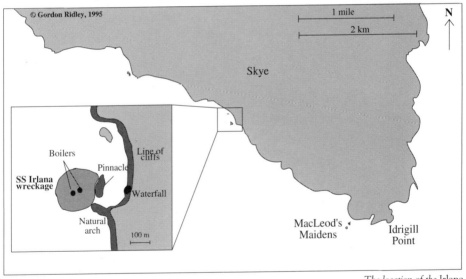

The location of the Irlana

CAROLINE ?

Wreck No : 300
Latitude : 57 22 10 N PA
Decca Lat : 5722.17 N
Location : Damsel Rocks, W side of Skye
Type : Steamship
Length : 157.0 ft.   **Beam :**   ft.
How Sunk : Ran aground

Date Sunk : 21 01 1887
Longitude : 06 42 24 W PA
Decca Long : 0642.40 W
Area : Skye
Tonnage : 516 gross
Draught :   ft.
Depth :   metres

Damsel Rocks lie about 150 yards off the cliffs at Hoe Point, on the North side of Lorgill Bay, about 4 miles South east of Neist Point in the West of Skye.

Large iron hoops have been found on the rocky shore. This may be the remains of the 380 ton wooden steamship *Caroline*, (ex-*Ansgarius*) which was built at Carlskrona by C. Grondahl in 1873. She was lost in Lorgill Bay on 21st January 1887. The wreck is reported to be broken into at least four pieces and spread out over 600 yards.

Very close to the above position, a ship's lifeboat lies well above the high water mark, but it is thought that this lifeboat is of much more recent vintage than the *Caroline*, and may possibly have come from the *Irlana*.

UNKNOWN - PRE-1978

Wreck No : 301
Latitude : 57 24 15 N
Decca Lat : 5724.25 N
Location : Sgeir Ghoblach, Poll Creadha
Type : Trawler
Length : ft.   **Beam :**   ft.
How Sunk : Ran aground

Date Sunk :
Longitude : 05 49 04 W
Decca Long : 0549.07 W
Area : Skye
Tonnage :   gross
Draught : ft.
Depth : 1 metres

This position is close to the shore about 2 miles South of Applecross Bay. The wreck, which is a small trawler, was reported to be high and dry.

INGER TOFT

Wreck No : 302
Latitude : 57 25 00 N PA
Decca Lat : 5725.00 N
Location : Little Minch, W of Skye
Type : Steamship
Length : 285.6 ft.   **Beam :** 41.5 ft.
How Sunk : Torpedoed by *U-722*

Date Sunk : 16 03 1945
Longitude : 06 52 00 W PA
Decca Long : 0652.00 W
Area : Skye
Tonnage : 2190 gross.
Draught : 19.9 ft.
Depth :   metres

The British steamship *Inger Toft*, (ex-*Elphinston*), built in 1920 by Swan Hunter, was torpedoed by *U-722* (Reimers), at 9.20 am on 16th March 1945. The position was given as 270°, 3 miles from Neist Point. Thirty survivors were picked up by the anti-submarine trawler *Grenadier*. The position is as given in German records, and also in *British Vessels Lost at Sea 1939-45*. *Lloyds World War 2 Losses* gives the latitude as 572530N. She had been en route from Reykjavik to Loch Ewe and London with a cargo of 604 tons of herring meal and 281 tons of cod liver oil. A number of barrels of cod liver oil were recovered in the Western Highlands.

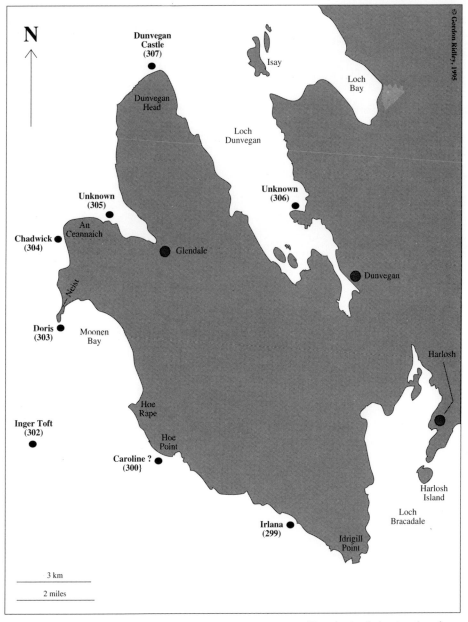

N

Dunvegan
Castle
(307)

Isay

Loch
Bay

Dunvegan
Head

Loch
Dunvegan

Unknown
(305)

Unknown
(306)

An
Ceannaich

Chadwick
(304)

Glendale

Dunvegan

Neist

Doris
(303)

Moonen
Bay

Harlosh

Inger Toft
(302)

Hoe
Rape

Hoe
Point

Caroline ?
(300}

Harlosh
Island

Loch
Bracadale

Irlana
(299)

Idrigill
Point

3 km

2 miles

© Gordon Ridley, 1995

*Chart showing the location of wrecks on
the far West of Skye*

DORIS

Wreck No : 303
Latitude : 57 25 15 N
Decca Lat : 5725.25 N
Location : Moonen Bay, NW Skye

Date Sunk : 12 07 1909
Longitude : 06 47 25 W
Decca Long : 0647.42 W
Area : Skye

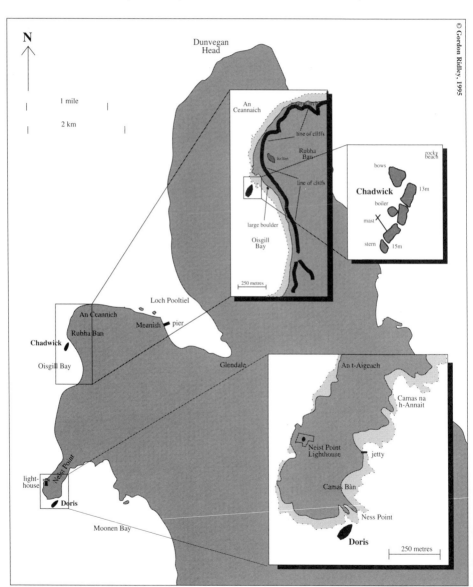

© Gordon Ridley, 1995

The location of the Chadwick and the Doris

Type : Steamship	**Tonnage** : 1381 gross.
Length : 255.0 ft. **Beam** : 36.0 ft.	**Draught** : 15.7 ft.
How Sunk : Ran aground	**Depth** : 24 metres

En route from Liverpool to Stettin, the 844 tons net Norwegian steel steamship *Doris* ran on to the rocks at Neist Point, Glendale, Skye on 12th July 1909. She was built in 1900 by Wood, Skinner of Newcastle, engine by N. E. Marine of Sunderland.

The wreck was located in 1970 close in to the South east corner of the Neist Promontory, below the lighthouse on Neist Point. (The lighthouse is on the top of the cliffs at the western edge of the Neist Promontory, just to the North of Neist Point..)

The position has also been recorded as 572510N, 064704W.

The wreck is steel, with an iron propeller, and is now completely broken up, lying on a slope of rock and sand in 6-24 metres of water.

CHADWICK

Wreck No : 304	**Date Sunk** : 02 07 1892
Latitude : 57 27 05 N PA	**Longitude** : 06 47 00 W PA
Decca Lat : 5727.08 N	**Decca Long** : 0647.00 W
Location : S of An Ceannaich, L Pooltiel	**Area** : Skye
Type : Steamship	**Tonnage** : 1463 gross.
Length : 247.5 ft. **Beam** : 35.0 ft.	**Draught** : 18.0 ft.
How Sunk : Ran aground	**Depth** : 25 metres

The 917 tons net iron steamship *Chadwick* was a collier built by Swan Hunter in 1882. She ran aground with a cargo of coal from the Clyde to St. Petersburg in July 1892, and lies below a large boulder at the foot of the cliff of Rubha Ban at the North end of Oisgill Bay, about 30 metres off the gullies and low rocks. Least depth to the wreck is 17 metres. The position has also been recorded as 572712N, 064706W.

UNKNOWN - PRE-1970

Wreck No : 305	**Date Sunk** :
Latitude : 57 27 30 N PA	**Longitude** : O6 45 10 W PA
Decca Lat : 5727.50 N	**Decca Long** : 0645.17 W
Location : W of Meanish, Loch Pooltiel	**Area** : Skye
Type :	**Tonnage** : gross
Length : ft. **Beam** : ft.	**Draught** : ft.
How Sunk :	**Depth** : metres

Charted as a wreck. Chains and steel plates have been found in Loch Pooltiel, West of

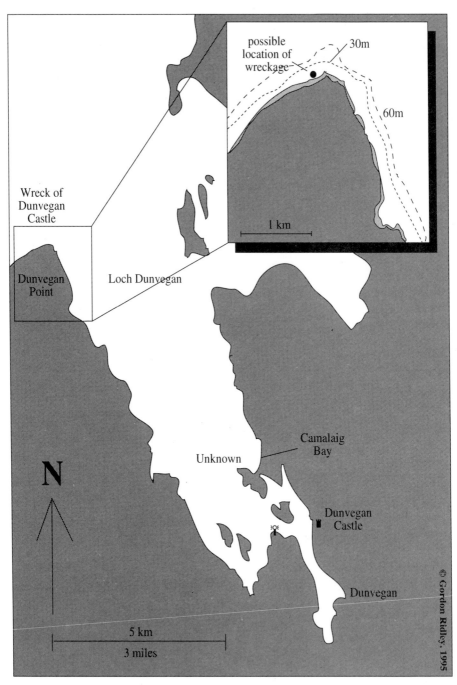

The location of the Dunvegan Castle

Meanish at NG 151508. This may be part of the *Chadwick*, but this wreck is known locally as the *salt boat*, which suggests the remains may be part of another vessel which carried a cargo of salt.

UNKNOWN

Wreck No : 306
Latitude : 57 27 44 N
Decca Lat : 5727.73 N
Location : Camalaig Bay, Loch Dunvegan
Type :
Length : 70.0 ft.   Beam : 20.0 ft.
How Sunk :

Date Sunk :
Longitude : 06 36 57 W
Decca Long : 0636.95 W
Area : Skye
Tonnage :   gross
Draught :   ft.
Depth :   metres

This is the wreck of a wooden vessel located in 1970, just to the South of drying rocks in the centre of the bay. This suggests the vessel ran aground.

DUNVEGAN CASTLE

Wreck No : 307
Latitude : 57 30 48 N PA
Decca Lat : 5730.80 N
Location : Dunvegan Point
Type : Steamship
Length :   ft.   Beam :   ft.
How Sunk : Ran aground

Date Sunk : 21 10 1874
Longitude : 06 43 00 W PA
Decca Long : 0643.00 W
Area : Skye
Tonnage : 149 gross.
Draught :   ft.
Depth :   metres

The 149 tons net iron steamship *Dunvegan Castle* was dashed ashore on Dunvegan Point in a North west hurricane, Force 12, on 21st October 1874. The vessel was en route from Tarbert to Glasgow with a general cargo and six passengers. According to a report in the *Highlander* newspaper of 11th September 1875, the wreck has been removed.

SHIELA

Wreck No : 308
Latitude : 57 35 00 N PA
Decca Lat : 5735.00 N
Location : Rubha na Fearn, Loch Torridon
Type : Steamship
Length :   ft.   Beam :   ft.

Date Sunk : 01 01 1927
Longitude : 05 50 30 W PA
Decca Long : 0550.50 W
Area : Skye
Tonnage : 280 gross.
Draught :   ft.

How Sunk : Ran aground   **Depth :**   metres

The MacBrayne steamship *Shiela* ran aground just South of the entrance to Loch Torridon in the early hours of New Years Day 1927, while making for Applecross Bay. No lives were lost, but the vessel became a total loss.

573400N, 055100W may be a more accurate position for Fearn na More Point.

VISCOUNT

Wreck No : 309   **Date Sunk :** 17 02 1924
Latitude : 57 35 05 N   **Longitude :** 05 50 20 W
Decca Lat : 5735.08 N   **Decca Long :** 0550.33 W
Location : Murchadh Breac, Loch Torridon   **Area :** Skye
Type : Steamship   **Tonnage :**   gross
Length :   ft.   **Beam :**   ft. **Draught :** ft.
How Sunk : Ran aground   **Depth :** 15 metres

This position is near Rubha na Fearn at the entrance to Loch Torridon.

NORMAN

Wreck No : 310   **Date Sunk :** 10 10 1903
Latitude : 57 36 30 N   **Longitude :** 06 38 00 W
Decca Lat : 5736.50 N   **Decca Long :** 0638.00 W
Location : Vaternish Point   **Area :** Skye
Type : Barque   **Tonnage :** 830 gross.
Length :   ft.   **Beam :**   ft. **Draught :** ft.
How Sunk : Ran aground   **Depth :**   metres

The 830 tons net Norwegian barque *Norman*, en route from Glasgow to Christiania with a cargo of coal, was lost on Vaternish Point, Skye on 10th October 1903.

BEN AIGEN

Wreck No : 311   **Date Sunk :** 19 07 1978
Latitude : 57 36 55 N   **Longitude :** 06 29 37 W
Decca Lat : 5736.92 N   **Decca Long :** 0629.62 W
Location : Loch Snizort, E of Ascrib Is.   **Area :** Skye
Type : Trawler   **Tonnage :**   gross
Length :   ft.   **Beam :**   ft. **Draught :** ft.

How Sunk :   **Depth :** 65 metres

The *Mary Croan* was also lost close to this position on 18th March 1980, but she was raised by the Elder brothers of Gairloch.

UNKNOWN

Wreck No : 312	**Date Sunk :** 1588
Latitude : 57 38 30 N PA	**Longitude :** 06 12 00 W PA
Decca Lat : 5738.50 N	**Decca Long :** 0612.00 W
Location : Staffin Island	**Area :** Skye
Type : Armada vessel	**Tonnage :** gross
Length : ft. **Beam :** ft.	**Draught :** ft.
How Sunk : Ran aground?	**Depth :** metres

There is reputed to be an Armada wreck somewhere around Staffin Island.

RHODESIA

Wreck No : 313	**Date Sunk :** 09 04 1915
Latitude : 57 41 14 N	**Longitude :** 06 20 45 W
Decca Lat : 5741.23 N	**Decca Long :** 0620.75 W
Location : At the S of Tulm Island	**Area :** Skye
Type : Trawler	**Tonnage :** 193 gross.
Length : 100.0 ft. **Beam :** 21.0 ft.	**Draught :** 14.0 ft.
How Sunk : Ran aground	**Depth :** 6 metres

Rhodesia was an armed Naval trawler, (iron screw ketch), built by Cochranes of Selby in 1899, engine by C. D. Holmes of Hull. Despite the shallow depth, (part of the wreck protrudes 1 metre above the surface at low water), she is reported to be intact and covered in kelp. The funnel is missing, and the mast and a winch lie on the seabed adjacent to the wreck.

ALEXANDERS

Wreck No : 314	**Date Sunk :** 29 01 1974
Latitude : 57 43 27 N	**Longitude :** 06 17 42 W
Decca Lat : 5743.45 N	**Decca Long :** 0617.70 W
Location : S side of Eilean Trodday	**Area :** Skye
Type : Trawler	**Tonnage :** gross
Length : ft. **Beam :** ft.	**Draught :** ft.

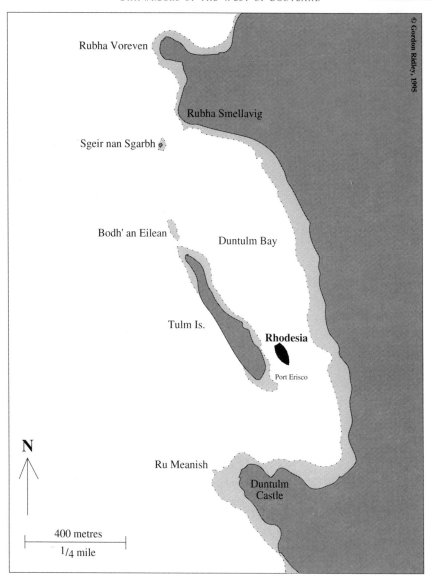

The location of the Rhodesia.

How Sunk : Ran aground   **Depth :** 2 metres

Alexanders was a Dutch motor fishing vessel with a wooden hull. The wreck is scattered amongst the rocks at the South side of Eilean Trodday. The position has also been recorded as 574328N, 061810W.

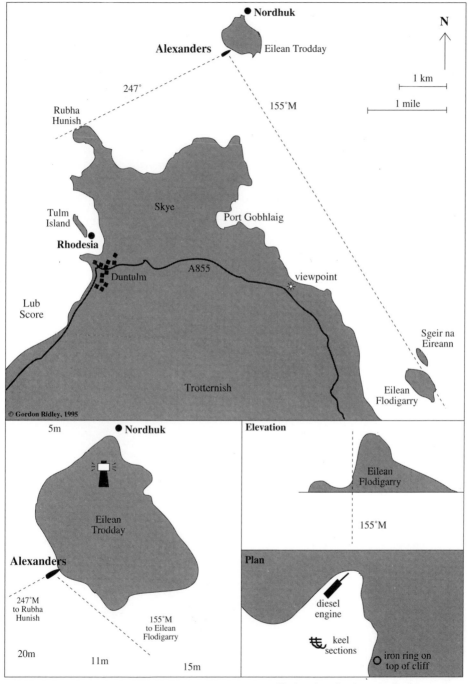

The location of and transits for the
Alexanders.

NORDHUK

Wreck No : 315
Latitude : 57 43 48 N
Decca Lat : 5743.80 N
Location : NE side of Eilean Trodday
Type : Motor vessel
Length : 225.0 ft.   **Beam :** 39.0 ft.
How Sunk : Ran aground

Date Sunk : 02 05 1976
Longitude : 06 17 48 W
Decca Long : 0617.80 W
Area : Skye
Tonnage : 1359 gross.
Draught : 12.2 ft.
Depth : 28 metres

Nordhuk (ex-*Meteor*), was a German coaster. While carrying a cargo of grain from Gothenburg to Liverpool, she was running South through the Minch on automatic pilot when she ran aground below the lighthouse on the north east side of Eilean Trodday, off the north of Skye. Her propeller was subsequently salvaged, and the wreck has gradually

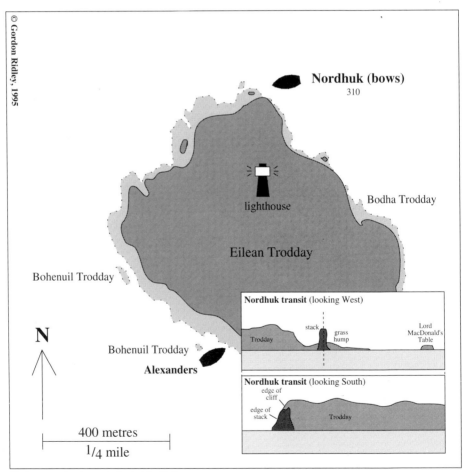

The location of and transits for the Nordhuk.

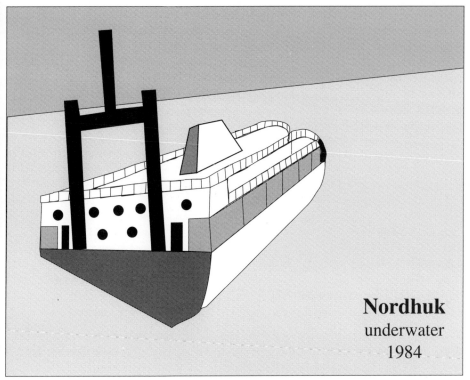

Nordhuk
underwater
1984

Sketch of the bows of the Nordhuk *seen underwater in 1984.*

broken up in 28 metres, although the stern third of the vessel is still fairly intact and stands up 10 metres from the bottom. The wreck lies at right angles to the cliffs, 100-150 metres off. Slack water is essential for diving, as there are otherwise strong tidal streams running NW/SE in this area.

APOLLO

Wreck No : 316
Latitude : 57 44 21 N
Decca Lat : 5744.35 N
Location : SW end of Fladda Chuain
Type : Motor vessel
Length : 247.5 ft.　　**Beam :** 36.0 ft.
How Sunk : Ran aground

Date Sunk : 21 09 1971
Longitude : 06 25 51 W
Decca Long : 0625.85 W
Area : Skye
Tonnage : 1274 gross.
Draught : 13.7 ft.
Depth : 10 metres

The wreck is reported to be lying on her starboard side and breaking up. She lies about

30 metres out from the shore. Other parts of the wreck lie at the West end of Fladda Chuain at 574442N, 062630W. It has also been suggested that this may be part of the remains of a vessel named *Ofela* or *Ophelia*, but this may have been due to a mistranslation of the Greek lettering for *Apollo*. Another position given is 574424N, 062542W. The *Apollo* was built in Holland, but was Cypriot-owned at the time of loss. She was carrying a cargo of salt. More wreckage lies at the North end of Fladda Chuain in only 1 metre of water, and may be part of the *Apollo*, but is more likely to be from the Liberty ship *Frederick Bartholdi* (q.v.).

FREDERICK BARTHOLDI

Wreck No : 317	**Date Sunk :** 25 12 1943
Latitude : 57 44 48 N	**Longitude :** 06 26 30 W
Decca Lat : 5744.80 N	**Decca Long :** 0626.50 W
Location : At N end of Fladda Chuain	**Area :** Skye
Type : Steamship	**Tonnage :** 7000 gross.
Length : 441.5 ft. **Beam :** 57.0 ft.	**Draught :** 27.8 ft.
How Sunk : Ran aground/refloated	**Depth :** 1 metres

Wreckage which was obviously from a vessel of welded construction was found here in 1980, and it was estimated that the wreckage had been here for at least 10 years. This may be the very broken remains of a small vessel, but it is more likely to be the remains of wreckage from the Liberty ship *Frederick Bartholdi* which ran aground here on 25th December 1943 while en route from Jacksonville to London with a general cargo. The position was given as 5744N, 0626W PA.

She came to rest with her bow and stern perched on the rocks, but with her centre section unsupported, she broke her back, virtually splitting in two. Her cargo was removed with great difficulty as the surrounding rocks made it impossible for other vessels to get alongside. It was not possible to refloat her with compressed air without rejoining the separated ends of her double bottom, and the usual method of patching was unsuitable, because a rigid patch would be displaced as the vessel regained her shape as buoyancy was achieved. To overcome the problem, a rubber patch was fastened to each side of the breaks in the hull, and this flexed as compressed air was pumped into the sealed compartments and the two ends of the ship realigned themselves as she floated off the rocks. The ship was then towed to the sandy beach at Uig Bay where further patching work was carried out before the vessel was towed to the Clyde. Her damage was found to be too great to justify permanent repairs, and she was beached and scrapped at Kames Bay in the Clyde in September 1944.

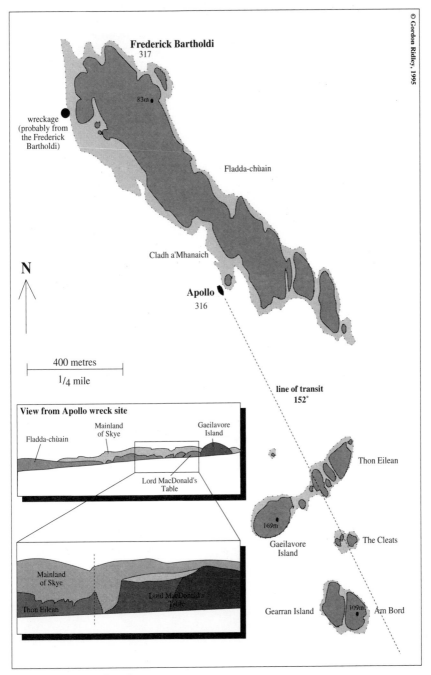

The locations of the Apollo *and*
the Frederick Bartholdi.

CHAPTER 10

THE WRECKS OF THE MINCH, LOCH EWE, LOCH BROOM

Introduction

The creation of the beautiful Inverewe Garden, at the head of Loch Ewe was started in 1862 by Osgood MacKenzie, and became his life's work. Although it is on the same latitude as Hudsons Bay, Moscow and Siberia, the climate allows a wide variety of plants and trees to grow here - species which would in many cases be expected to flourish only in more southerly, warmer latitudes - e.g. palm trees and bamboo. The garden has been under the care of the National Trust for Scotland since 1952, and any trip to this area would be the poorer for not spending time in making a visit here.

Gruinard Bay, between Loch Ewe and Loch Broom, contains the mile-long Gruinard Island which was infected with anthrax in a biological experiment during the Second World War. Landing was prohibited here for about 50 years, and notices warning of the danger were posted at intervals along the coastal road round Gruinard Bay. The island would have remained dangerous to humans and animals for about 100 years had it not been decontaminated, at considerable expense, only two or three years ago. After being declared safe, it was sold back to its original owner for £500, which was the amount of compensation he was given when it was requisitioned during the war.

Loch Ewe was the main marshalling point in Britain for the Russian Convoys during that war, and there is still a NATO refuelling base at Aultbea, on the North shore of the loch.

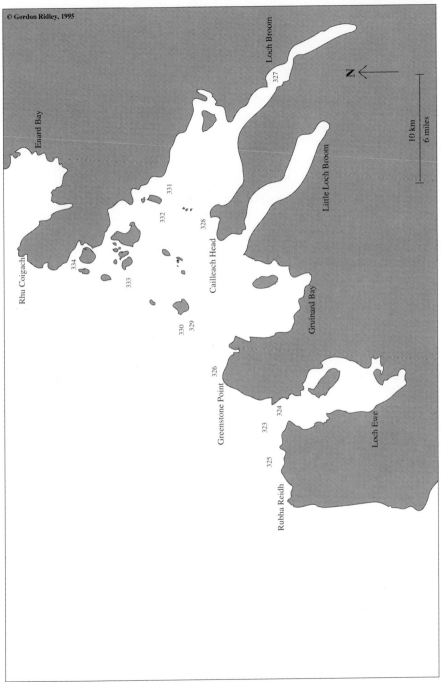

© Gordon Ridley, 1995

Loch Broom

327

N

10 km
6 miles

Einard Bay

Little Loch Broom

331

332

328

334

333

Rhu Coigach

Cailleach Head

Gruinard Bay

330

329

326

Greenstone Point

324

323

Loch Ewe

325

Rubha Reidh

Chart showing the location of wrecks lying off the coast of Loch Ewe and Loch Broom

THE WRECKS

KONDOR

Wreck No : 318
Latitude : 58 02 30 N PA
Decca Lat : 5750.00 N
Location : 10 miles S of Stornoway
Type : Motor vessel
Length :   ft.   **Beam :**   ft.
How Sunk : Foundered under tow

Date Sunk : 25 04 1990
Longitude : 06 18 00 W PA
Decca Long : 0650.00 W
Area : Minch
Tonnage : 2650 gross.
Draught : ft.
Depth : 105 metres

En route from Ullapool to Falmouth, the Bulgarian fishing ship (factory ship?) *Kondor* ran aground at Ushinish, North west Skye on 24th April 1990. Although she was holed, she was towed off the rocks after all 28 crew members had been taken off by Stornoway lifeboat. While still under tow towards Stornoway for repairs, the towing line had to be cut as the stricken vessel foundered about 14 miles South of Stornoway. The wreck is thought to lie about 10 miles South of Stornoway at 580230N, 061800W, PA in 105 metres.

UNKNOWN

Wreck No : 319
Latitude : 58 12 26 N
Decca Lat : 5812.43 N
Location : Off the Point of Stoer
Type :
Length : 108.0 ft.   **Beam :**   ft.
How Sunk :

Date Sunk :
Longitude : 05 32 41 W
Decca Long : 0532.68 W
Area : Minch
Tonnage :   gross
Draught : ft.
Depth : 112 metres

The wreck at 581226N, 053241W is apparently 108 ft long, and it was suggested that it may be part of *U-1021*. An examination of the sonar traces, however, cast doubt about the validity of that suggestion.

NORMANNVIK

Wreck No : 320
Latitude : 58 12 49 N
Decca Lat : 5812.82 N
Location :
Type : Motor ship
Length : 184.0 ft.   **Beam :** 31.0 ft.
How Sunk : Foundered

Date Sunk : 18 01 1970
Longitude : 05 43 08 W
Decca Long : 0543.13 W
Area : Minch
Tonnage : 499 gross.
Draught : 12.0 ft.
Depth : 69 metres

The Norwegian motor vessel *Normannvik* was en route from Norway to Runcorn with a cargo of felspar (stone). In heavy seas on 18th January 1970, the cargo shifted, and the vessel capsized and sank. The crew were rescued by a fishing boat. The wreck lies WNW/ESE and has a least depth of 69 metres in a general depth of 86 metres.

UNKNOWN

Wreck No : 321	Date Sunk :
Latitude : 58 12 52 N	Longitude : 05 43 53 W
Decca Lat : 5812.87 N	Decca Long : 0543.88 W
Location :	Area : Minch
Type :	Tonnage : gross
Length : 390.0 ft. Beam : ft.	Draught : ft.
How Sunk :	Depth : 88 metres

This wreck was found during a sonar sweep in 1970. From side scan sonar images, it appears to be a two-funnelled passenger ship, 390 ft long. The wreck lies NW/SE and stands up about 14 metres from the bottom which is at 103 metres.

U-1021

Wreck No : 322	Date Sunk : 30 03 1945
Latitude : 58 19 30 N	Longitude : 05 32 00 W
Decca Lat : 5819.50 N	Decca Long : 0532.00 W
Location : 6 miles West of Point of Stoer	Area : Minch
Type : Submarine	Tonnage : 769 gross
Length : 221.4 ft. Beam : 20.5 ft.	Draught : 15.8 ft.
How Sunk : Depth-charged	Depth : metres

U-1021 (KL Holpert), was depth-charged and sunk by the RN ships *Rupert, Deane* and *Conn* at 581900N, 053100W in the Minch on 30th March 1945. A strong smell of diesel followed this attack. In a subsequent depth-charge attack on a bottom contact at 581930N, 053200W, a large quantity of diesel fuel and wreckage came to the surface.

GLEN ALBYN

Wreck No : 323	Date Sunk : 23 12 1939
Latitude : 57 52 30 N	Longitude : 05 39 52 W
Decca Lat : 5752.50 N	Decca Long : 539.87 W
Location : Entrance to Loch Ewe	Area : Lochewe
Type : Drifter	Tonnage : 82 gross.

Length : ft. **Beam :** ft. **Draught :** ft.
How Sunk : Mined **Depth :** 40 metres

HM drifter *Glen Albyn* was lost in the entrance to Loch Ewe on 23rd December 1939 when she detonated a magnetic mine laid almost two months previously by the U-31 on 28th October 1939. The date and cause of the *Glen Albyn*'s loss are given in *British Vessels Lost at Sea 1939-45*, and in Rohwer's *Axis Submarine Successes 1939-45*. Curiously, *Lloyds World War 2 Losses* gives the date as 23rd December 1940, exactly one year later, and says *"sunk by Admiralty in secret circumstances."* In the German grid system, U-Boat records give the position of the mines laid as AM 3826. This would appear to equate to a position of about 581500N, 054100W, in the Minch, some distance North of Loch Ewe, but in fact 18 TMB mines were laid in a line, just outside the entrance to the loch, 8.5 cables 289° from Leacan Donna. *U-31* (Habekost), had apparently intended to lay his mines inside Loch Ewe, but was prevented from entering the loch by the anti-submarine boom across the entrance.

On 4th December 1939, the 33950 ton battleship HMS *Nelson* was damaged by one of the magnetic mines laid there by *U-31* on 28th October. The cause of the damage, and indeed the fact that the *Nelson* had been damaged at all were kept secret, even from the Commonwealth Prime Ministers. The *Nelson* was taken to the lee of Ewe Island, where she lay 7.5 ft down by the bow, and with a slight list to starboard. The cruiser HMS *Cairo* was despatched to Loch Ewe to provide anti-aircraft cover until the *Nelson* could be patched up.

At that time, urgent efforts were being made to find a successful method of dealing with this new type of mine. HMS *Borde* was a collier hurriedly converted to a mine destructor vessel by fitting it with an enormous electro - magnet weighing 400-500 tons. The core of the magnet was a bundle of railway lines 200 ft long! The idea was to create a powerful magnetic field around the ship to cause the mines to detonate at a safe distance from the vessel. According to one report it detonated its first mine on 24th December 1939. Another report gives the date as 4th January 1940. The force of the explosion close to the vessel was such that the crew had to stand on thick rubber mats to avoid broken ankles, and the ship itself was badly shaken.

I do not know where this trial took place, but the drifters *Glen Albyn* and *Promotive* were used to try out one of several other approaches to the magnetic mine problem. They were wound around with coils of copper wire, and towed about in the entrance to Loch Ewe to find and detonate magnetic mines. Neither vessel had any crew aboard. The coils of copper wire were probably energised by power from a generator on board the towing vessel. Magnetic mines were found, and successfully detonated, but at the expenditure of the two drifters which were sunk by the explosions.

Their wrecks now lie half a mile apart, and part of the copper coils have been recovered. Where better to test a new minesweeping method than in a remote location, away from prying eyes, and where the presence of magnetic mines had so recently been established by the nature of the damage to HMS *Nelson*? Secrecy surrounding the circumstances of the loss would be understandable, as it was important to avoid giving the Germans any hint of the British efforts to counter the menace of these mines.

It was obviously impractical to continue expending vessels in this way, and finally, a satisfactory solution to the problem was developed. This was the *Double Longitudinal*, or *Double L* sweep, which consisted of two wooden vessels steaming on a parallel course about 300 yards apart, each vessel towing two lengths of floating cable. One cable was much longer than the other. Synchronised positive electrical pulses were sent down one of the cables, and negative pulses down the other. The salt water between the electrodes at the ends of the cables completed the circuit, creating an intense magnetic field over a wide area, exploding any magnetic mines, without damaging either the cables or the towing vessels. By this continuous process, a broad channel was quickly swept. The first floating cable was delivered on 18th January 1940, and the system became fully operational from May 1940, and continued until after the end of the war.

PROMOTIVE

Wreck No : 324	**Date Sunk :** 23 12 1939
Latitude : 57 52 40 N	**Longitude :** 05 40 44 W
Decca Lat : 5752.67 N	**Decca Long :** 0540.73 W
Location : Entrance to Loch Ewe	**Area :** Lochewe
Type : Drifter	**Tonnage :** 78 gross.
Length : ft. **Beam :** ft.	**Draught :** ft.
How Sunk : Mined	**Depth :** 46 metres

HM drifter *Promotive* was lost in the entrance to Loch Ewe on 23rd December 1939 when she detonated one of the magnetic mines laid by the *U-31* on 28th October 1939.

WILLIAM H WELCH

Wreck No : 325	**Date Sunk :** 26 02 1944
Latitude : 57 52 33 N	**Longitude :** 05 43 03 W
Decca Lat : 5752.55 N	**Decca Long :** 0543.05 W
Location : Nr. Cove, entrance to Loch Ewe	**Area :** Lochewe
Type : Steamship	**Tonnage :** 7200 gross.
Length : 423.0 ft. **Beam :** 57.1 ft.	**Draught :** 34.8 ft.
How Sunk : Ran aground	**Depth :** metres

William H Welch was an American Liberty ship built by Bethlehem Fairfield yard in March 1943. While en route, in ballast from London to New York, she was second in line in a convoy of ten ships seeking the shelter of Loch Ewe in a storm in the early hours of 26th February 1944. In the darkness, she missed the entrance to the Loch, and at 04.20 hrs ran aground at Black Bay, at the West of the entrance to Loch Ewe, and broke in two.

Flares fired at 06.00 hrs were seen, and despite the blizzard conditions, local crofters set out across several miles of rough moorland with blankets and tea to find and help the

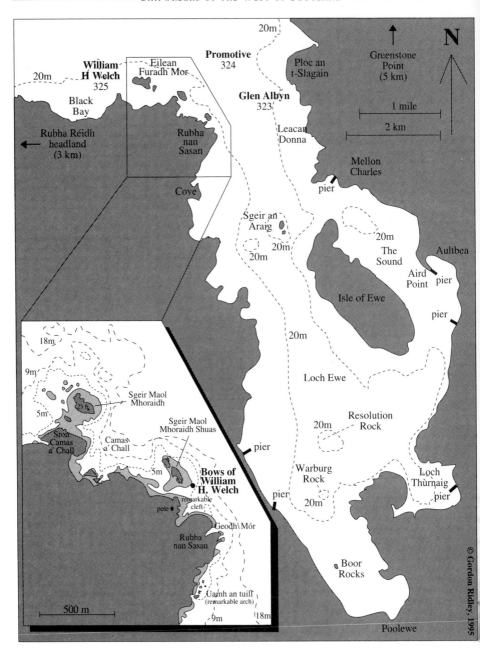

Chart showing the location of wrecks lying in or near Loch Ewe together with the position of the bows of the steamship William H Welch.

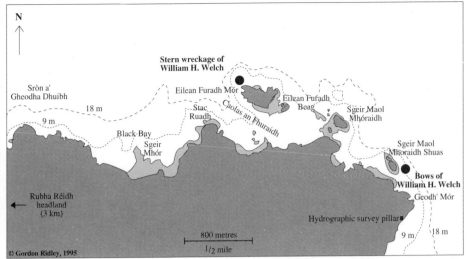

The locations of the bow and stern wreckage of the steamship
William H Welch *near the mouth Loch Ewe*

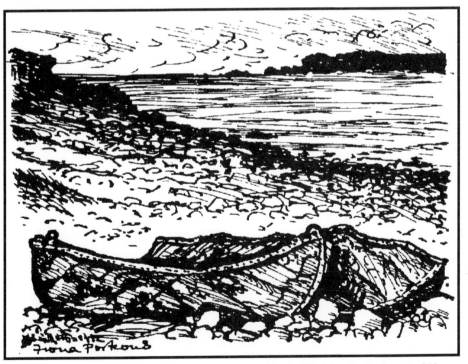

*Sketch of Black Bay showing the rusting lifeboats
from the steamship* William H Welch
(*Drawing courtesy of Fiona Porteous*).

crew. The two keepers from Ruadh Reidh lighthouse also set off across one of the wildest, snow-covered rocky areas in Scotland to assist. Only 28 bodies and 12 survivors were recovered from the crew of 74. Two of those washed ashore still had sufficient strength to stagger for two hours towards Cove, where the defensive guns were situated. As the crofters spoke Gaelic, a language unknown to the American crew, the survivors imagined they had been wrecked somewhere on the Russian coast.

The stern section of the wreck now lies broken up and scattered over a wide area close to the shore, 40 metres off the West of Eilean Furadh Mor, just outside the entrance to Loch Ewe at 575233N, 054303W. Only the bow section remains reasonably intact at 575204N, 054105W, just off the rocky islet of Sgeir Maol Mhoraidh Shuas, near the former gun positions at Rubha nan Sasan, near Cove.

Two rusting lifeboats from the *William H Welch* still lie where they were washed up by the huge waves on the rocky shore south of Eilean Furadh Mor. The crew had been unable to use them in the raging conditions at the time of stranding.

Loch Ewe was the main marshalling point for the Russian convoys during the Second World War. There is a fair amount of ship debris, including bottles, portholes and bells lying around the bottom of the loch, left behind after the wartime activities there.

GRATITUDE

Wreck No : 326
Latitude : 57 55 36 N
Decca Lat : 5755.60 N
Location : Greenstone Point

Date Sunk : 15 11 1958
Longitude : 05 36 48 W
Decca Long : 0536.80 W
Area : Lochewe

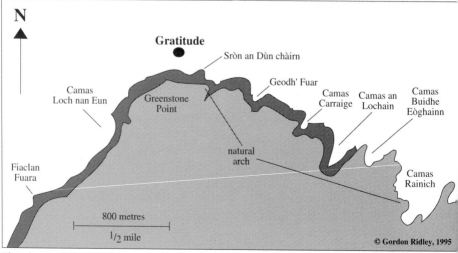

Chart showing the location of the wreck of the Gratitude

Type : Trawler   **Tonnage :** gross
Length : ft.   **Beam :** ft.   **Draught :** ft.
How Sunk : Ran aground   **Depth :** 20 metres

356° 400 metres from the triangulation mark on Greenstone Point.

UNKNOWN

Wreck No : 327   **Date Sunk :**
Latitude : 57 53 45 N   **Longitude :** 05 09 20 W
Decca Lat : 5753.75 N   **Decca Long :** 0509.33 W
Location : Ullapool Harbour, E of Pier   **Area :** Broom
Type : Trawler   **Tonnage :** gross
Length : ft.   **Beam :** ft.   **Draught :** ft.
How Sunk :   **Depth :** 15 metres

According to an article in the May 1967 edition of *Underwater World* magazine, there is wreckage from more than one trawler in 50 ft of water near the jetty at Ullapool.

INNISJURA

Wreck No : 328   **Date Sunk :** 10 01 1921
Latitude : 57 56 14 N   **Longitude :** 05 21 33 W
Decca Lat : 5756.23 N   **Decca Long :** 0521.55 W
Location : Iolla Carn Dearg   **Area :** Broom
Type : Puffer   **Tonnage :** 127 gross
Length : 74.0 ft.   **Beam :** 21.0 ft.   **Draught :** 0.0 ft.
How Sunk : Ran aground   **Depth :** 0 metres

The *Innisjura* was built at Alloa in 1913, and was diesel powered. She was presumably a very similar vessel to the *Ballista*.

On 10th January 1921, while carrying a cargo of telegraph poles, she stranded high and dry on Iolla Carn Dearg. Salvage was started, but a SW gale blew up after a week and she disappeared. The wreck now lies 50 metres out from a U-shaped mini bay which faces North, at Iolla Carn Dearg, West of Cailleach Head, between Loch Broom and Little Loch Broom.

The wreck of the MFV *Fairweather V*, which was lost in the late 1980s, lies about 100 metres from the *Innisjura*.

GUIDING STAR

Wreck No : 329	**Date Sunk :** 09 12 1964
Latitude : 57 57 25 N	**Longitude :** 05 30 58 W
Decca Lat : 5757.42 N	**Decca Long :** 0530.97 W
Location : SW Priest Island	**Area :** Broom
Type : Trawler	**Tonnage :** 39 gross.
Length : ft. **Beam :** ft.	**Draught :** ft.
How Sunk : Collision?	**Depth :** 8 metres

The fishing vessels *Guiding Star* and the *Silver Reward* both ran aground on Priest Island on the same day. This suggests fog prevailed over the area on that day.

SILVER REWARD

Wreck No : 330	**Date Sunk :** 09 12 1964
Latitude : 57 57 45 N	**Longitude :** 05 31 18 W
Decca Lat : 5757.75 N	**Decca Long :** 0531.30 W
Location : SW Priest Island	**Area :** Broom
Type : Trawler	**Tonnage :** 50 gross.
Length : ft. **Beam :** ft.	**Draught :** ft.
How Sunk : Collision?	**Depth :** 20 metres

SILVER SPRAY

Wreck No : 331	**Date Sunk :** 07 12 1965
Latitude : 57 58 32 N	**Longitude :** 05 20 14 W
Decca Lat : 5758.53 N	**Decca Long :** 0520.23 W
Location : 300 metres SE of Iolla Mhor	**Area :** Broom
Type : Trawler	**Tonnage :** 40 gross.
Length : 66.0 ft. **Beam :** ft.	**Draught :** ft.
How Sunk : Ran aground	**Depth :** 36 metres

Silver Spray was a wooden fishing vessel 66 ft long.

UNKNOWN

Wreck No : 332
Latitude : 57 59 00 N PA
Decca Lat : 5759.00 N
Location : Horse Island
Type : Armada Vessel
Length : ft.   **Beam :** ft.
How Sunk :

Date Sunk : 1588
Longitude : 05 21 00 W PA
Decca Long : 0521.00 W
Area : Broom
Tonnage : gross
Draught : ft.
Depth : metres

A Spanish gold coin has been found on Horse Island, reputedly from an Armada vessel.

UNKNOWN

Wreck No : 333
Latitude : 58 00 45 N PA
Decca Lat : 5800.75 N
Location : Tanera More Anchorage
Type : Trawler
Length : ft.   **Beam :** ft.
How Sunk :

Date Sunk :
Longitude : 05 24 00 W PA
Decca Long : 0524.00 W
Area : Broom
Tonnage : gross
Draught : ft.
Depth : 22 metres

Reportedly sunk in the 1980s.

UNKNOWN

Wreck No : 334
Latitude : 58 03 00 N PA
Decca Lat : 5803.00 N
Location : Bo Bhuiridh Bay, Isle Ristol
Type : Armada vessel
Length : ft.   **Beam :** ft.
How Sunk :

Date Sunk : 1588
Longitude : 05 26 00 W PA
Decca Long : 0526.00 W
Area : Broom
Tonnage : gross
Draught : ft.
Depth : metres

There is a local legend of an Armada vessel that was wrecked in the northern bay off Bo Bhuiridh on Isle Ristol. This links interestingly with the Horse Island information. (G. Ridley, *Dive North West Scotland*).

CHAPTER 11

THE WRECKS OF ENARD BAY, EDDRACHILLIS BAY, KYLESKU AND CAPE WRATH

Introduction

The scenery in this area is absolutely stunning, with many bays, inlets and islets, and 30 metres underwater visibility is not uncommon. Because of the clarity of the water, marine life in this area is outstandingly prolific. For divers visiting by car and towing an inflatable, there are numerous launching places. The two largest centres of population are the fishing villages of Lochinver and Kinlochbervie, where trawlers may be hired.

Cape Wrath is the *Land's End* of the North west of the British mainland. It is not an easy place to reach, as the nearest public road stops 12 miles away. The remoteness and isolation of Cape Wrath is part of its appeal. One way to visit Cape Wrath is to leave your car at Oldshoremore, about four miles West of Kinlochbervie, and walk North for some four miles along a peat track to the beautiful and isolated mile long Sandwood Bay, reputed to be the hauling-out point of mermaids. Cross the shallow Sandwood river which flows over the beach, then continue for about another five miles as the crow flies (although, as it is impossible to walk in a straight line, the actual distance to be walked is about three times as far) following the coast along the cliff tops, through a wilderness of bogs and rough uninhabited moorland, stopping frequently to rest and admire the scenery. The silence in this desolated, trackless wilderness (called the Parph) is audible.

The lighthouse, which is hidden from view until the last few hundred yards, was built in 1828. It sits atop a 370 ft cliff , and its beam is visible for 27 miles. On a clear day, Lewis can be seen fifty miles to the South west as a long, low line on the horizon. Sixty three miles East, the 1140 ft high cliffs of Hoy in the Orkneys can be seen. Due to atmospheric refraction, North Rona, which rises 355 ft can be seen 45 miles to the North west, towards Iceland. To the North, there is no land between Cape Wrath and the North Pole. There is no land there either. The nearest land in a straight line in that direction is actually 3000 miles away on the North coast of North east Russia, near the

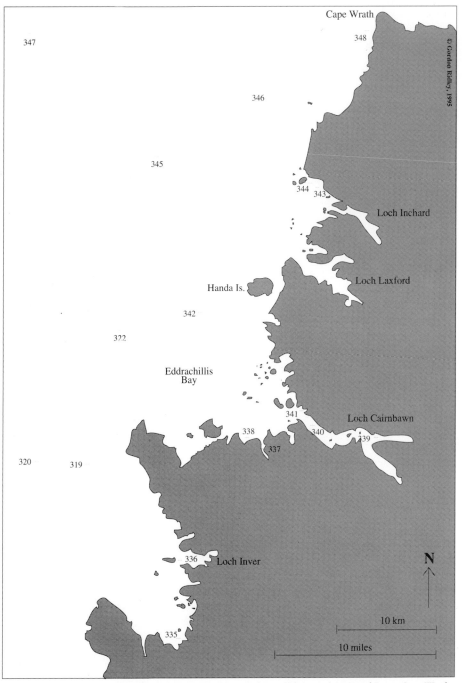

Cape Wrath

348

347

346

345

344 343

Loch Inchard

Loch Laxford

Handa Is.

342

322

Eddrachillis
Bay

341

Loch Cairnbawn

338 340

320   319   337   339

336   Loch Inver

N

335

10 km

10 miles

© Gordon Ridley, 1995

Chart showing the location of wrecks lying off the coast from Enard Bay to Cape Wrath

Bering Strait, at the other side of the world! (I did say Cape Wrath was a remote place!) Looking South, down the coast, Sandwood Bay and the tall red sandstone sea stack Am Buchaille (The Herdsman), is visible about 10 miles away.

You could retrace your steps back to your car, but having made the effort to come this far you may prefer to walk 12 miles eastward along the Northern Lighthouse Commission's private road across more rolling moorland of the Parph to the Kyle of Durness. Unless you are an ardent masochist, by this time you will probably consider there is never likely to be another chance of this walk; alternatively, you can take the minibus which operates during the summer months. Cross the sea inlet by the small passenger ferry that night, (the ferryman lives on the West side), and either camp at the roadside until the postbus comes along in the morning to take you back to Kinlochbervie, or continue for a further seven miles to Durness for the night. Alternatively, arrange for someone to meet you with a car on the mainland side of the Kyle of Durness. You are unlikely to forget this trip!

THE WRECKS

GOTFREDE

Wreck No : 335	**Date Sunk :** 06 10 1882
Latitude : 58 04 30 N PA	**Longitude :** 05 17 00 W PA
Decca Lat : 5804.50 N	**Decca Long :** 0517.00 W
Location : Inverpolly	**Area :** Enard
Type : Steamship	**Tonnage :** 116 gross.
Length : ft. **Beam :** ft.	**Draught :** ft.
How Sunk : Ran aground	**Depth :** metres

Gotfrede was a Danish wooden steamship which was lost by stranding at Inverpolly in a Force 6 south-westerly on 6th October 1882. Inverpolly Lodge is close to Polly Bay, a small inlet at the South east corner of Enard Bay. The wreck is presumably close to the shore in Polly Bay.

LOCH ERISORT

Wreck No : 336	**Date Sunk :** 27 03 1981
Latitude : 58 08 15 N PA	**Longitude :** 05 18 00 W PA
Decca Lat : 5808.20 N	**Decca Long :** 0518.00 W
Location : 1 mile W of Kirkaig Point	**Area :** Enard
Type : Trawler	**Tonnage :** 37 gross.
Length : 57.0 ft. **Beam :** ft.	**Draught :** ft.
How Sunk : Ran aground	**Depth :** 10 metres

The wreck of the wooden trawler *Loch Erisort* lies upside down about a mile West of Kirkaig Point, near the mouth of Loch Inver. She ran aground off Soyea Island, then later sank off Kirkaig Point, Loch Inver. Two of the crew of four were lost.

UNKNOWN

Wreck No : 337	**Date Sunk :** 1936
Latitude : 58 14 45 N	**Longitude :** 05 10 20 W
Decca Lat : 5814.75 N	**Decca Long :** 0510.33 W
Location : Loch Nedd	**Area :** Enard
Type : Drifter	**Tonnage :** gross
Length : ft. **Beam :** ft.	**Draught :** ft.
How Sunk :	**Depth :** 10 metres

The wreck of a drifter, blown up but full of scrap, presumably from the liner *Bermuda*, lies about ! / 3 of the distance up Loch Nedd from the sea. A wreck is charted on the West shore near the head of Loch Nedd. The wreck of the *Bermuda* itself seems to have been picked clean of goodies, but there may be some worthwhile pickings from the cargo of this drifter, in addition to any trophies from the drifter itself. The hull of the wreck is about 90 ft long, made of wood, and is partially buried in sand. Apparently it is usually buoyed by the local fishermen as it is a hazard to other vessels because it comes so close to the surface. The position has been recorded as 581417N, 051009W.

BERMUDA

Wreck No : 338	**Date Sunk :** 30 04 1933
Latitude : 58 15 01 N	**Longitude :** 05 11 31 W
Decca Lat : 5815.02 N	**Decca Long :** 0511.52 W
Location : Eddrachillis Bay	**Area :** Enard
Type : Steamship	**Tonnage :** 19086 gross.
Length : 525.9 ft. **Beam :** 74.1 ft.	**Draught :** 45.0 ft.
How Sunk : Ran aground	**Depth :** 12 metres

The liner *Bermuda* was built in 1927 by Workman Clark of Belfast for Furness Withy Lines. She caught fire at Bermuda on 17th June 1931, and the following month, under her own power, was taken to Belfast for repairs by her builders.

On 19th November 1931, in Workman Clark's yard at Belfast, she caught fire again, and sank alongside the wharf. The burned hulk was raised and her intact engines were removed before the hulk was sold to Metal Industries Ltd. for about £8000.

Under tow by the tugs *Seaman* and *Superman* she left Belfast on 27th April 1933 for Rosyth, to be broken up. The tow parted en route, and the *Bermuda* drifted into

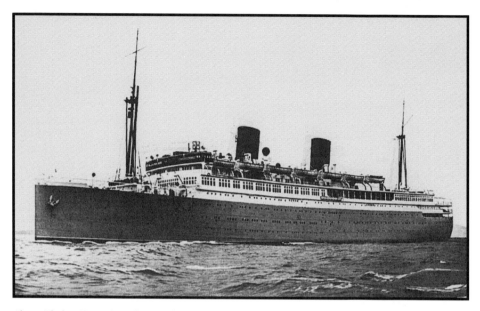

Above: The liner Bermuda *as she was in her prime (photograph courtesy of the World Ship Society). Below: As she became after going aground (photograph courtesy of the World Ship Society).*

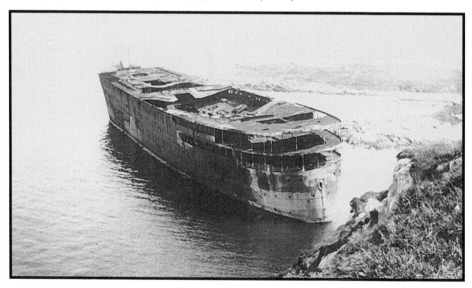

Eddrachillis Bay, hitting Sgeir Liath, before finally going aground at the South side of Eddrachillis Bay, between Culkein Drumbeg and the entrance to Loch Nedd. She was unable to be refloated, and was extensively salvaged where she lay. A puffer vessel engaged in this salvage work was lost nearby.

The wreck is now in three massive sections close ashore, with some of the wreckage

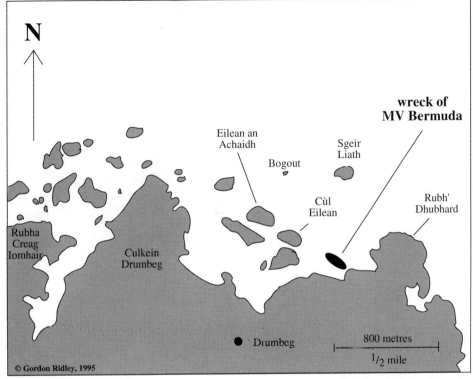

The location of the liner Bermuda.

lying visible on the rocks. The clarity of the water in this area is of gin quality, with lots of life and huge kelp fronds attached to the wreckage. The bottom is sandy, with underwater rocky islets, making this a very scenic wreck dive both above and below water.

CROWN

Wreck No : 339
Latitude : 58 15 24 N
Decca Lat : 5815.40 N
Location : Creag Ruadh, Loch Glendhu
Type : Drifter
Length :   ft.   **Beam :**   ft.
How Sunk : Fire

Date Sunk : 1924
Longitude : 04 56 50 W
Decca Long : 0456.83 W
Area : Kylesku
Tonnage :   gross
Draught : ft.
Depth : 15 metres

The drifter *Crown* sank in 1924, after a fire in her engine room.

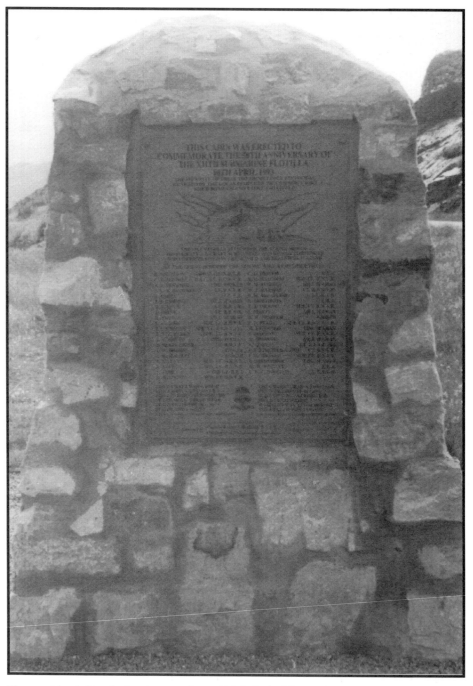

The memorial to the X-craft submariners near the new Kylesku Bridge (Photograph: Bob Baird).

WELMAN 10

Wreck No : 340
Latitude : 58 15 36 N
Decca Lat : 5815.60 N
Location : In Loch Cairnbawn
Type : Midget submarine
Length : 17.3 ft.   **Beam :** 3.5 ft.
How Sunk : Foundered

Date Sunk : 09 09 1943
Longitude : 05 04 45 W
Decca Long : 0504.75 W
Area : Kylesku
Tonnage : 3 gross.
Draught :   ft.
Depth : 65 metres

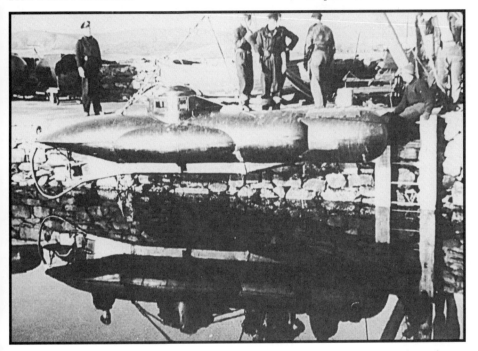

Above:A Welman midget submarine being lowered into the water. Below: Diagram of a Welman submarine.
(With acknowledgement to the Royal Naval Submarine Museum, Gosport).

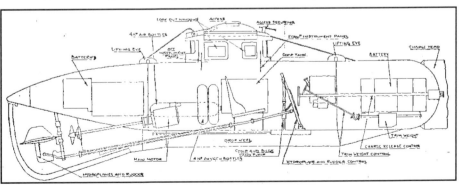

Welman submarines were one-man operated submarines which measured 17.25 ft long without the detachable explosive charge, and 20.5 ft long with the charge attached.

Welman 10 sank alongside the depot ship HMS *Bonaventure*, in Loch Cairnbawn. There were apparently two midget submarines sunk in Loch Cairnbawn, one of them with the crewman inside. This would presumably be *Welman 10*. I believe the other midget submarine was a *Chariot*. They are charted in 65 metres near the centre of the loch at National Grid References NC 193342 and NC 194342. Unlike X-craft, there was no facility to allow the crewman to leave the *Welman* while submerged.

HMS *Bonaventure* (ex-*Clan Davidson*), 10423 tons gross, 457 x 62.75 x 28.5 ft carried the six XE-Craft to Australia on her deck in February 1945, for use against the Japanese. These six were eventually scrapped in Australia.

UNKNOWN

Wreck No : 341	Date Sunk :
Latitude : 58 16 45 N	Longitude : 05 06 30 W
Decca Lat : 5816.75 N	Decca Long : 0506.50 W
Location : Loch Shark, Edrachillis Bay	Area : Kylesku
Type :	Tonnage : gross
Length : ft. Beam : ft.	Draught : ft.
How Sunk :	Depth : 5 metres

The wreck of a small vessel lies in 5 metres at the mouth of Loch Shark. The position has also been given as 581642N, 050636W.

W A MASSEY

Wreck No : 342	Date Sunk : 11 03 1918
Latitude : 58 22 00 N PA	Longitude : 05 20 00 W PA
Decca Lat : 5823.00 N	Decca Long : 0520.00 W
Location : 5 miles W of Creag a Mhail	Area : Wrath
Type : Drifter	Tonnage : 96 gross.
Length : ft. Beam : ft.	Draught : ft.
How Sunk : Mined	Depth : metres

Charted PA 5 miles West of Creag a Mhail, Handa Island, with at least 28 metres of water over it. Depths in the area range from 60-100 metres. Four miles W by N of Handa Island.

WINCHESTER

Wreck No : 343	Date Sunk : 06 04 1933
Latitude : 58 28 00 N PA	Longitude : 05 05 00 W PA
Decca Lat : 5828.00 N	Decca Long : 0505.00 W

Location : N of Eilean a Connaidh   **Area :** Wrath
Type : Drifter   **Tonnage :** 94 gross.
Length : 86.0 ft.   **Beam :** 18.6 ft.   **Draught :** 8.7 ft.
How Sunk : Ran aground   **Depth :** 20 metres

Winchester was a Peterhead steam drifter (steel screw ketch), built in 1907 by Dundee S. B. Co., engine by A. Shanks & Son, Arbroath. One report puts the position of loss as North of Eilean a Connaidh, while another suggests she went ashore half a mile North west of Loch Alsh. (Presumably Kyle of Lochalsh). Both reports agree on the date of loss. According to Lloyds she ran aground on rocks West of Cape Wrath, then slipped off and sank in deep water.

VALONIA

Wreck No : 344   **Date Sunk :** 06 10 1975
Latitude : 58 28 10 N   **Longitude :** 05 05 10 W
Decca Lat : 5828.17 N   **Decca Long :** 0505.17 W
Location : ½ m W of Eilean an Roin Beag   **Area :** Wrath
Type : Trawler   **Tonnage :**   gross
Length : ft.   **Beam :** ft.   **Draught :** ft.
How Sunk : Ran aground   **Depth :** 35 metres

The fishing vessel *Valonia* ran aground one mile North of Kinlochbervie on 6th October 1975 and became a total loss. The crew were all saved.

NOREEN MARY

Wreck No : 345   **Date Sunk :** 05 07 1944
Latitude : 58 30 59 N   **Longitude :** 05 33 24 W
Decca Lat : 5830.98 N   **Decca Long :** 0533.40 W
Location : Off Kinlochbervie   **Area :** Wrath
Type : Trawler   **Tonnage :** 207 gross.
Length : ft.   **Beam :** ft.   **Draught :** ft.
How Sunk : Submarine - gunfire   **Depth :** metres

The length of this vessel has been estimated at about 150 ft. The steam trawler *Noreen Mary* was sunk by gunfire from *U-247* (Matschulat), who gave the position as 5830N, 0523W.

MAJORKA

Wreck No : 346   **Date Sunk :** 14 08 1917
Latitude : 58 34 00 N PA   **Longitude :** 05 13 40 W PA
Decca Lat : 5834.00 N   **Decca Long :** 0513.67 W

Location : 3 miles NW of Am Balg
Type : Sailing vessel
Length : 259.5 ft.   Beam : 38.2 ft.
How Sunk : By submarine

Area : Wrath
Tonnage : 1684 gross.
Draught : 23.1 ft.
Depth : 30 metres

The *Majorka* was an iron sailing ship built in 1882 by R. Duncan, Port Glasgow, and registered in Drammen, Norway. She was sunk by a submarine on 14th August 1917. *Lloyds War Losses* gives the position of attack as 5830N, 0520W. Decca co-ordinates are E52.65, B22.30.

The wreck lies WNW/ESE in 50 metres, and stands up 3.75 metres from the bottom. According to one report, a mast used to show at low water, but this seems hardly credible in view of her depth!

U-965

Wreck No : 347
Latitude : 58 35 31 N
Decca Lat : 5835.52 N
Location : 23 miles W of Cape Wrath
Type : Submarine
Length : 221.4 ft.   Beam : 20.5 ft.
How Sunk : Depth-charged

Date Sunk : 27 03 1945
Longitude : 05 46 06 W
Decca Long : 0546.10 W
Area : Wrath
Tonnage : 769 gross.
Draught : 15.8 ft.
Depth : 130 metres

U-965 (KL Unverzagt), was depth-charged and sunk by the RN frigate *Conn* in the Minch, 23 miles West of Cape Wrath at 12.58 hrs on 27th March 1945. There were no survivors. This position is also about 28 miles North east of the Butt of Lewis. *U-965*

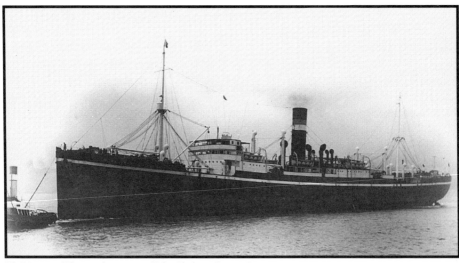

The *Manipur (Photograph courtesy of John Clarkson, Longton)*

was a Type VIIC Atlantic U-Boat, 769 tons surfaced, 871 tons submerged. Her maximum diving depth was 309 ft.

SUNNYVALE

Wreck No : 348	**Date Sunk** : 16 12 1971
Latitude : 58 36 30 N PA	**Longitude** : 05 00 30 W PA
Decca Lat : 5836.50 N	**Decca Long** : 0500.50 W
Location : ½ mile S of Am Bodach	**Area** : Wrath
Type : Trawler	**Tonnage** : gross
Length : ft. **Beam** : ft.	**Draught** : ft.
How Sunk : Ran aground	**Depth** : 30 metres

The name has also been recorded as *Sunnydale*, a MFV, 1 mile South of Cape Wrath.

MANIPUR

Wreck No : 349	**Date Sunk** : 17 07 1940
Latitude : 58 41 17 N	**Longitude** : 05 11 43 W
Decca Lat : 5841.28 N	**Decca Long** : 0511.72 W
Location : 8 miles NW of Cape Wrath	**Area** : Wrath
Type : Steamship	**Tonnage** : 8652 gross.
Length : 473.0 ft. **Beam** : 64.0 ft.	**Draught** : 37.0 ft.
How Sunk : Torpedoed by *U-57*	**Depth** : 68 metres

The British steamship *Manipur* was torpedoed by *U-57* (Topp), on 17th July 1940 while en route from Baltimore and Halifax, Nova Scotia to London.

Some salvage was carried out by Risdon Beazley/Ulrich Harms in 1971, and the wreck was reported to be very broken up. One is bound to wonder what the nature of the cargo was to make salvage worthwhile some 31 years after she sank?

INGER

Wreck No : 350	**Date Sunk** : 23 08 1941
Latitude : 58 58 00 N PA	Longitude 07 50 00 W PA
Decca Lat : 5858.0 N	**Decca Long** : 0750.0 W
Location :	**Area** : Wrath
Type : Steamship	**Tonnage** :1418 gross.
Length : 249.8 ft. **Beam** : 38.0 ft.	**Draught** : 15.7 ft.
How Sunk : Torpedoed by *U-143*	**Depth** : metres

The Norwegian steamship *Inger*, built in Trondheim in 1930, was torpedoed by the *U-143* (Gelhaus) just before midnight on 23rd August 1941.

Appendix 1

Loss Analysis

Excluding those whose cause of loss is not known, and can therefore only be speculation, an analysis of the causes of loss of the vessels included in this book reveals the following:

Ran aground	208	68.6%	
Foundered	26	8.6%	
By submarine	23	7.6%	(Includes torpedoes and gunfire)
Collision	15	5.0%	
Mined	10	3.3%	
Depth-charged	8	2.6%	
Fire/explosion	5	1.7%	
By aircraft	3	1.0%	(Includes bomb, torpedoes and gunfire)
Gunfire by surface ship	2	0.7%	
Crashed into the sea	2	0.7%	(These are aircraft)
Scuttled	1	0.3%	
Jammed under pier	1	0.3%	
Total war causes	46	15.2%	

It is interesting to compare the above statistics with *Lloyds Casualty Report* for 1991, which lists 258 ships of 100 tons gross and above, lost world-wide during that year. The total tonnage lost amounted to 1.5 million tons, and 1204 lives were lost, proving that modern technology has not eliminated shipping losses.

Foundered	111	43.0%	
Ran aground	45	17.4%	
Fire/explosion	37	14.3%	
Collision	36	14.0%	
War losses	13	5.0%	(Includes the Gulf war and Yugoslavia)
Contact	13	5.0%	
Missing	3	1.2%	

Appendix 2

Diving Information

Diving

Very few of the wrecks can be considered as shore dives. Boats are required to reach almost all of them. Even those which were lost through running aground close to the shore are in positions which are inaccessible from the land, either because there is no road nearby, or they are at the bottom of a cliff, or off islands or off-lying rocks.

Some of the wrecks are such a great distance offshore that it would be prudent to visit them only in company with several seaworthy RIBs equipped with marine VHF, or by hiring a trawler or other large specialist offshore dive boat. Even then, it would be a good idea to have an attendant RIB, manned by very experienced divers.

Weather Information (24 hours):

H.M.Coastguard: Clyde Area (01475 729988), Oban Area (01631 563720), Kyle of Lochalsh (01599 4438), Mallaig (01687 2336)
MARINECALL provides a 24-hour recorded two-day forecast for Mull of Kintyre to Ardnamurchan Point (01891 500463) and Ardnamurchan Point to Cape Wrath (01891 500464).
The current weather in these areas can also be obtained for Mull of Kintyre to Ardnamurchan Point (01891 226463) and Ardnamurchan Point to Cape Wrath (01891 226464).

Dive Centres / Shops / Air / Equipment / Accommodation

There a number of diving centres within the area covered by this book. Apart from compressed air, they will also be able to provide equipment, boats, and accommodation, either from their own resources, or know where these may be obtained locally.

Some useful names, addresses and telephone numbers are listed below:

Campbeltown Branch, SSAC. Donald Fairgray (01586 553589; evenings) or Calum Buchanan (01586 81202; evenings)
Sport Dive Islay, 10, Charlotte Street, Port Ellen, Islay. (01496 302441)
Oban Divers, Laggan, Glenshellach, Oban. (01631 562755 or 566618)

Nervous Wreck, Ganavan Sands, Oban. (01631 566000 or 566126)
Mull Diving Centre, The Pier, Salen, Mull. (016803 411)
Seafare, Portmore Place, Tobermory, Mull. (01688 2277)
Tobermory Diving Centre, Main Street, Tobermory, Mull.
Camasnagaul Dive Centre, Sail Mhor Croft, Dundonnel, by Garve, Little Loch Broom, Rossshire. (0185483 224)
Wester Ross Marine, South Erradale, Gairloch. Elder Bros., The Pier, Gairloch.
Barry Todd, Ullapool. (01854 2036)
Glen Uig Inn, by Lochailort (016877 219)
Skye Diving Centre, Harlosh, Dunvegan, Skye. (0147022 366)
Portree Diving Services, 5, Achachork, Portree, Skye. (01478 2274)

Boat Charterers

These usually also supply compressed air. Some of the boat charterers are based in the area virtually all year round, while others are seasonal, and their operating areas tend to vary throughout the year.

The following list is not exhaustive, but includes some of the moreregular operators:

MV *Kylebhan*, Jim Kilcullen, 3, Dal-an-Aiseig, North Connel, Oban. (01389 77028)
MV *Amidas*, Charlie Laverty, Tobermory. (01688 2048)
Jim Laverty, Tobermory. (01688 2083)
MV *Harry Slater*, North West Charters, Oban. (01631 20 6543)
MV *Gaelic Rose*, Bob Jones, Kirk Brae, Lochaline. (01967 421654)
MV *Lady Margaret*, Oban. (01631 572562)
MV *Porpoise*, Dave Ainsley, Balvicar, Argyll. (01852 300203)
MV *Heron*, Ullapool. (01854 622261)
MV *Cuma*, Minch Charters, Mallaig. (01687 2304)
Jim Crooks, 6, Inver Park, Lochinver, Sutherland. (015714 362)

APPENDIX 3

BIBLIOGRAPHY

The following is a list of publications and sources that were used for reference:

The Admiralty Hydrographic Department, Taunton.
All the World's Fighting Ships 1922-1946, pub. by Conway Maritime Press, 1980.
Argyll Shipwrecks, by Peter Moir and Ian Crawford, pub. by Moir Crawford, 1994.
Axis Submarine Successes 1939-45, by Jurgen Rowher, pub. by Patrick Stephens, 1983.
British Vessels Lost at Sea 1914-18 and 1939-45, pub. by Patrick Stephens, 1988.
BSAC Wreck Register
Court of Enquiry Reports (Various)
Dictionary of Disasters at Sea in the Age of Steam, by C.Hocking, pub. by Lloyd's, 1989.
Dive West Scotland, by Gordon Ridley, pub. by Underwater World Publications, 1984.
Dive North West Scotland, by Gordon Ridley, pub. by Underwater World Publications, 1985.
Jane's Book of Fighting Ships
Lloyds List of Shipping Losses
Lloyds Register of Shipping
Lloyds War Losses
The *Oban Times*
Parliamentary Papers (Various)
Royal Naval Submarines 1901-1982, by M.P.Cocker, pub. by Frederick Warne.
The *Scots Magazine*, pub. by D.C.Thompson.
Shipwrecks Around Britain, by Leo Zanelli, pub. by Kaye & Ward, 1970.
Submarines of World War 2, by Erminio Bagnasco pub. by Arms and Armour Press.
Unknown Shipwrecks Around Britain, by Leo Zanelli, pub. by Kaye & Ward, 1974.
The U-Boat, by Eberhard Rossler pub. by Arms & Armour Press, 1981.
The U-Boat Offensive 1914-1945, by V.E.Tarrant, pub. by Arms & Armour Press, 1989.
Warship Losses of WW2, by David Brown, pub. by Arms & Armour Press, 1990.

APPENDIX 4

SCOTTISH PLACE NAMES

A good idea of the nature of a place can be often be gained from its Gaelic name, which usually describes its most prominent feature(s). The following selection of Gaelic words, often associated with island or seashore names or features, may be useful. Spellings tend to vary slightly, and depend on whether singular or plural, masculine or feminine; so look for possible alternatives.

To the uninitiated, Gaelic words often seem to be unpronounceable. Consonants followed by an h are not often pronounced. *Bh* or *Mh* is pronounced *V*. *Fh* is mute. *C* is always hard, as *K*. At the end of a word *-aidh* is pronounced as the *y* in *my*, *-idh* as the *y* in *ferry*. In the middle of a word *ea* is usually pronounced as the *e* in *well*, *ao* as the *oo* in *pool*.

A, Am, An, An t-	The	Gleann	Valley
Acairseid	Anchorage	Gorm, Ghorm	Blue (green if applied to foliage)
Aline	Meadow, green place	Holm	Small island
Aidh, Aigh	Place of	Iar	West, western
Ail, Aileach	Rock, a stony place	Inch, Innis	Island
Aird, Ard	Promontory	Inver	Mouth of river
Allt, Ault	Stream	Iolaire	Eagle
Bagh, Baigh	Bay	Iomallach	Remote area
Ban	Fair, white (also woman)	Kin..(Ceann)	Head of
Bealach	Narrow passage	Knap	Knob, lump, hillock
Beg, Beag	Small, little	Kyle	Strait, firth
Beul, Bel	Mouth of	Laimhrige	Landing place, harbour
Blaven	Blue	Leac	Scree, flat stone, slab
Bodach	Old man	Leathann	Broad
Bogha, Bodha, Bo'	Detached rock which uncovers	Liath	Grey
Borro, Borg	Castle, fort	Lic, Lice	Flat stone, slab
Buchaille	Shepherd, herdsman	Linn, Linne	Pool
Buidhe, Bhuide	Yellow	Machair	Plain, level country
Cailleach	Old woman, hag	Maoile	Brow of hill
Cala	Harbour	Mara	Sea
Camas	Channel, Bay	Meall	Rounded hill
Caol, Caolas	Sound, strait	Monadh	Mountain
Casteil	Castle	Mor, Mhor	Big, Large
Ceann, Cinn, Kin..	Head	Muc, Muck	Pig (sea-pig = porpoise, whale)
Cille	Church, cemetery	Mull	Promontory
Cnoc, Cnap	Knob, Lump, Hillock	Na, Nan, Nam, Na h-	Of the
Coire	Hollow, whirlpool	Nish, Ness	Promontory, point
Craobh	Tree	Ob, Oban	Bay
Creag	Cliff, rock	Oitir	Shallows, drying rock
Croin	Tree, mast	Poll, Phuill	Pool
Cumhainn	Narrows	Reamhar	Thick
Dearg	Red (bright)	Reidh	Level, smooth
Deas	South	Rhu	Promontory
Dobhar	Water	Righ (pron. Ree)	King
Doirlinn	Neck of land left dry at low	Ron, Roinn	Seal
	tide, beach	Ruadh	Red (brownish)
Domhain, Dhomhain	Deep	Rubha, Rudha, Ru	Headland
Donn	Brown	Ruinn, Rinn	Sharp point, promontory
Dorch(a)	Dark	Sgeir	Rock in the sea
Dorus	Door, opening	Sgurr	Rocky peak
Dun	Castle, fort	Sron	Nose (headland)
Dubh	Black	Sruth	Current
Ear, Earrair	East, Eastern	Stac	Pinnacle
Eas, Easa, Easan	Waterfall	Strome	Current, stream
Eilean, Eileanan	Island, Islands	Stron, Strone	Nose, point
Fada	Long	Tarbert	Narrow isthmus
Faoilinn	Beach	Teas, Thais	Heat, warm
Fionn	White, fair	Tigh	House
Fearn, Fearna	Alder tree	Tob	Bay
Fuar, Fuaire	Cold	Tober	Well
Gabhar, Gobhair	Goat	Tolm, Tuilm	Island near shore
Gailbheach	Stormy, furious	Tor, Torr	Round hill
Gair	Short	Traigh	Sandy beach
Gaoth	Windy	Tuath	North
Gamhainn, Gamhna	Calf	Tulm, Tuilm	Islet
Gaineamh, Gaimheach	Sand	Uaine, Uinn	Green
Garbh	Rough	Uamh(a)	Cave
Geal, Gheal	White	Uig	Bay
Glas	Grey or Green	Uisge	Water

Appendix 5

U-boat Reference Grid

U-boat captains used a confusing grid for position reporting in WW2. This is shown right and should enable some sense to be made of these position reports when studying accounts of WW2 actions and sinkings.

Squared chart of British waters used by U-boat captains for grid references. (Redrawn from WW2 German records.)

Die Gewässer um England

NAME INDEX

Name	Latitude	Longitude	Area	Wreck	Page
Chadwick	57 27 12 N	06 47 06 W	Skye	304	239
Chevalier	55 48 00 N PA	06 30 00 W PA	W Islay	109	87
Chevalier	55 53 00 N PA	05 50 00 W PA	Jura	130	104
Christine Rose	55 53 04 N	05 41 27 W	W.Kintyre	51	50
City of Simla	55 55 00 N PA	08 20 00 W PA	NW Islay	121	94
Clansman	55 17 00 N PA	05 36 00 W PA	S.Kintyre	8	27
Clydesdale	56 26 40 N	05 37 00 W	Oban	159	125
Colonial	55 29 04 N	05 31 01 W	E.Kintyre	34	41
Colonial Empire	55 47 00 N PA	06 28 00 W PA	W Islay	105	85
Comet	56 07 44 N	05 36 24 W	Jura	132	106
Cormoran	55 44 42 N	06 29 06 W	W Islay	96	77
Cossack	55 39 10 N PA	06 03 50 W PA	SE Islay	70	64
Craigenroan	57 00 00 N PA	05 49 40 W PA	Mallaig	283	221
Crane	56 38 48 N PA	06 01 18 W PA	Mull	211	176
Cretan	56 29 17 N	06 07 08 W	Mull	225	183
Criscilla	55 47 37 N	06 03 58 W	E Islay	75	66
Crown	58 15 24 N	04 56 50 W	Kylesku	339	267
Crystaline	57 12 57 N	05 40 05 W	Skye	289	225
Culzean	55 56 20 N PA	05 50 45 W PA	Jura	131	105
Cygnet	56 52 00 N PA	05 45 00 W PA	Mallaig	277	218
Dalton	55 44 08 N	06 29 54 W	W Islay	94	76
Dartmouth	56 30 12 N	05 41 59 W	Mull	189	155
Davaar	55 17 00 N PA	05 32 30 W PA	E.Kintyre	28	38
Deerpark?	57 13 30 N PA	05 38 30 W PA	Skye	291	227
Doris	57 25 15 N	06 47 25 W	Skye	303	238
Duchess	55 22 00 N PA	06 02 00 W PA	W.Kintyre	42	46
Duchess of Lancaster	55 17 00 N PA	05 48 00 W PA	S.Kintyre	9	27
Dunvegan Castle	57 30 48 N PA	06 43 00 W PA	Skye	307	241
Earl Lennox			E.Islay	74	66
Earl of Carrick	56 27 36 N	05 17 30 W	Oban	162	129
Edith Morgan	55 47 44 N	06 03 26 W	E Islay	76	66
Eileen M	55 34 46 N	06 17 37 W	SE Islay	54	54
Eli	56 09 30 N PA	06 54 00 W PA	Mull	215	177
Elisabeth	55 21 30 N	05 31 12 W	E.Kintyre	30	38
Ellida ?	55 35 10 N	06 18 55 W	SE Islay	60	57
Embrace	57 09 30 N	05 47 12 W	Skye	287	225
Empire Adventure	55 55 00 N PA	07 25 00 W PA	NW Islay	120	94
Ena	55 35 00 N PA	06 20 00 W PA	SE Islay	59	56
Evelyn Rose	56 31 08 N	05 45 24 W	Mull	193	159
Exit	56 27 36 N PA	05 17 30 W PA	Oban	163	130
Exmouth	55 49 50 N	06 27 30 W	W Islay	111	88
Exmouth Castle	55 51 10 N PA	06 27 20 W PA	W Islay	112	89
Fair Morn	56 58 30 N	05 53 30 W	Mallaig	282	220
Fairy Queen	55 25 00 N PA	05 46 00 W PA	W.Kintyre	46	48
Fanny	55 20 25 N	05 30 35 W	E.Kintyre	29	38
Faraday	56 33 38 N PA	06 41 33 W PA	Coll	255	201
Fisher Queen	56 32 30 N PA	06 46 45 W PA	Tiree	249	196
Floristan	55 45 06 N	06 28 07 W	W Islay	97	78
Forest Chief	55 46 30 N PA	06 28 00 W PA	W Islay	101	84
Frederick Bartholdi	57 44 48 N	06 26 30 W	Skye	317	248
Gaul	56 31 30 N PA	06 57 30 W PA	Tiree	245	195
General Consul Elissejeff	56 37 45 N	06 29 29 W	Coll	262	206
Girl Sandra	56 29 45 N	05 42 42 W	Mull	184	151
Glen Albyn	57 52 30 N	05 39 52 W	Lochewe	323	253
Glen Holme	55 50 36 N	06 05 20 W	E Islay	78	68
Glen Rosa	56 19 31 N	05 47 29 W	Mull	172	146
Glenhead	55 27 06 N	05 31 12 W	E.Kintyre	33	41
Godetia	55 19 12 N	06 05 42 W	N.Channel	1	24
Golden Gift	56 25 00 N	05 28 32 W	Oban	151	120
Golden Gleam			Mull	180	150

Name	Latitude	Longitude	Area	Wreck	Page
Maid of Lorne	56 17 48 N	06 25 40 W	Mull	220	180
Maine	56 18 38 N	05 50 20 W	Mull	170	144
Majorka	58 34 00 N PA	05 13 40 W PA	Wrath	346	271
Malve	56 31 57 N	06 52 15 W	Tiree	251	197
Manipur	58 41 17 N	05 11 43 W	Wrath	349	273
Mardi Dan	56 29 38 N	05 36 48 W	Mull	178	149
Martha	56 35 45 N	05 23 20 W	Oban	168	140
Mary Stuart	56 30 07 N	06 48 14 W	Tiree	242	193
Meldon	56 19 32 N	05 55 33 W	Mull	173	146
Midas	57 03 30 N PA	06 21 00 W PA	Rum	275	217
Milewater	55 35 00 N	06 15 42 W	SE Islay	56	55
Mobeka	55 18 18 N	05 42 18 W	S.Kintyre	18	32
Mon Cousu	55 42 38 N	05 39 49 W	Gigha	128	102
Mona	55 59 48 N PA	06 18 00 W PA	Oronsay	134	107
Morning Star	56 34 57 N	05 57 34 W	Mull	204	170
Mount Park	55 52 00 N PA	06 06 00 W PA	E Islay	80	69
Mountaineer	56 26 40 N	05 37 00 W	Oban	158	124
Myrtle	55 16 30 N PA	05 36 00 W PA	S.Kintyre	7	27
Nellie	56 56 30 N	06 07 45 W	Mallaig	280	219
Nessmore	56 33 36 N	06 41 37 W	Coll	254	200
Nevada II	56 41 24 N	06 29 27 W	Coll	264	209
New Blessing	56 27 30 N PA	05 39 12 W PA	Mull	182	150
New Sevilla	55 54 05 N	07 29 54 W	NW Islay	119	94
New York	55 17 24 N	05 45 24 W	S.Kintyre	15	30
Niels-Rossing-Parelius	55 19 24 N	05 33 12 W	S.Kintyre	25	36
Nils Gorthon	55 47 00 N PA	07 00 00 W PA	W Islay	106	86
Nordhuk	57 43 48 N	06 17 48 W	Skye	315	246
Noreen Mary	58 30 59 N	05 33 24 W	Wrath	345	271
Norman	55 40 00 N PA	06 39 00 W PA	SW Islay	84	70
Norman	57 36 30 N	06 38 00 W	Skye	310	242
Normannvik	58 12 49 N	05 43 08 W	Minch	320	252
Norval	56 18 27 N	05 40 26 W	Oban	144	117
Nyland	56 14 18 N	06 27 39 W	Mull	217	178
Ocean	55 45 18 N	06 28 28 W	W Islay	98	79
Osprey	55 31 00 N PA	05 45 00 W PA	W.Kintyre	50	50
Ostende	56 19 18 N	06 15 50 W	Mull	221	180
Otranto	55 45 46 N	06 28 40 W	W Islay	99	80
Pansy	56 25 30 N	05 29 32 W	Oban	156	124
Parthenia	55 10 00 N	05 40 30 W	S.Kintyre	3	25
Pattersonian	55 34 43 N	06 16 44 W	SE Islay	55	55
Pecten	56 22 00 N PA	07 55 00 W PA	Tiree	236	191
Pelican	56 37 14 N	06 02 50 W	Mull	208	173
Perelle	55 12 00 N PA	05 48 00 W PA	S.Kintyre	4	26
Plover	56 35 30 N PA	05 24 00 W PA	Oban	167	140
Port Hobart	55 32 00 N PA	06 44 00 W PA	SW Islay	82	69
Port Napier	57 15 59 N	05 41 12 W	Skye	294	228
Portaferry	57 15 00 N	05 39 00 W	Skye	290	227
Promotive	57 52 40 N	05 40 44 W	Lochewe	324	255
Protesilaus	56 22 13 N	07 15 29 W	Mull	223	182
Quebec	55 59 48 N PA	06 18 00 W PA	Oronsay	135	108
Quesada	55 22 18 N	05 27 00 W	E.Kintyre	31	39
Rapid	55 19 24 N PA	05 33 12 W PA	S.Kintyre	26	36
Ravensheugh	56 25 00 N PA	07 05 00 W PA	Mull	224	182
Rhodesia	57 41 14 N	06 20 45 W	Skye	313	243
Riant	56 40 30 N PA	05 50 30 W PA	Mull	214	177
Riddha	56 32 00 N	06 53 00 W	Tiree	246	195
River Tay	56 30 10 N	05 42 00 W	Mull	187	155
Robert Hewett			Mull	179	149
Robert Limbrick	56 38 02 N	06 13 40 W	Mull	231	187
Rondo	56 32 17 N	05 54 40 W	Mull	199	162

Name	Latitude	Longitude	Area	Wreck	Page
Ros Guill	56 39 42 N	06 07 12 W	Mull	213	176
Rosebud II	56 14 00 N PA	06 25 00 W PA	Mull	216	177
Rotche	56 57 32 N	05 55 00 W	Mallaig	281	220
Rothesay Castle	55 53 36 N	06 21 48 W	NW Islay	117	92
Saint Conon	55 19 24 N	05 33 12 W	S.Kintyre	24	34
San Sebastian	55 38 03 N	06 04 40 W	SE Islay	67	61
Sanda	56 22 00 N PA	05 42 00 W PA	Mull	174	148
Saxon	56 31 20 N PA	07 01 00 W PA	Tiree	243	193
Scomber	57 21 00 N PA	05 51 00 W PA	Skye	298	234
Seavar	55 46 00 N PA	06 35 00 W PA	W Islay	100	84
Serb	55 37 38 N	06 04 42 W	SE Islay	66	61
Shackleton Aircraft	56 30 25 N	05 44 05 W	Mull	191	158
Shiela	57 35 00 N PA	05 50 30 W PA	Skye	308	241
Shuna	55 39 05 N	06 02 25 W	SE Islay	69	64
Shuna	56 33 24 N	05 54 48 W	Mull	201	166
Signal	55 17 55 N PA	05 47 40 W PA	S.Kintyre	17	32
Silver Reward	57 57 45 N	05 31 18 W	Broom	330	260
Silver Spray	57 58 32 N	05 20 14 W	Broom	331	260
Solway Firth	56 26 30 N PA	05 34 00 W PA	Oban	157	124
South Esk	56 52 39 N PA	06 07 36 W PA	Eigg	268	212
Spindrift	57 19 53 N	06 03 50 W	Skye	296	233
Ssafa	56 35 10 N	06 34 50 W	Coll	260	205
St. Brandan	56 40 46 N	06 31 12 W	Coll	263	207
St. Clair	56 32 24 N	06 40 00 W	Coll	252	198
St. Joseph	56 28 30 N	05 36 45 W	Oban	165	131
St. Kilda	55 17 00 N PA	05 48 00 W PA	S.Kintyre	10	28
St. Tudwal	55 34 00 N PA	06 15 00 W PA	SE Islay	53	54
Staffa	55 39 42 N	05 47 12 W	Gigha	126	99
Steam Dredger No.285	55 17 15 N PA	05 34 18 W PA	S.Kintyre	12	28
Stina	56 48 00 N PA	06 30 00 W PA	Coll	265	209
Stirling Castle	56 43 20 N PA	05 14 30 W PA	Oban	169	141
Stormlight	55 50 01 N	05 56 09 W	Jura	129	103
Strathbeg	56 36 44 N	06 02 00 W	Mull	206	172
Sturdy	56 29 00 N	06 59 00 W	Tiree	237	191
Sunnyvale	58 36 30 N PA	05 00 30 W PA	Wrath	348	273
Surprise	55 39 18 N	06 02 52 W	SE Islay	71	65
Swan (or Speedwell?)	56 29 45 N	05 39 19 W	Mull	183	151
Tapti	56 33 40 N	06 37 53 W	Coll	256	201
Tarbert Castle	55 58 00 N PA	05 20 30 W PA	E.Kintyre	37	44
Tartar	56 49 40 N PA	06 13 30 W PA	Muck	266	212
Teunika	56 35 42 N	06 23 36 W	Mull	227	184
Thalia	56 28 09 N	05 31 24 W	Oban	164	131
Thesis	56 30 02 N	05 41 26 W	Mull	185	151
Thomas	55 40 18 N	06 30 52 W	SW Islay	85	70
Tobago	55 42 22 N	06 30 00 W	SW Islay	90	73
Triton	57 10 00 N PA	05 59 30 W PA	Skye	288	225
Tuscania	55 36 30 N	06 26 24 W	SE Islay	62	57
U-1014	55 17 00 N PA	06 44 00 W PA	W.Kintyre	41	46
U-1021	58 19 30 N	05 32 00 W	Minch	322	253
U-296 ?	55 25 48 N	06 19 48 W	W.Kintyre	48	49
U-482	55 30 00 N PA	05 53 00 W PA	W.Kintyre	49	50
U-484	56 30 00 N PA	07 40 00 W PA	Tiree	240	192
U-722	57 09 00 N PA	06 55 00 W PA	Skye	286	224
U-965	58 35 31 N	05 46 06 W	Wrath	347	272
UB-82	55 13 00 N PA	05 55 00 W PA	S.Kintyre	5	26
Udea	55 39 42 N	05 47 12 W	Gigha	125	99
Unknown	55 17 21 N	05 33 12 W	S.Kintyre	13	29
Unknown	55 18 00 N	05 31 00 W	S.Kintyre	19	33
Unknown	55 19 01 N	05 27 47 W	S.Kintyre	22	34
Unknown	55 39 27 N	06 04 27 W	SE Islay	72	65

Name	Latitude	Longitude	Area	Wreck	Page
Unknown	55 46 58 N	06 27 30 W	W Islay	104	85
Unknown	55 49 18 N	06 36 26 W	W Islay	113	90
Unknown	55 49 23 N	06 36 37 W	W Islay	114	90
Unknown	55 57 52 N	05 42 14 W	W.Kintyre	52	51
Unknown	56 19 16 N	05 35 29 W	Oban	145	117
Unknown	56 21 48 N	06 05 06 W	Mull	222	181
Unknown	56 23 33 N	05 30 47 W	Oban	146	117
Unknown	56 24 30 N	05 29 50 W	Oban	149	118
Unknown	56 29 12 N	06 52 24 W	Tiree	238	191
Unknown	56 36 54 N PA	06 21 48 W PA	Mull	230	186
Unknown	57 15 45 N	05 43 24 W	Skye	293	228
Unknown	57 27 44 N	06 36 57 W	Skye	306	241
Unknown	57 38 30 N PA	06 12 00 W PA	Skye	312	243
Unknown	57 53 45 N	05 09 20 W	Broom	327	259
Unknown	57 59 00 N PA	05 21 00 W PA	Broom	332	261
Unknown	58 00 45 N PA	05 24 00 W PA	Broom	333	261
Unknown	58 03 00 N PA	05 26 00 W PA	Broom	334	261
Unknown	58 12 26 N	05 32 41 W	Minch	319	252
Unknown	58 12 52 N	05 43 53 W	Minch	321	253
Unknown	58 14 45 N	05 10 20 W	Enard	337	265
Unknown	58 16 45 N	05 06 30 W	Kylesku	341	270
Unknown - Aircraft?	56 24 25 N	05 30 10 W	Oban	148	118
Unknown - Hafton?	56 24 36 N	05 37 30 W	Mull	175	148
Unknown - Jason?	56 33 00 N	06 28 00 W	Mull	226	183
Unknown - Meldon?	56 15 12 N	05 45 15 W	Oban	140	112
Unknown - Nydalen?	56 36 52 N	06 30 33 W	Coll	261	206
Unknown - Pre-1919	56 04 00 N PA	06 10 00 W PA	Colonsay	138	109
Unknown - Pre-1922	55 55 02 N	06 04 48 W	E Islay	81	69
Unknown - Pre-1932	56 37 21 N	06 03 53 W	Mull	209	175
Unknown - Pre-1947	56 32 22 N	05 56 50 W	Mull	200	164
Unknown - Pre-1957	55 46 37 N	06 16 18 W	W Islay	103	85
Unknown - Pre-1966	55 52 15 N	05 24 17 W	E.Kintyre	36	44
Unknown - Pre-1970	57 27 30 N PA	06 45 10 W PA	Skye	305	239
Unknown - Pre-1978	57 24 15 N	05 49 04 W	Skye	301	236
Unknown - Pre-1982	56 54 35 N	05 51 57 W	Mallaig	279	219
Unknown - Stately?	55 17 42 N	05 43 24 W	S.Kintyre	14	30
Unknown - U-722?	56 58 45 N	06 39 48 W	Rum	273	216
Unknown U-Boat	55 16 48 N	05 59 27 W	W.Kintyre	40	45
Unknown U-Boat	55 24 12 N	06 29 40 W	W.Kintyre	43	47
Unknown U-Boat	55 25 00 N	06 19 10 W	W.Kintyre	45	48
Unknown U-Boat	55 25 00 N	06 25 51 W	W.Kintyre	44	48
Untamed	55 20 00 N PA	05 30 00 W PA	S.Kintyre	27	37
Valonia	58 28 10 N	05 05 10 W	Wrath	344	271
Vandal	55 43 48 N	05 22 24 W	E.Kintyre	35	43
Veni	55 55 18 N	06 17 30 W	NW Islay	122	95
Viscount	57 35 05 N	05 50 20 W	Skye	309	242
Vivo	56 31 21 N	06 57 31 W	Tiree	248	196
W A Massey	58 22 00 N PA	05 20 00 W PA	Wrath	342	270
Welman 10	58 15 36 N	05 04 45 W	Kylesku	340	269
Westerbotten	55 35 10 N	06 18 55 W	SE Islay	61	57
Wharfinger			Mull	181	150
White Head	56 34 18 N PA	05 58 53 W PA	Mull	202	168
Wilhelm Aberg	56 12 00 N PA	05 41 00 W PA	Jura	133	107
William H Welch	57 52 33 N	05 43 03 W	Lochewe	325	255
Winchester	58 28 00 N PA	05 05 00 W PA	Wrath	343	270
Wyre Majestic	55 52 58 N	06 07 12 W	W Islay	91	74
Wyre Victory	56 54 06 N	06 36 00 W	Mallaig	278	219
Young Fisherman	56 25 00 N PA	05 30 00 W PA	Oban	152	121

LATITUDE INDEX

Latitude	Longitude	Name	Area	Wreck	Page
55 35 00 N PA	06 20 00 W PA	Hoheluft	SE Islay	57	56
55 35 00 N PA	06 20 00 W PA	Ena	SE Islay	59	56
55 35 10 N	06 18 55 W	Ellida ?	SE Islay	60	57
55 35 10 N	06 18 55 W	Westerbotten	SE Islay	61	57
55 36 30 N	06 26 24 W	Tuscania	SE Islay	62	57
55 37 04 N	06 11 40 W	Limelight	SE Islay	63	58
55 37 16 N	06 11 08 W	Islay	SE Islay	64	60
55 37 30 N	06 05 42 W	Luneda	SE Islay	65	60
55 37 38 N	06 04 42 W	Serb	SE Islay	66	61
55 38 00 N PA	07 39 00 W PA	Justicia	W Islay	92	75
55 38 03 N	06 04 40 W	San Sebastian	SE Islay	67	61
55 38 10 N	06 05 30 W	John Strachan	SE Islay	68	62
55 38 18 N	05 45 19 W	Aska	W.Kintyre	124	98
55 39 05 N	06 02 25 W	Shuna	SE Islay	69	64
55 39 10 N PA	06 03 50 W PA	Cossack	SE Islay	70	64
55 39 18 N	06 02 52 W	Surprise	SE Islay	71	65
55 39 27 N	06 04 27 W	Unknown	SE Islay	72	65
55 39 42 N	05 47 12 W	Udea	Gigha	125	99
55 39 42 N	05 47 12 W	Staffa	Gigha	126	99
55 40 00 N PA	06 39 00 W PA	Norman	SW Islay	84	70
55 40 03 N	06 01 10 W	Guethary	SE Islay	73	65
55 40 18 N	06 30 52 W	Thomas	SW Islay	85	70
55 41 00 N PA	06 31 00 W PA	Anida	SW Islay	88	73
55 41 36 N	06 31 57 W	Blythville	SW Islay	86	72
55 42 00 N PA	06 32 00 W PA	Ida Adams	SW Islay	87	72
55 42 06 N	06 30 36 W	Agios Minas	SW Islay	89	73
55 42 10 N	05 44 45 W	Kartli	Gigha	127	101
55 42 22 N	06 30 00 W	Tobago	SW Islay	90	73
55 42 38 N	05 39 49 W	Mon Cousu	Gigha	128	102
55 43 11 N	06 30 10 W	Agate	W Islay	93	75
55 43 48 N	05 22 24 W	Vandal	E.Kintyre	35	43
55 44 08 N	06 29 54 W	Dalton	W Islay	94	76
55 44 30 N PA	06 22 30 W PA	Henry Clay	W Islay	95	76
55 44 42 N	06 29 06 W	Cormoran	W Islay	96	77
55 45 06 N	06 28 07 W	Floristan	W Islay	97	78
55 45 18 N	06 28 28 W	Ocean	W Islay	98	79
55 45 46 N	06 28 40 W	Otranto	W Islay	99	80
55 46 00 N PA	06 35 00 W PA	Seavar	W Islay	100	84
55 46 30 N PA	06 28 00 W PA	Forest Chief	W Islay	101	84
55 46 30 W PA	06 28 00 W PA	La Plata	W Islay	102	84
55 46 37 N	06 16 18 W	Unknown - Pre-1957	W Islay	103	85
55 46 58 N	06 27 30 W	Unknown	W Islay	104	85
55 47 00 N PA	06 28 00 W PA	Colonial Empire	W Islay	105	85
55 47 00 N PA	07 00 00 W PA	Nils Gorthon	W Islay	106	86
55 47 26 N	06 59 50 W	Lexington?	W Islay	107	86
55 47 37 N	06 03 58 W	Criscilla	E Islay	75	66
55 47 37 N	06 54 04 W	Jacksonville	W Islay	108	86
55 47 44 N	06 03 26 W	Edith Morgan	E Islay	76	66
55 48 00 N PA	06 30 00 W PA	Chevalier	W Islay	109	87
55 48 48 N	06 27 38 W	Graph	W Islay	110	87
55 49 18 N	06 36 26 W	Unknown	W Islay	113	90
55 49 23 N	06 36 37 W	Unknown	W Islay	114	90
55 49 50 N	06 27 30 W	Exmouth	W Islay	111	88
55 50 00 N PA	06 06 00 W PA	Kay D	E Islay	77	68
55 50 00 N PA	08 03 00 W PA	Brittany	W Islay	115	90
55 50 01 N	05 56 09 W	Stormlight	Jura	129	103
55 50 06 N	06 27 26 W	Belford	W Islay	116	91
55 50 36 N	06 05 20 W	Glen Holme	E Islay	78	68
55 51 10 N PA	06 27 20 W PA	Exmouth Castle	W Islay	112	89
55 52 00 N PA	06 06 00 W PA	Lily Melling	E Islay	79	68

Latitude	Longitude	Name	Area	Wreck	Page
56 25 00 N PA	07 05 00 W PA	Ravensheugh	Mull	224	182
56 25 02 N	05 29 42 W	Hyacinth	Oban	154	122
56 25 15 N	05 29 37 W	Calum Cille	Oban	155	123
56 25 18 N PA	05 39 00 W PA	Accord	Mull	177	149
56 25 30 N	05 29 32 W	Pansy	Oban	156	124
56 26 30 N PA	05 34 00 W PA	Solway Firth	Oban	157	124
56 26 40 N	05 37 00 W	Mountaineer	Oban	158	124
56 26 40 N	05 37 00 W	Clydesdale	Oban	159	125
56 27 10 N	05 33 40 W	Appletree	Oban	160	126
56 27 22 N	05 29 14 W	Madam Alice	Oban	161	126
56 27 30 N PA	05 39 12 W PA	New Blessing	Mull	182	150
56 27 36 N	05 17 30 W	Earl of Carrick	Oban	162	129
56 27 36 N PA	05 17 30 W PA	Exit	Oban	163	130
56 28 09 N	05 31 24 W	Thalia	Oban	164	131
56 28 30 N	05 36 45 W	St. Joseph	Oban	165	131
56 28 33 N	05 25 00 W	Breda	Oban	166	132
56 29 00 N	06 59 00 W	Sturdy	Tiree	237	191
56 29 12 N	06 52 24 W	Unknown	Tiree	238	191
56 29 17 N	06 07 08 W	Cretan	Mull	225	183
56 29 38 N	05 36 48 W	Mardi Dan	Mull	178	149
56 29 45 N	05 39 19 W	Swan (or Speedwell?)	Mull	183	151
56 29 45 N	05 42 42 W	Girl Sandra	Mull	184	151
56 29 57 N	07 01 36 W	Cairnsmuir	Tiree	241	192
56 29 58 N	06 48 02 W	Lady Isle	Tiree	239	192
56 30 00 N PA	07 40 00 W PA	U-484	Tiree	240	192
56 30 02 N	05 41 26 W	Thesis	Mull	185	151
56 30 07 N	06 48 14 W	Mary Stuart	Tiree	242	193
56 30 10 N	05 41 59 W	Ballista	Mull	186	153
56 30 10 N	05 42 00 W	River Tay	Mull	187	155
56 30 10 N	05 42 00 W	Alexander	Mull	188	155
56 30 12 N	05 41 59 W	Dartmouth	Mull	189	155
56 30 15 N	05 44 28 W	Buitenzorg	Mull	190	157
56 30 25 N	05 44 05 W	Shackleton Aircraft	Mull	191	158
56 30 30 N PA	05 44 00 W PA	Jane Shearer	Mull	192	159
56 31 08 N	05 45 24 W	Evelyn Rose	Mull	193	159
56 31 12 N	05 37 06 W	Janet	Mull	194	160
56 31 20 N PA	07 01 00 W PA	Saxon	Tiree	243	193
56 31 20 N PA	07 01 00 W PA	Ardandhu	Tiree	244	195
56 31 21 N	06 57 31 W	Vivo	Tiree	248	196
56 31 22 N	05 51 12 W	Cessna 150 Aircraft	Mull	195	160
56 31 30 N PA	06 57 30 W PA	Gaul	Tiree	245	195
56 31 52 N	05 46 57 W	Johanna	Mull	196	161
56 31 55 N	05 46 58 W	Logan	Mull	197	161
56 31 57 N	06 52 15 W	Malve	Tiree	251	197
56 32 00 N	05 48 16 W	John Preston	Mull	198	162
56 32 00 N	06 53 00 W	Riddha	Tiree	246	195
56 32 04 N	06 56 00 W	Ingrid	Tiree	247	196
56 32 17 N	05 54 40 W	Rondo	Mull	199	162
56 32 20 N	06 40 05 W	Hurlford	Coll	253	198
56 32 22 N	05 56 50 W	Unknown - Pre-1947	Mull	200	164
56 32 24 N	06 40 00 W	St. Clair	Coll	252	198
56 32 30 N PA	06 46 45 W PA	Fisher Queen	Tiree	249	196
56 32 30 N PA	07 26 30 W PA	Adamton ?	Tiree	250	197
56 33 00 N	06 28 00 W	Unknown - Jason?	Mull	226	183
56 33 24 N	05 54 48 W	Shuna	Mull	201	166
56 33 36 N	06 41 37 W	Nessmore	Coll	254	200
56 33 38 N PA	06 41 33 W PA	Faraday	Coll	255	201
56 33 40 N	06 37 53 W	Tapti	Coll	256	201
56 33 42 N	06 38 00 W	Arnold	Coll	257	201
56 34 18 N PA	05 58 53 W PA	White Head	Mull	202	168

Latitude	Longitude	Name	Area	Wreck	Page
57 20 00 N PA	06 00 00 W PA	Irishman	Skye	297	234
57 21 00 N PA	05 51 00 W PA	Scomber	Skye	298	234
57 21 19 N	06 39 20 W	Irlana	Skye	299	235
57 22 10 N PA	06 42 24 W PA	Caroline ?	Skye	300	235
57 24 15 N	05 49 04 W	Unknown - Pre-1978	Skye	301	236
57 25 00 N PA	06 52 00 W PA	Inger Toft	Skye	302	236
57 25 15 N	06 47 25 W	Doris	Skye	303	238
57 27 12 N	06 47 06 W	Chadwick	Skye	304	239
57 27 30 N PA	06 45 10 W PA	Unknown - Pre-1970	Skye	305	239
57 27 44 N	06 36 57 W	Unknown	Skye	306	241
57 30 48 N PA	06 43 00 W PA	Dunvegan Castle	Skye	307	241
57 35 00 N PA	05 50 30 W PA	Shiela	Skye	308	241
57 35 05 N	05 50 20 W	Viscount	Skye	309	242
57 36 30 N	06 38 00 W	Norman	Skye	310	242
57 36 55 N	06 29 37 W	Ben Aigen	Skye	311	242
57 38 30 N PA	06 12 00 W PA	Unknown	Skye	312	243
57 41 14 N	06 20 45 W	Rhodesia	Skye	313	243
57 43 27 N	06 17 42 W	Alexanders	Skye	314	243
57 43 48 N	06 17 48 W	Nordhuk	Skye	315	246
57 44 21 N	06 25 51 W	Apollo	Skye	316	247
57 44 48 N	06 26 30 W	Frederick Bartholdi	Skye	317	248
57 52 30 N	05 39 52 W	Glen Albyn	Lochewe	323	253
57 52 33 N	05 43 03 W	William H Welch	Lochewe	325	255
57 52 40 N	05 40 44 W	Promotive	Lochewe	324	255
57 53 45 N	05 09 20 W	Unknown	Broom	327	259
57 55 36 N	05 36 48 W	Gratitude	Lochewe	326	258
57 56 14 N	05 21 33 W	Innisjura	Broom	328	259
57 57 25 N	05 30 58 W	Guiding Star	Broom	329	260
57 57 45 N	05 31 18 W	Silver Reward	Broom	330	260
57 58 32 N	05 20 14 W	Silver Spray	Broom	331	260
57 59 00 N PA	05 21 00 W PA	Unknown	Broom	332	261
58 00 45 N PA	05 24 00 W PA	Unknown	Broom	333	261
58 02 30 N PA	06 18 00 W PA	Kondor	Minch	318	252
58 03 00 N PA	05 26 00 W PA	Unknown	Broom	334	261
58 04 30 N PA	05 17 00 W PA	Gotfrede	Enard	335	264
58 08 15 N PA	05 18 00 W PA	Loch Erisort	Enard	336	264
58 12 26 N	05 32 41 W	Unknown	Minch	319	252
58 12 49 N	05 43 08 W	Normannvik	Minch	320	252
58 12 52 N	05 43 53 W	Unknown	Minch	321	253
58 14 45 N	05 10 20 W	Unknown	Enard	337	265
58 15 01 N	05 11 31 W	Bermuda	Enard	338	265
58 15 24 N	04 56 50 W	Crown	Kylesku	339	267
58 15 36 N	05 04 45 W	Welman 10	Kylesku	340	269
58 16 45 N	05 06 30 W	Unknown	Kylesku	341	270
58 19 30 N	05 32 00 W	U-1021	Minch	322	253
58 22 00 N PA	05 20 00 W PA	W A Massey	Wrath	342	270
58 28 00 N PA	05 05 00 W PA	Winchester	Wrath	343	270
58 28 10 N	05 05 10 W	Valonia	Wrath	344	271
58 30 59 N	05 33 24 W	Noreen Mary	Wrath	345	271
58 34 00 N PA	05 13 40 W PA	Majorka	Wrath	346	271
58 35 31 N	05 46 06 W	U-965	Wrath	347	272
58 36 30 N PA	05 00 30 W PA	Sunnyvale	Wrath	348	273
58 41 17 N	05 11 43 W	Manipur	Wrath	349	273
58 58 00 N PA	07 50 00 W PA	Inger	Wrath	350	273
		Earl Lennox	E.Islay	74	66
		Robert Hewett	Mull	179	149
		Golden Gleam	Mull	180	150
		Wharfinger	Mull	181	150

Forthcoming Nekton Books titles

For publication in 1996:
St. Kilda : A Submarine Guide, 3rd edition, Gordon Ridley, 180 pages
Merchant Ships lost in Scottish Waters 1816-1945, Gordon Ridley, 400 pages
The Outer Hebrides : A Submarine Guide, Gordon Ridley, 192 pages

For publication in 1996/7:
The Loss of Submarine K13, Ian Johnston & Gordon Ridley, 160 pages
Shipwrecks the North & North East of Scotland, Bob Baird, 224 pages
Shipwrecks & Other Dive Sites of Mull, Iain Maclean, 224 pages
Shipwrecks of the Western Isles, Bob Baird & Gordon Ridley, 192 pages

For publication in 1997:
The Hebridean Outliers : A Submarine Guide, Gordon Ridley, 128 pages
Freshwater Diving in Scotland : A Submarine Guide, Gordon Ridley, 128 pages
Submarines Lost in Scottish Waters, Gordon Ridley, 192 pages

Research is well advanced on all the above titles but all information will still be welcome. Please contact the authors via the Publisher. Page numbers are approximate.

A further series of dive guides to all Scottish waters is planned for publication by the Millenium. These will be a comprehensive development of Gordon Ridley's books published by Underwater World Publications Ltd.

Please place me on your mailing list / send me further information on:

☐ Nekton Books dive guide series

☐ Nekton Books wreck guide series

☐ Other Nekton publications about Scottish wrecks & dive sites

Please supply ____ copies of Bob Baird's first book *Shipwrecks of the Forth* at £13.70 each, including p & p. Payment by means of cheque, postal order or cash (registered) should be included.

Name: Telephone:

Address:

My particular interests are:

I have more information on these areas:

Send these details to Nekton Books, 94 Brownside Road, Cambuslang, Glasgow, G72 8AG.

A companion volume to
"Shipwrecks of the West of Scotland"

The definitive
guide to the
shipwrecks in
this popular
diving area.

Written by
Bob Baird, the
acknowledged
expert.

Published by
Nekton Books.

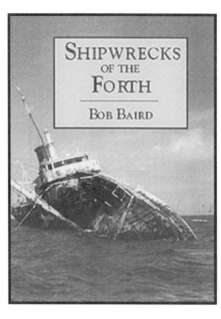

SHIPWRECKS
OF THE
FORTH

BOB BAIRD

- 214 pages
- 320 wrecks
- ship data
- descriptions
- sinkings
- photographs
- maps
- locations
- transits
- drawings
- analysis
- diving data
- bibliography
- name index
- latitude index

Bob is a well-known Scottish diver who spent 15 years researching his first love shipwrecks in the Forth. This book is the culmination of his work and describes wrecks, many for the first time, sunk during the period 1745 - 1980.

Shipwrecks of the Forth has received very flattering reviews and is the first of its kind. It is invaluable to both wreck diving enthusiasts and shipping historians.

The Forth has been one of several important Scottish shipping areas for many centuries. The early coastal trade was not as prolific as that of the West Coast, but it was still important in its day. Trade with Scandinavia has always featured in Forth shipping, in particular much of the Baltic wood trade came to Bo'ness and other Forth ports. The movement of coal by sea was central to early British trade and industry. Many ships also traded with the British Empire, the export of whisky being especially important. There has also been large amounts of naval shipping using the Forth for many years.

For much of the maritime history of the Forth, there were no lights or lighthouses and, furthermore, ships were at the mercy of the wind. The plethora of modern electronic navigation aids were a thing of the distant future. Many fine ships were lost to the above trades due to these circumstances. For instance, some 500 were lost between 1850 and 1900 alone. Earlier records are incomplete and elusive and many more vessels must have been lost.

More recently, by far the most common causes of shipwrecks are running aground and collisions, while during both wars, submarine torpedoes, mines, and attack by aircraft were additional hazards which accounted for a substantial number of the wrecks. In fact, the Forth has the unenviable distinction of having been the scene of both the first and the last enemy attacks on the British mainland during the Second World War.

Price £12.95, p&p 75p

Available from: Nekton Books, 94 Brownside Road, Cambuslang, Glasgow, G72 8AG
Tel / Fax : 0141 641 4200